COVID-19 and Psychologi Distress in Africa

This timely book draws on unique African experiences to explore the intersection between mental health and African communitarianism in the context of COVID-19, giving voice to the perspectives of vulnerable populations facing pre-existing challenges such as depression, anxiety, and stress.

Advancing knowledge and contributing to the global debate about the effects of the pandemic on the psychological well-being of African people, chapters critique the role of media, information, misinformation, and disinformation during this period on individual- and community-based mental health. Using a holistic approach, the book highlights the need to prioritise the localising of mental health systems and clinical services to provide a better standard of care and comprehensive, context-specific mental health interventions that consider the heterogeneity within and between African regions. The book demonstrates through nuanced evidence and analysis that communitarian perspectives allow African societies to balance collective solidarity with individual well-being to benefit overall mental health.

Ultimately drawing on communal values and localised knowledge to cultivate resilience to fight the psychosocial impacts of COVID-19 in Africa, the book will be of interest to scholars, postgraduate students and researchers exploring psychology, philosophy of mental health, and public health policy more broadly, as well as and cultural studies and the sociology of pandemics.

Yamikani Ndasauka is Associate Professor in Department of Philosophy, University of Malawi, Malawi.

Routledge Research in Psychology

This series offers an international forum for original and innovative research being conducted across the field of psychology. Titles in the series are empirically or theoretically informed and explore a range of dynamic and timely issues and emerging topics. The series is aimed at upper-level and post-graduate students, researchers, and research students, as well as academics and scholars.

Recent titles in the series include:

Multidisciplinary Perspectives on Representational Pluralism in Human Cognition
Tracing Points of Convergence in Psychology, Science Education, and Philosophy of Science
Edited by Michel Bélanger, Patrice Potvin, Steven Horst, Eduardo Fleury Mortimer, and Andrew Shtulman

Unitary Developmental Theory and Psychological Development Across the Lifespan, Volume 1
A Model of Developmental Learning for Psychological Maturation and Recovery
Myles Sweeney

Unitary Developmental Theory and Organization Development, Volume 2
A Model of Developmental Learning for Change, Agility and Resilience
Myles Sweeney

Alan Watts in Late-Twentieth-Century Discourse
Commentary and Criticism from 1974–1994
Edited by Peter J. Columbus

COVID-19 and Psychological Distress in Africa
Communitarian Perspectives
Edited by Yamikani Ndasauka

COVID-19 and Psychological Distress in Africa

Communitarian Perspectives

Edited by Yamikani Ndasauka

Routledge
Taylor & Francis Group
LONDON AND NEW YORK

First published 2024
by Routledge
4 Park Square, Milton Park, Abingdon, Oxon OX14 4RN

and by Routledge
605 Third Avenue, New York, NY 10158

Routledge is an imprint of the Taylor & Francis Group, an informa business

© 2024 selection and editorial matter, Yamikani Ndasauka; individual chapters, the contributors

The right of Yamikani Ndasauka to be identified as the author of the editorial material, and of the authors for their individual chapters, has been asserted in accordance with sections 77 and 78 of the Copyright, Designs and Patents Act 1988.

Trademark notice: Product or corporate names may be trademarks or registered trademarks, and are used only for identification and explanation without intent to infringe.

British Library Cataloguing-in-Publication Data
A catalogue record for this book is available from the British Library

Library of Congress Cataloging-in-Publication Data
Names: Ndasauka, Yamikani, editor, author.
Title: COVID-19 and psychological distress in Africa : communitarian perspectives / edited by Yamikani Ndasauka.
Other titles: Routledge research in psychology.
Description: New York : Routledge, 2024. | Series: Routledge research in psychology | Includes bibliographical references and index.
Identifiers: LCCN 2023042048 (print) | LCCN 2023042049 (ebook) | ISBN 9781032546308 (hardback) | ISBN 9781032546315 (paperback) | ISBN 9781003425861 (ebook)
Subjects: LCSH: Mental health—Social aspects—Africa, Sub-Saharan. | COVID-19 Pandemic, 2020—Africa, Sub-Saharan—Psychological aspects. | Communitarianism—Africa, Sub-Saharan.
Classification: LCC RA790.7.A357 C685 2024 (print) | LCC RA790.7.A357 (ebook) | DDC 362.204250967—dc23/eng/20230906
LC record available at https://lccn.loc.gov/2023042048
LC ebook record available at https://lccn.loc.gov/2023042049

ISBN: 978-1-032-54630-8 (hbk)
ISBN: 978-1-032-54631-5 (pbk)
ISBN: 978-1-003-42586-1 (ebk)

DOI: 10.4324/9781003425861

Typeset in Galliard
by Apex CoVantage, LLC

Contents

Contributors

Alex Zumazuma is a psychiatrist working as a clinical lecturer in the Mental Health and Psychiatry Department at Kamuzu University of Health Sciences (KUHES). His research interests are psychosis, mood disorders, psychotherapy, translational research, and neurosciences.

Atipatsa Chiwanda Kaminga is an educationist and epidemiologist with a PhD in public health and preventive medicine, teaching at Mzuzu University.

Daniel Chikatentha is a Master's in development studies student in the Faculty of Social Sciences at the University of Malawi. His research interests are mental health, child development and protection, gender, and social behaviour change.

Demoubly Kokota is a psychology lecturer at the University of Malawi. He is a Doctoral fellow in mental health at the Kamuzu College of Health Sciences. His main research interests are task shifting and integrating mental health into African primary healthcare.

Donya Rahimi is a global health programme director with 19 years of experience supporting, leading, and designing international development programmes, including regional and global programmes across Central Asia, Africa, and Central and South America.

Drinney Labanna holds a BA in English and African languages and linguistics from Mzuzu University in Malawi. Her research interests are the media and forensic linguistics.

Eckhard Kleinau, PhD, is a Senior Advisor in the Centre for Innovation Solutions Development at the University Research Co. (URC). He has 30 years of experience strengthening health systems and the workforce through innovative approaches and technologies and generating evidence through monitoring, evaluation, and implementation research. Orcid: https://orcid.org/0000-0003-0304-1644.

Edister S. Jamu is a senior lecturer in the Department of Psychology and Medical Humanities at the University of Malawi. His research interests focus on talent management, higher education, digital technologies, mental health, and social inclusion.

Felix Chimera Nyika holds a PhD from Mzuzu University. He is the lead Pastor of Kairos Christian Centre Lilongwe with its Leadership Institute and Theological Seminary.

Flemmings Fishani Ngwira is Senior Lecturer at Malawi University of Business and Applied Sciences in the Department of Language and Communication Studies. His research interests are health communication, behavioural change communication, psychology, and human behaviour. He is an editor of the *Malawi Journal of Applied Sciences and Innovation* (MJASI).

Foster Gondwe is Senior Lecturer in the Education Foundations department at the University of Malawi. His research fields include instructional technology, international and comparative education. He is also the Book Reviews Editor of the *Journal of Interactive Media in Education*.

Gowokani Chijere-Chirwa is Associate Professor in the Department of Economics at the University of Malawi. His research interests are in Health economics and Microeconometrics. He is the editor of the *Malawi Journal of Economics and Frontiers in Economics*.

Hellen Jepkemoi Magut is a librarian at the University of Eastern Africa Baraton-Kenya. Her research interests are in library automation, information literacy and e-learning.

Jimmy Kainja is Senior Lecturer at the University of Malawi. His research interests are media and communication policy, journalism, new media, digital rights, freedom of expression, access to information and the intersection of media, democracy and development.

Jones Mawerenga is Senior Lecturer in Systematic Theology & Christian Ethics, University of Malawi and a Research Fellow in the Department of Practical Theology and Mission Studies at the University of Pretoria.

Joshua Isaac Kumwenda is Senior Lecturer of African Literature in the Department of Language, Cultural and Creative Studies at Mzuzu University. He holds a PhD in African literature from the University of the Witwatersrand.

Joyce Dainess Mlenga teaches in the Department of Theology and Religious Studies at Mzuzu University. Her research interests include religion and culture, Christian education, and gender and religion. She is Associate Editor for Africa of the *On Knowing Humanity Journal*.

Katy Gorentz is a global health monitoring and evaluation specialist. She currently works as Senior M&E Specialist at Chemonics International and holds experience in health systems strengthening, health workforce, and health market development.

Lazarus Sauti holds an MA in media and communication studies from the University of Zimbabwe (UZ). His research focuses on media, conflict resolution and transformation, digital media cultures, political communication, cultural productions, human rights, peace, democracy, and governance.

Limbika Maliwichi is Senior Lecturer of Psychology and former Deputy Dean of the Faculty of Social Science at the University of Malawi. Her research interests are in child and adolescent mental health.

Mary Ooko holds PhD in distance education. She is the director of the Distance Education Department at the University of Pretoria.

Michael Kapps is a health and technology entrepreneur based out of Brazil. He founded Vitalk, a chat-based mental health tool that was acquired by Gympass in 2022. He is currently the founder of Sanii, a company focused on improving elderly care and longevity in Brazil.

Nick Mdika Tembo is Associate Professor in the Department of Literary Studies at the University of Malawi. His teaching and research interests are in trauma and memory studies, holocaust and genocide studies, childhood studies, and African life writing.

Pascal Newbourne Mwale is Senior Lecturer in the Department of Philosophy at the University of Malawi. His research interests include media ethics, politics and media, science in public, science communication, public understanding of science, phenomenology, and critical theory.

Peter J. O. Aloka holds PhD in educational psychology from the University of the Western Cape. He is Senior Lecturer at the Wits School of Education, University of the Witwatersrand, South Africa.

Peter Mhagama is Associate Professor in the Department of Language and Communication at the Malawi University of Business and Applied Sciences. His research interests are communication for development, media audiences, and social and behavioural change communication.

Rachel Chimbwete-Phiri is Senior Media and Communication Studies Lecturer at the University of Malawi. Her research interests include media genres, professional discourse, and social and behavioural change communication.

Rachel NyaGondwe Fiedler is Associate Professor at Mzuzu University. She holds a PhD from the University of the Free State.

Rhodian Munyenyembe is a theological educator holding a PhD in church history from the University of the Free State (2016). He is the head of department (Theology and Religious Studies) at Mzuzu University.

Richard Guto is a lecturer in the Social Sciences Department at Chuka University. His research interests are records and archive management, knowledge management, and informatics.

Tendai Makaripe is a practising journalist and a politics and international relations researcher. His work focuses on Zimbabwean politics, governance, political communication, alternative media and conflict management, insurgency, and terrorism in Africa.

Tilinao Lamba is a counselling psychologist registered with the Malawi Association of Counsellors and a lecturer in the Department of Psychology and Medical Humanities at The University of Malawi. Her research interests include youth mental health advocacy and mental health literacy.

Wanda Jaskiewicz is a project director for Credence Management Solutions' USAID Global Health Training, Advisory and Support Contract (GHTASC). She brings over 25 years of workforce development experience, leading global human resources for health and capacity-building programmes, performance improvement, and training and workforce motivation and retention efforts.

Wasilat Opeoluwa Lasisi is an early-career researcher and an assistant lecturer at the Department of Philosophy at Lagos State University. Her research interests are in logic, philosophy of science, and ethics.

Wellman Kondowe is a senior lecturer in the Department of Languages and Literature at the Mzuzu University. He is currently co-editing a book on Multilingualism in Southern Africa: Issues and Perspectives to be published by Routledge.

Yamikani Ndasauka is an associate professor in the Department of Philosophy at the University of Malawi. His research interests are in philosophy, applied ethics, and mental health. He is also the editor of the *Journal of Humanities*.

Preface

This book provides empirical and theoretical foundations to inform pandemic responses by spotlighting diverse disciplinary perspectives on intersections of culture, technology, media, gender, age, and locality with mental health in Africa during COVID-19. As this book demonstrates, foregrounding lived experiences while engaging critically with communitarian notions reveals a complex reality requiring multifaceted policy and programming. Thus, seeking convergence between traditional communal practices and emerging biomedical paradigms can imbue interventions with richness, relevance, and sensitivity to support collective flourishing.

The COVID-19 pandemic has profoundly impacted mental health across Africa. As the virus spread, it threatened physical health and exacerbated existing mental health conditions and risk factors, leading to a rising prevalence of psychological distress across countries (Kola et al., 2021). African nations faced a unique convergence of disease-related stressors alongside disruptions to livelihoods, support systems, and access to care resulting from lockdowns and containment efforts (Ajayi et al., 2021). These mounting pressures have tested the resilience of African communities already facing systemic challenges around poverty, social services, and infrastructure.

Amidst this crisis, the role of African cultural values and communal coping strategies in addressing rising mental health burdens has gained attention. In particular, the philosophy of communitarianism, which emphasises collective identity, mutual support, and relational well-being, has been proposed as a grounding framework to strengthen mental health responses (Kainja et al., 2022). African communitarianism recognises human beings' fundamental interconnectedness, arguing that personhood and fulfilment derive from participation in a communal network of reciprocal rights and duties (Mbiti, 1970; Gyekye, 1997). This contrasts with Western individualism and may foster environments where mental health problems are addressed through shared burdens rather than isolation.

However, critiques note that communitarianism has limitations, including the potential to suppress individual rights or allow inequities if improperly applied (Gyekye, 1997). Thus, calls have been made for a moderate communitarian approach balanced with personal clinical care (Egbe et al., 2014). Integrating communal practices like peer counselling and cultural rituals with evidence-based treatment can render interventions locally resonant while upholding standards.

As Africa continues responding to COVID-19's mental health impacts, leveraging communitarian assets while addressing systemic gaps remains vital. This collection contributes nuanced perspectives to this task by investigating mental health experiences across diverse African contexts, foregrounding community-based capacities alongside vulnerabilities requiring external intervention. A complex biopsychosocial picture reveals how disruptions to communitarian structures during COVID-19 exacerbated risks, but reimagining social obligations and relationships could help mitigate harm.

As calls to improve after COVID-19 prompt reimagining mental healthcare landscapes, the Afrocentric ethic of care, relationality, and mutual responsibility underpinning communitarianism remain a vital touchstone. By bridging communities and clinical services; leveraging arts, technology, and communication; and upholding equity, these chapters illuminate strategic priorities for localising mental health systems to nurture resilience as Africa navigates persistent uncertainty. This work contributes nuanced evidence and analysis to advance a context-specific understanding of COVID-19's psychological impacts and culturally grounded responses that leave no one behind.

In this book, Chapter 1 discusses how COVID-19 exacerbated mental health challenges across Africa, with factors like poverty, unemployment, and isolation increasing risks of depression and anxiety. It analyses these issues through the lens of African communitarianism, arguing that this philosophy's emphasis on collective identity and mutual support provides strengths for mental healthcare, but limitations like stigma and inadequate resources persist. Calls are made for balanced, context-specific interventions combining communal coping strategies and clinical, evidence-based practices. Chapter 2 also examines mental health during COVID-19, finding heterogeneous sociodemographic factors associated with increased depression in Malawi that underscore the importance of tailored, multifaceted mental health interventions.

A few chapters focus on the acute mental health impacts of the pandemic on women and youth. For instance, Chapter 3 reports that Malawian women suffered less psychological distress than men during COVID-19, attributing this to reduced involvement in leadership roles and isolation policies disrupting women's caregiving responsibilities. However, Chapter 12 conversely discusses devastating mental health effects for African women from surges in online gender-based violence and economic uncertainties of the pandemic. Chapter 4 explores the vulnerabilities of African youth to mental health consequences of the COVID-19 infodemic, like teenage pregnancies and the inability to sift through misinformation.

Finally, Chapters 5 and 6 reveal workplace mental health impacts, with university academics and journalists reporting heightened stress, anxiety, and burnout during the pandemic from shifting work norms, heavy workloads, isolation, and economic uncertainties. Both advocate organisational change and strengthen mental health support systems for these groups.

Several chapters illuminate the significant role of information, misinformation, and framing during COVID-19. Chapters 7, 8, and 9 examine how media coverage set negative frames that potentially amplified public fear and anxiety. Chapter 10 explores the complexities of social media as both a space for collective coping and a conduit for misinformation that heightened distress. Chapters 10 and 11 investigate the processing of COVID-19 (mis) information through sociocultural lenses, with Chapter 11 specifically arguing that Africans' interpretation of information through hybridity contributed to psychological impacts.

Several chapters emphasise the value of culture-centred interventions. Chapter 13 recommends tackling vaccine hesitancy by addressing its sociocultural roots. Chapters 4 and 8 argue that African communal philosophies could help frame positive messaging and culture-based coping strategies. Specific cultural resources identified include integrating traditional healing systems (Chapter 13), leveraging the arts for awareness and collective healing (Chapter 8), and supporting youth networks (Chapter 4).

Finally, a unifying theme is the double-edged potential of technology for mental health during COVID-19. Chapter 16 comprehensively synthesises this "pharmakon" perspective, analysing how increased digital connectivity enabled social support but also spread misinformation. At the same time, shifts to remote learning expanded educational access but increased isolation and stress. It advocates balanced tech policies to leverage benefits while mitigating risks. While Chapter 14 assesses a mental health app, showing that digital literacy and cost constraints inhibited the uptake of this potentially helpful technology, Chapter 15 argues that the use of social media proliferated depression and anxiety among individuals during the COVID-19 pandemic.

These chapters and this book highlight the complex psychosocial impacts of COVID-19 in Africa and the need for holistic, context-specific responses leveraging culture, technology, and mental healthcare systems to support well-being collectively and individually. While challenges persist, insights emerge on cultivating resilience by drawing on communal values and localised knowledge.

References

Ajayi, K. V., Wachira, E., Bolarinwa, O. A., & Suleman, B. D. (2021). Maternal mental health in Africa during the COVID-19 pandemic: A neglected global health issue. *Epidemiology Health*, *43*, e2021078.

Egbe, C. O., Brooke-Sumner, C., Kathree, T., Selohilwe, O., Thornicroft, G., & Petersen, I. (2014). Psychiatric stigma and discrimination in South Africa: Perspectives from key stakeholders. *BMC Psychiatry*, *14*(1), 1–10. https://doi.org/10.1186/s12888-014-0191-x

Gyekye, K. (1997). *Tradition and modernity: Philosophical reflections on the African experience*. Oxford University Press.

Kainja, J., Ndasauka, Y., Mchenga, M., Kondowe, F., M'manga, C., Maliwichi, L., & Nyamali, S. (2022). Umunthu, Covid-19 and mental health in Malawi. *Heliyon*, *8*(11), e11316. https://doi.org/10.1016/j.heliyon.2022.e11316

Kola, L., Kohrt, B. A., Hanlon, C., Naslund, J. A., Sikander, S., Balaji, M., Benjet, C., Cheung, E., Eaton, J., Gonsalves, P., Haq, I. U., Honikman, S., Joska, J. A., Luitel, N., Lund, C., Patel, V., Rahman, A., Silove, D., van Ommeren, M., . . . Ventevogel, P. (2021). COVID-19 mental health impact and responses in low-income and middle-income countries: Reimagining global mental health. *The Lancet Psychiatry*, *8*(6), 535–550. https://doi.org/10.1016/S2215-0366(21)00025-0

Mbiti, J. S. (1970). *Concepts of god in Africa*. Society for Promoting Christian Knowledge.

Acknowledgements

I sincerely thank all contributors for making this work possible. Huge thanks should go to members of the COVID-19 and Mental Health in Malawi Project team – Jimmy Kainja, Simunye Nyamali, Martina Mchenga, Chilungamo M'manga, Fiskani Kondowe, and Limbika Maliwichi for your inspiration and encouragement.

This book was produced and funded under the COVID-19 Africa Rapid Grant Fund (COV19200603527586), supported under the auspices of the Science Granting Councils Initiative in sub-Saharan Africa (SGCI) and administered by South Africa's National Research Foundation (NRF) in collaboration with Canada's International Development Research Centre (IDRC), the Swedish International Development Cooperation Agency (Sida), South Africa's Department of Science and Innovation (DSI), the Fonds de Recherche du Quebec (FRQ), the United Kingdom's Department of International Development (DFID), United Kingdom Research and Innovation (UKRI) through the Newton Fund, and the SGCI participating councils across 15 countries in sub-Saharan Africa.

1 COVID-19 and Mental Health in Africa

A Communitarian Perspective

Yamikani Ndasauka

1.1 Introduction

The chapter aims to explore the effect of the COVID-19 pandemic on psychological wellbeing in Africa. The study on which this chapter is based adopted an African communitarian perspective. The World Health Organization (WHO) declared COVID-19 a pandemic when it started claiming lives in 2020. Many people succumbed to the pandemic and much happened due to its spread. The media, health practitioners, and scholars explored the various effects COVID-19 had as a result of its escalating reach. The COVID-19 pandemic significantly affected mental health worldwide; Africa is no exception. The pandemic also brought about a range of challenges that have affected the mental well-being of individuals across the continent (see M'manga et al., 2023). Depression, stress, and anxiety, among other mental problems brought about by COVID-19, were coupled with poverty, unemployment, and living standards in Africa.

African communitarianism is a philosophical and sociopolitical ideology emphasising the importance of community and collective well-being within African societies (Gyekye, 1997). It is based on the belief that individuals are inherently interconnected and that their identities and values are shaped by their participation in communal relationships. In African communitarianism, the community is viewed as the primary unit of social organisation, and individual identity and fulfilment are closely tied to the community's well-being (Menkiti, 1984). This philosophy emphasises that individuals have social responsibilities and obligations to their families and extended kinship networks, including the larger community. African communitarianism has influenced various aspects of African societies, such as social structures, governance systems, and approaches to conflict resolution. Communitarianism often contrasts with individualistic ideologies prevalent in Western societies, as the former emphasises collective identities and social harmony (Kayange, 2020).

African communitarianism has implications for mental health within African societies. On the negative side, there are challenges and limitations, such as the potential for social pressure, stigma, and the lack of access to specialised mental health services. Additionally, globalisation and modernisation have influenced changes in African societies, leading to shifts in traditional community

DOI: 10.4324/9781003425861-1

structures and practices. However, African communitarianism may be a panacea for mental health (Kainja et al., 2022). The emphasis on community and collective well-being provides a supportive environment for individuals' mental health. Section 1.2 discusses in depth the effect of the pandemic on mental health in Africa; section 1.3 expounds on African communitarianism; section 1.4 considers mental health in the light of African communitarianism; and the final section 1.5 discusses the nuances between and within African countries.

1.2 COVID-19 and Mental Health in Africa

The COVID-19 pandemic took a toll on mental health in Africa. The fear of contracting the virus, uncertainty about the future, and the effect of lockdowns and restrictions led to heightened anxiety and stress among many Africans. The pandemic disrupted people's lives, causing financial strain, loss of livelihoods, and social isolation, all contributing to mental health issues (Duby et al., 2022). In contexts where poverty and mental health stressors already interact to affect the most vulnerable populations negatively, COVID-19 has worsened these effects. Duby et al. (2022) examined the socioeconomic and mental health effects of COVID-19 on South African adolescent girls and young women to understand how additional challenges brought on by COVID-19 have intersected with existing challenges, compounding the young women's vulnerabilities. Numerous pre-existing problems affect the mental health of adolescent girls and young women, and the effects of COVID-19 have worsened their impact. Mudiriza and Lannoy (2020) equally explored the effects of COVID-19 on mental health, focusing on the youth of South Africa. Depressive factors with which the child is challenged, such as unemployment and poverty, were exacerbated by the pandemic. The prevalent problems affect the youth's mental health (Mudiriza & Lannoy, 2020).

The pandemic affected vulnerable populations, such as impoverished people, refugees, and internally displaced persons (see Joska et al., 2020; Bantjes et al., 2023). These individuals often face additional stressors and limited access to healthcare and support systems, exacerbating their mental health challenges. An increase in depression at one school was consistent, and prevalence rates of common mental disorders among learners increased steadily with the advent of COVID-19 (Bantjes et al., 2023). Joska et al. (2020) looked at the individual-level consequences of COVID-19 on the mental health of women living with HIV. The mental health and well-being of this group of the South African population were at increased risk. The early stages of the COVID-19 pandemic in South Africa exerted deleterious mental health effects on women living with HIV, something which rekindled the trauma related to restrictions applied to specific communities under apartheid and increased anxieties related to potential infection with a fatal virus (Joska et al., 2020).

Gyasi (2020) studied the effects of COVID-19 on the mental health of older persons in Africa. With the propensity of seeing a second wave and the potential for flare-ups of the pandemic, a critical evaluation of cost-effective therapies and interventions to respond to the mental health needs of older people required integrated attention (Haag et al., 2022). Gyasi (2020) argues that, at the time of his study, there was a need to strengthen cognitive and psychiatric health services and prepare for the inevitably precipitated challenges of the pandemic in sub-Saharan Africa. Shared responsibility was urgently needed to effectively address the substantial mental health and well-being effects of COVID-19 among older people in sub-Saharan Africa. Regional and country-specific development policy agendas had to include post-COVID-19 health recovery and cognitive rehabilitation programmes for older people (Gyasi, 2020).

Falgas-Bague et al. (2023), Dawood et al. (2022), and Robertson et al. (2020) also examined the mental health influence of COVID-19 on health workers in Africa. Robertson et al. (2020) found that infectious disease outbreaks caused high psychosocial stress among healthcare workers in South Africa, which may negatively affect workplace functioning. Depression, anxiety, post-traumatic stress, and other mental health conditions are prevalent among healthcare workers exposed to COVID-19 and other outbreaks (Haag et al., 2022). Similarly, in their study of healthcare workers in KwaZulu-Natal (South Africa), Dawood et al. (2022) observed that health workers in KwaZulu-Natal experienced high depression, anxiety, stress, and traumatic stress combined with poor perceptions of employer support.

Before the pandemic, mental health services in Africa were often inadequate, with limited resources and infrastructure (WHO, 2021). The COVID-19 crisis further strained these services, making it even more challenging for individuals to access the support they need. There is a shortage of mental health professionals, especially in rural areas, and mental health stigma persists in many communities today (Durizo et al., 2023). Many African mental health programmes and initiatives have been disrupted or redirected to address the immediate health crisis posed by COVID-19. This redirection has reduced focus on pre-existing mental health issues, further affecting the mental well-being of individuals. Sodi et al. (2021) analysed existing mental health policies in four African countries (Ghana, Kenya, South Africa, and Zimbabwe). They demonstrated that, at the time, all four countries lacked the capacity of these legislative provisions to enable psychology professionals to deal with psychosocial problems brought about by COVID-19.

Africa has weak health systems, poor mental health policies and infrastructure, high poverty rates, and unreliable maternal care (Ajayi et al., 2021). In addition, the pandemic had dire consequences on maternal mental health in the region (Ajayi et al., 2021). Multipronged mental health interventions and strategies should be developed considering the heterogeneity within and between African areas. Maternal mental health must be prioritised to achieve the United Nations' Sustainable Development Goals by 2030 and close the widening gap caused by the COVID-19 pandemic. Understanding the heterogeneity between and within the African region is critical for employing context-specific mental health initiatives to mitigate the pandemic's adverse maternal mental health consequences on pregnant women and new mothers. Rethinking approaches to maternal mental health to reduce the effects of the pandemic and provide a blueprint for future public health emergencies would benefit Africa (Ajayi et al., 2021).

1.3 African Communitarianism

Communitarianism is a philosophy that undergirds the connection between the individual and society (Mbiti, 1970). According to communitarianism, one's social identity and personality are greatly influenced by community relationships. The theory rejects the hegemony of individual rights and instead argues for the common good and the responsibility of all community members to achieve it (Kalumba, 2020). Communitarianism opposes extreme individualism and a laissez-faire approach, which deprioritises the stability of the overall community (Etzioni, 2014). The theory of communitarianism stipulates that an individual being cannot be a person on their own but by others, among others, and by being in a polis or community (Cohen, 2000). Communities must therefore be emphasised rather than individuals. Our very being is derived from our community's existence (Cohen, 2000). This means that personhood and all it involves depend on society, and one cannot be a person without the community.

African communitarianism emphasises the community (Mbiti, 1970; Menkiti, 1984). Menkiti (1984) articulates a communitarian ethos and argues that the community has priority over the individual in Africa. He distinguishes the Western and African views, claiming that the Western theory holds that a person is independent of the community. In contrast, the African view holds that a person is defined by reference to the surrounding community. Mbiti's (1970) maxim "I am because we are, and since we are, therefore I am" buttresses this view. According to Menkiti (1984), from an African point of view, the reality of the communal world takes precedence over the existence of individual life histories. He argues that the collective ethos has ontological and epistemological priority on biological and social grounds because an individual comes from a shared gene pool and belongs to a linguistic community. An individual becomes a person through social and ritual incorporation. The community defines the person as a person, not some isolated static quality of rationality, will, or memory. The African view supports the notion of personhood as acquired, not merely granted, as a consequence of birth and that as far as African societies are concerned, personhood is something individuals could fail (Oyowe, 2015).

Mbiti (1970) argues that the direct influence of the community in forming the individual is taken to mean the supremacy of the community over the individual. The community is the primary reference point for social and human existence (Mbiti, 1970). All forms of social utilities needed for human flourishing are seen from the lens of the collective. This implies that the essence of the individual cannot be understood outside the nature of the community. Individuals owe their existence and meaning to their normative standing in the community. This emphasis on the community in the Afro-communitarian debate suggests that all that can be known of the individual only concerns the community (Adeate, 2023).

Gyekye (1997) departs from other Afro-communitarians by claiming moderate communitarianism. He rejects the moral subordination of the individual to the community (also see Kalumba, 2020). Gyekye (1997) thus laments that the individual and the community have the status of equal moral standing, challenging other radical communitarians who emphasise the priority of the community over the individual. He argues that rationality, virtue, evaluation of moral judgements, and choice are critical in determining personhood in Africa. Gyekye (1995) uses an Akan proverb, "a person is not a palm tree to survive alone" to highlight human interdependence. Gyekye (1996) argues that individual capacities, talents, goals, and needs are met in interaction with those of others in a community. He challenges the notion that puts an individual's existence before the community. Citing another Akan proverb, "one tree does not make a forest," Gyekye (1997) argues that a community derives from an individual and their relationship. The reality of the community is derivative, not primary, and individuals choose whether they want to belong to a community (Gyekye, 1995).

African moderate communitarianism is not a widely recognised or established term or concept. However, as argued by Gyekye (1995), it is possible to explore the idea of a moderate approach to communitarianism within an African context. Moderate communitarianism is a perspective that acknowledges the value of the community and collective well-being while recognising the importance of individual rights, autonomy, and diversity within the community. It seeks a balanced approach that avoids extreme collectivism or individualism (see Gyekye, 1997; Kayange, 2020). Moderate Communitarianism acknowledges the importance of community cohesion and cooperation for the well-being of individuals while respecting the rights and autonomy of individuals within the community. It recognises that individual flourishing could contribute to the overall strength and prosperity of the community (Kayange, 2020). Moderate communitarianism recognises and embraces the diversity of individuals within the community, including differences in perspectives, beliefs, and values, as it promotes inclusivity, tolerance, and respect for individual choices, provided they do not harm others or undermine the common good.

1.4 Mental Health through African Moderate Communitarianism Lens

Extreme poverty, unemployment, toxic masculinity, community expectations, and responsibilities have been reported to be the leading causes of the surge in mental illness in Africa (Ajayi et al., 2021). Unlike individualistic societies,

African cultures help reduce the risk of cognitive issues because of their communitarian nature, as espoused in Nyanja proverbs, such *as mutu umodzi suzenza denga* meaning "one head does not support a roof" (Kayange, 2020). The saying demonstrates the togetherness in African communities, such that when faced with a problem, one should share it or ask for help but not keep the pain to oneself. In times of dire stress and depression, among other mental issues, the African community envisions these problems as communal and not individual problems.

The communitarian nature of African societies provides social support and connectedness that can buffer individuals against mental health challenges. According to the stress-buffering hypothesis, social support can intervene between stressful events and physiological stress reactions by attenuating perceptions of stress, increasing one's ability to cope, and restoring feelings of self-worth (Cohen, 2000). Among African cultures, community connectedness has been associated with lower rates of anxiety and depressive symptoms (Kinyanda et al., 2013). The communal worldview encourages collective responsibility, whereby the community shares the burden of caring for members experiencing mental health issues (Egbe et al., 2014).

However, the COVID-19 pandemic threatened traditional communitarian values in Africa. Preventive measures, particularly self-isolation of COVID-19-positive individuals, social distancing, and limitations on gatherings, challenged collectivist ideals like *Ubuntu* and Umunthu that have been crucial in alleviating mental health issues (Kainja et al., 2022). For instance, the restriction of hospital visitations during COVID-19 affected family caregivers' mental health and eroded caregiving concepts centred on togetherness (Mulaudzi et al., 2022). Not only were hospital visits curtailed, but home-based patients faced increased isolation. Loneliness spiked, even in the comfort of home. This contradicted the African emphasis on communal coping and caregiving.

Beyond hospital settings, COVID-19 mitigation policies limited social gatherings and interactions in communities more broadly. Mandates to avoid direct contact hampered engagement in cultural rituals and ceremonies that bolster social ties and community identity. Funerals, weddings, and religious gatherings were constrained. This likely elevated mental strain, as participation in collective rituals can improve psychological well-being by reinforcing shared values, providing comfort through grieving processes, and giving meaning to life experiences (Sorsdahl et al., 2009). With COVID-19 disruptions to cultural practices, many Africans lost critical outlets for affirming their belonging, reducing distress, and upholding Ubuntu.

At the national level, lockdowns and curfews to control COVID-19 transmission further isolated individuals and fragmented communities. Mobility restrictions and economic shutdowns disrupted livelihoods and support networks, elevating poverty, uncertainty, and family stress – key risk factors for mental illness (Jenkins et al., 2013). Simultaneously, access to formal mental health services declined due to health system strains and fear of contagion in clinical settings (Kola et al., 2021). This combination of increasing risk factors and reduced care options likely contributed to rising mental health burdens, as studies show an increased prevalence of depression, anxiety, and post-traumatic stress during the pandemic in multiple African nations (see review by Chen et al., 2021).

Bolstering communitarian ideologies like Ubuntu could help Africa address the mental health repercussions of COVID-19 (Kainja et al., 2022; Chima-konam & Ogbonnaya, 2022). Ubuntu emphasises compassion, solidarity, and relational well-being over individual interests – principles that could foster collective healing from pandemic trauma. This framework can guide public health messaging and interventions to promote social reconnection and collective coping after heightened isolation. Additionally, communal self-help groups and peer counselling networks could be leveraged to provide mental health support and build resilience where clinical services are scarce (Abas et al., 2016). Such community-driven efforts to jointly bear burdens could mitigate the spikes in individual mental illness.

However, reconceptualising mental health as a collective concern also risks unduly burdening already marginalised groups. The COVID-19 pandemic intensified pre-existing gender inequalities as women bore heightened domestic duties while facing greater violence – key stressors affecting African women's mental health (Mahlangu et al., 2022). Thus, the rhetoric around communal coping should not absolve duty-bearers like the state and expect women to shoulder collective burdens alone. Similarly, youth struggled under school closures, economic constraints, and isolation – underscoring the need for targeted mental health outreach for this demographic.

While moderate communitarian frameworks hold promise to address COVID-19's mental health burdens, implementing these approaches involves overcoming persistent social and systemic challenges. Long-standing barriers related to stigma, access, awareness, and resources continue to hinder mental healthcare in Africa, potentially limiting communitarian strategies. Reflecting critically on these obstacles illuminates areas requiring continued advocacy and reform. One significant barrier is the mental illness stigma that remains prevalent in some African communities. A qualitative South African study found that cultural beliefs about supernatural causes of mental disorders contributed to stigma from faith healers, families, and community members (Egbe et al., 2014). The cultural emphasis on communal harmony may pressure individuals to hide mental health struggles that could ostensibly disturb the balance. Similarly, a study in Nigeria identified stigmatising attitudes wherein mental illness was associated with weakness of character or divine punishment (James et al., 2012). Breaking stigma through a communitarian approach requires shifting perceptions of mental healthcare as a communal responsibility rather than individual weakness.

Access barriers also continue to impede mental healthcare in resource-constrained settings. A Ugandan study highlighted shortages of mental health professionals, prescription drugs, and inpatient facilities, with most care concentrated in urban centres (Miller et al., 2021). Patients' communitarian support networks are limited if clinical services remain geographically inaccessible or unaffordable. Integrating mental healthcare into primary facilities and national health coverage could help address these gaps. Telepsychiatry holds promise but requires infrastructure investments.

Moreover, a lack of mental health awareness persists in some communities, leading to delays in help-seeking. A study in Ethiopia revealed that many respondents had limited knowledge about mental illness, often conflating these conditions with substance abuse (Jarso et al., 2022). This contributed to preferences for informal healers over psychiatrists. Improving mental health literacy through a communitarian approach would emphasise collective education to share knowledge, combat misconceptions, and encourage supportive social norms around care-seeking.

Finally, poverty and unmet social needs, directly and indirectly, impact mental health but may not be fully addressed through a communitarian model alone. Food insecurity, housing instability, and lack of social safety nets elevate mental health risks. While communitarianism promotes mutual aid, government action is essential to ensure universal access to education, income, social services, and poverty reduction programmes. This highlights that addressing mental health requires multisectoral efforts across public health, policymaking, and socioeconomic domains. Africa's communitarian philosophies contain tremendous potential for addressing the mental health impacts of COVID-19 but must be enacted carefully. Bolstering communal coping and social connectedness could alleviate psychosocial distress heightened by the pandemic. However, this approach must avoid overburdening vulnerable groups or substituting for strengthened mental health systems. COVID-19 has tested African communities' resilience; leveraging togetherness ideologies could foster healing, but implementation must be thoughtful and avoid reinforcing inequalities.

1.5 Nuances between and Within African Countries

While this chapter has focused broadly on Africa, it is essential to note the immense diversity across and within African countries regarding culture, resources, policies, and COVID-19 impacts. There is no uniform African experience. Applying communitarian perspectives to mental healthcare must consider contextual heterogeneity at local levels.

At the country level, the extent of COVID-19 mental health impacts varied. For instance, a population survey in Nigeria indicated significant escalations in depression, anxiety, and stress compared to pre-pandemic prevalence (Aborode et al., 2022). However, a Kenyan study found no statistically significant increases in common mental disorders during COVID-19, potentially attributable to robust family support systems (Jenkins et al., 2013). Structural country differences in social protections may explain some of these contrasts. Even within nations, differences emerged – one study found that rural

Nigerian communities experienced more mental health decline than urban areas under lockdowns (Aborode et al., 2022).

There were also variations in mental healthcare resources and capacities. South Africa has the most extensive mental health policies and mental hospital facilities on the continent but still faces stigma and access issues in rural locales (Ajayi et al., 2021). By contrast, most African countries have minimal mental health leadership and specialists for their population sizes, constraining service delivery (Kola et al., 2021). These systems gaps require tailored strengthening efforts attuned to local needs. Applying communitarian approaches would imply leveraging extended family and communal networks to differing extents based on existing formal service availability and cultural variations.

Furthermore, the impact of COVID-19 disruption on cultural practices important for mental health likely differed across groups. Quantitative data from South Africa indicated that preventing gatherings for rites of passage ceremonies and burial rituals negatively impacted psychological well-being (Ajayi et al., 2021). In Muslim communities across Africa, banning Friday prayer gatherings and communal mourning rituals under COVID-19 severed critical cultural coping outlets, potentially heightening isolation and grief (Vahed, 2020). Restoring these practices through a communitarian lens would necessitate considering local cultural nuances. Overall, heterogeneity between and within African nations reinforces arguments against monolithic characterisations and the need for context-specific mental healthcare grounded in particular community needs, values, and lived realities. Applying shared communitarian philosophies involves tailoring approaches to diverse settings with unique risks, resources, and cultural practices. No "one size fits all" model exists for realising communal mental health.

1.6 Conclusion

Individualism and communitarianism play positive and influential roles in mental health in Africa. As the current chapter has shown, COVID-19 hurt the mental health of people in Africa. Nevertheless, even though communitarianism might not be the sole panacea, community structures played a positive role in alleviating some mental health problems. Community-based initiatives and awareness campaigns were implemented to reduce the stigma of COVID-19 and increase mental health literacy. Additional efforts to address the mental health effects of the pandemic in Africa were to expand mental health services, train other mental health professionals, and integrate mental health support into primary healthcare systems. It is important to note that the situation might have varied across African countries due to variations in healthcare systems, resources, and socioeconomic factors.

Nonetheless, addressing African mental health needs remained crucial to ensure the overall well-being of individuals and communities affected by the COVID-19 pandemic. Promoting mental health within an African communitarian context requires a balance between preserving valuable cultural resources and incorporating evidence-based approaches to mental health care. It further required recognising the strengths of communal support systems while addressing gaps in resources, education, and awareness around mental health. Finally, by adopting a moderate communitarian approach to mental health, African societies could have balanced the values of communal solidarity and individual rights, recognising the interdependence of both aspects for the well-being of individuals and the community as a whole. This perspective provides a middle ground that promotes social cohesion and individual flourishing within the African context.

References

Abas, M., Ali, G. C., Nakimuli-Mpungu, E., & Chibanda, D. (2016). Depression in people living with HIV in sub-Saharan Africa: Time to act. *Tropical Medicine & International Health, 21*(12), 1392–1396.

Aborode, A. T., Corriero, A. C., Mehmood, Q., Nawaz, A., Aayush, Upadhyay, P., Badri, R., & Hasan, M. M. (2022). People living with mental disorder in Nigeria amidst COVID-19: Challenges, implications, and recommendations. *The International Journal of Health Planning and Management, 37*(3), 1191–1198. https://doi.org/10.1002/hpm.3394

Adeate, T. (2023). Mbiti on community in African political thought: Reconciling the "I" and the "we." *Phronimon, 24*(1). https://doi.org/10.25159/2413-3086/12205

Ajayi, K. V., Wachira, E., Bolarinwa, O. A., & Suleman, B. D. (2021). Maternal mental health in Africa during the COVID-19 pandemic: A neglected global health issue. *Epidemiology Health, 43*, e2021078.

Bantjes, J., Swanevelder, S., Jordaan, E., Sampson, N. A., Petukhova, M. V., & Lochner, C. (2023). COVID-19 and common mental disorders among university students in South Africa. *South African Journal of Science, 119*(1–2), article 13594. https://doi.org/10.17159/sajs.2023/13594

Chen, J., Farah, N., Dong, R. K., Chen, R. Z., Xu, W., Yin, J., Chen, B. Z., Delios, A. Y., Miller, S., Wan, X., Ye, W., & Zhang, S. X. (2021). Mental health during the COVID-19 crisis in Africa: A systematic review and meta-analysis. *International Journal of Environmental Research and Public Health, 18*(20), 10604. https://doi.org/10.3390/ijerph182010604

Chimakonam, J. O., & Ogbonnaya, L. U. (2022). Can Afro-communitarianism be useful in combating the challenge of human interaction posed by the COVID-19 pandemic? *International Journal of Environmental Research and Public Health, 19*(21), 14255.

Cohen, A. J. (2000). Does communitarianism require individual independence? *The Journal of Ethics, 4*(3), 283–305. www.jstor.org/stable/25115648

Dawood, B., Tomita, A., & Ramlall, S. (2022). "Unheard", "uncared for" and "unsupported": The mental health impact of Covid-19 on healthcare workers in KwaZulu-Natal Province, South Africa. *PLOS One, 17*(5), e0266008. https://doi.org/10.1371/journal.pone.0266008

Duby, Z., Bunce, B., Fowler, C., Bergh, K., Jonas, K., Dietrich, J. J., Govindasamy, D., Kuo, C., & Mathews, C. (2022). Intersections between COVID-19 and socioeconomic mental health stressors in the lives of South African adolescent girls and young women. *Child and Adolescent Psychiatry and Mental Health, 16*(23). https://doi.org10.1186/s13034-022-00457-y

Durizo, K., Asiedu, E., Merwe, A., & Gunther, I. (2023). Economic recovery but stagnating mental health during a global pandemic? Evidence from Ghana and South Africa. *The Review of Income and Wealth, 28*(2). https://doi.org/10.1111/roiw/12587

Egbe, C. O., Brooke-Sumner, C., Kathree, T., Selohilwe, O., Thornicroft, G., & Petersen, I. (2014). Psychiatric stigma and discrimination in South Africa: Perspectives from key stakeholders. *BMC Psychiatry, 14*(1), 1–10. https://doi.org/10.1186/s12888-014-0191-x

Etzioni, A. (2014). Communitarianism revisited. *Journal of Political Ideologies, 19*(3), 241–260.

Falgas-Bague, I., Thembo, T., Kaiser, J. L., Hamer, D. H., Scott, N. A., Ngoma, T., Paul, R., Juntunen, A., Rockers, P. C., & Fink, G. (2023). Trends in maternal mental health during the COVID-19 pandemic: Evidence from Zambia. *PLOS One, 18*(2), e0281091. https://doi.org/10.1371/journal. Pone.0281091

Gyasi, R. M. (2020). COVID-19 and mental health of older Africans: An urgency for public health policy and response strategy. *International Psychogeriatrics, 32*(10). https://doi.org/10.1017/S1041610220003312

Gyekye, K. (1995). *An essay on African philosophical thought: The Akan conceptual scheme*. Temple University Press.

Gyekye, K. (1996). *African cultural values: An introduction*. Sankofa.

Gyekye, K. (1997). *Tradition and modernity: Philosophical reflections on the African experience*. Oxford University Press.

Haag, K., Du Toit, S., Skeen, S., Steventon Roberts, K., Chideya, Y., Notholi, V., Sambudla, A., Gordon, S., Sherr, L., & Tomlinson, M. (2022). Predictors of COVID-related changes in mental health in a South African sample of adolescents and young adults. *Psychology, Health Medicine, 27*(S1), 239–255. https://doi.org/10.1080/13548506.2022.2108087

James, B. O., Omoaregba, J. O., & Okogbenin, E. O. (2012). Stigmatising attitudes towards persons with mental illness: A survey of medical students and interns from Southern Nigeria. *Mental Illness, 4*(1), e8. https://doi.org/10.4081/mi.2012.e8

Jarso, M. H., Debele, G. R., Gezimu, W., Nigatu, D., Mohammedhussein, M., Mamo, A., Dule, A., Hassen, M., & Jemal, K. (2022). Knowledge, attitude, and its correlates of the community toward mental illness in Mattu, South West Ethiopia. *Frontiers in Psychiatry, 13*, 1018440. https://doi.org/10.3389/fpsyt.2022.1018440

Jenkins, R., Othieno, C., Okeyo, S., Aruwa, J., Kingora, J., & Jenkins, B. (2013). Health system challenges to integration of mental health delivery in primary care in Kenya- perspectives of primary care health workers. *BMC Health Services Research, 13*(1), 368. https://doi.org/10.1186/1472-6963-13-368

Joska, J. A., Andersen, L., Rabie, S., Marais, A., Ndwandwa, E. S., Wilson, P., King, A., & Sikkema, K. J. (2020). Covid-19: Increased risk to the mental health and safety of women living with HIV in South Africa. *Aids and Behavior, 24*. https://doi.org/doi.org/10.1007

Kainja, J., Ndasauka, Y., Mchenga, M., Kondowe, F., M'manga, C., Maliwichi, L., & Nyamali, S. (2022). Umunthu, Covid-19 and mental health in Malawi. *Heliyon, 8*(11), e11316. https://doi.org/10.1016/j.heliyon.2022.e11316

Kalumba, K. M. (2020). A defence of Kwame Gyekye's moderate communitarianism. *Philosophical Papers, 49*(1), 137–158. https://doi.org/10.1080/05568641.2019.1684840

Kayange, G. M. (2020). *Capitalism and freedom in African political philosophy*. Palgrave Macmillan. https://doi.org/10.1007/978-3-030-44360-3

Kinyanda, E., Kizza, R., Abbo, C., Ndyanabangi, S., & Levin, J. (2013). Prevalence and risk factors of depression in childhood and adolescence in Uganda: A systematic review and meta-analysis. *Social Psychiatry and Psychiatric Epidemiology*, *48*(8), 1347–1360. https://doi.org/10.1007/s00127-013-0720-5

Kola, L., Kohrt, B. A., Hanlon, C., Naslund, J. A., Sikander, S., Balaji, M., Benjet, C., Cheung, E., Eaton, J., Gonsalves, P., Haq, I. U., Honikman, S., Joska, J. A., Luitel, N., Lund, C., Patel, V., Rahman, A., Silove, D., van Ommeren, M., . . . Ventevogel, P. (2021). COVID-19 mental health impact and responses in low-income and middle-income countries: Reimagining global mental health. *The Lancet Psychiatry*, *8*(6), 535–550. https://doi.org/10.1016/S2215-0366(21)00025-0

Mahlangu, P., Gibbs, A., Shai, N., Machisa, M., Nunze, N., & Sikweyiya, Y. (2022). Impact of COVID-19 lockdown and link to women and children's experiences of violence in the home in South Africa. *BMC Public Health*, *22*, 1029. https://doi.org/10.1186/s12889-022-13422-3

Mbiti, J. S. (1970). *Concepts of god in Africa*. Society for Promoting Christian Knowledge.

Menkiti, I. (1984). Person and community in African traditional thought. In R. Wright (Ed.), *African philosophy: An introduction*. University Press of America.

Miller, A. P., Ziegel, L., Mugamba, S., Kyasanku, E., Wagman, J. A., Nkwanzi-Lubega, V., Nakigozi, G., Kigozi, G., Nalugoda, F., Kigozi, G., Nkale, J., Watya, S., & Ddaaki, W. (2021). Not enough money and too many thoughts: Exploring perceptions of mental health in two Ugandan districts through the mental health literacy framework. *Qualitative Health Research*, *31*(5), 967–982. https://doi.org/10.1177/1049732320986164

M'manga, C., Ndasauka, Y., Kainja, J., Kondowe, F., Mchenga, M., Maliwichi, L., & Nyamali, S. (2023). The world is coming to an end! COVID-19, depression, and anxiety among adolescents in Malawi. *Frontiers in Psychiatry*, *13*, 1024793. https://doi.org/10.3389/fpsyt.2022.1024793

Mudiriza, G., & Lannoy, A. D. (2020). *Youth emotional well-being during the COVID-19-related lockdown in South Africa* (Working Paper No. 268). Southern Africa Labour and Development Research Unit.

Mulaudzi, F. M., Anokwuru, R. A., Du-Plessis, M. A. R., & Lebese, R. T. (2022). Reflections on the concomitants of the restrictive visitation policy during the COVID-19 pandemic: An ubuntu perspective. *Frontiers in Sociology*, *11*(6), 769199.

Oyowe, O. A. (2015). This thing called communitarianism: A critical review of Matolino's personhood in African philosophy. *South African Journal of Philosophy*, *34*(4), 504–515.

Robertson, L. J., Maposa, I., Samaroo, H., & Johnson, O. (2020). Mental health of healthcare workers during the COVID-19 outbreak: A rapid scoping review to inform provincial guidelines in South Africa. *South African Medical Journal Review*, *110*(10).

Sodi, T., Modipane, M., Oppong, K., Quarshie, E., Asatsa, S., Mutambara, J., & Khombo, S. (2021). Mental health policy and system preparedness to respond to COVID-19 and other health emergencies: A case study of four African countries. *South African Journal of Psychology*, *51*(2), 279–292.

Sorsdahl, K., Stein, D. J., Grimsrud, A., Seedat, S., Flisher, A. J., Williams, D. R., & Myer, L. (2009). Traditional healers in the treatment of common mental disorders in South Africa. *The Journal of Nervous and Mental Disease*, *197*(6), 434–441. https://doi.org/10.1097/NMD.0b013e3181a61dbc

Vahed, G. (2020). The contagious power of words: Muslim South Africans during the pandemic. *Transformation: Critical Perspectives on Southern Africa, 104,* 43–54. https://doi.org/10.1353/trn.2020.0031

World Health Organization. (2021). *COVID-19 continues to disrupt essential health services in 90% of countries.* www.who.int/news/item/23-04-2021-covid-19-continues-to-disrupt-essential-health-services-in-90-of-countries

Wright, J., & Jayawickrama, J. (2021). "We need other human beings to be human": Examining the indigenous philosophy of umunthu and strengthening mental health interventions. *Culture, Medicine, and Psychiatry, 45*(4), 613–628.

Part 1
The Heightened Burdens of COVID-19

2 Complex and Multifaceted Sociodemographic Depression Correlates in Malawi During COVID-19

Daniel Chikatentha, Edister S. Jamu, and Gowokani Chijere-Chirwa

2.1 Introduction

Mental health is the capacity of individuals and groups to interact with one another and the environment in ways that promote subjective well-being, the optimal development and use of cognitive, affective, and relational abilities, and the achievement of individual and collective goals consistent with justice (Rowling, 2002, p. 8). It implies that deficiency in any function is having what World Health Organization (WHO, 1992) refers to as a mental disorder, a broad term encompassing mental illness, intellectual disability, personality disorder, substance dependence, and adjustment to adverse life events.

Emerging literature on the relationship between the risk of mental health problems, such as depression, and the COVID-19 pandemic is high. A significant portion of this literature is from Asia, particularly China (such as Xiang et al., 2020), South Korea (such as Park & Park, 2020), Japan (such as Shigemura et al., 2020), but also from South America (Lima et al., 2020). A closer look at most of the mentioned literature revealed case studies highlighting how frontline workers and the general population are all at high risk of mental health after being subjected to quarantines and lockdowns. Research by DeLuca et al. (2020) shows the linkage between psychological stress, which poses a threat to mental health through home quarantines and an increase in symptoms of anxiety and depression.

A study by Barbisch et al. (2015) on the role of quarantine in combating infectious diseases such as severe acute respiratory syndrome (SARS) and Ebola in Africa found that subjecting people to quarantine could lead to severe psychological distress, which is worsened by fear and uncertainty of the disease. Quarantines could further lead to mass panic and problems in mental health simply because individuals are kept in small spaces for prolonged periods. Fiorillo and Gorwood (2020) contend that increased loneliness and reduced social interaction are a recipe for mental health disorders like schizophrenia and major depression. During the COVID-19 pandemic, there was reduced physical, social interaction and increased isolation, which, according to Fiorillo and Gorwood (2020), was a high risk for mental disorders, especially depression.

DOI: 10.4324/9781003425861-3

In Malawi, 128 cases of suicide occurred in the capital city, Lilongwe, between September 2018 and June 2019, as reported by the Malawi Police – most of them men. Between January 2022 and August of that year, the police reported 208 suicide cases, with 168 being male and 40 being female, indicating an increase from the same period in 2021 when they reported 160 suicide cases (Southern Africa Litigation Centre, 2022). It is on record that most of these suicides resulted from depression arising from either family challenges or economic hardships (Mweninguwe, 2019). Worse still, these statistics were recorded before the COVID-19 pandemic. Banda et al. (2021) argue that during the lockdown period (between April and September 2020) to mitigate the effect of the COVID-19 pandemic, Malawi witnessed a sharp increase in suicide cases, most resulting from financial hardships. Gordon et al. (2020) assert that the preventive measures in terms of social distancing and quarantines set due to COVID-19 brought about much stress because the government had crippled some sectors of the economy in the interest of public health. This eventually led to a loss of work and income. The link between this loss of income and fear and anxiety about the general well-being of family members makes the connection between mental health (depression) and COVID-19 obvious.

Udedi (2014) conducted a cross-sectional survey among patients attending the outpatient department at Matawale Health Centre in Zomba, where a total of 350 adults were randomly selected using systematic sampling, and found that the prevalence of depression among the selected patients was 30.3% while the detection rate of depression by the clinicians was 0%. Kutcher et al. (2017) conducted a similar study on adolescent depression. In this study, it was hypothesised that the onset of most depressive tendencies occurs during adolescence. The findings of the survey indicated that 75.4% of the patients received mental health-related diagnoses, 71.4% of the youth were diagnosed with depression, and 26% of the youth were diagnosed with other mental disorders. Muhia and Nanji (2021) recently examined mental health among East and Southern African youth during COVID-19. This latter study found that the most common mental health problems among the youth participating in the research were depression, anxiety, post-traumatic stress disorder (PTSD), generalised anxiety disorder, and harmful substance abuse. The study accurately demonstrated that COVID-19 had intensified these pressures. Lockdown measures, disruption of peer contact, and financial constraints played a role. The youth often opt for coping mechanisms that have worsened their mental well-being.

Literature on depression, locally and internationally, clarifies how damaging poor mental health can be (Kutcher et al., 2017; Muhia & Nanji, 2021; Ryff & Singer, 1998; Udedi, 2014; WHO, 2004, 2008). A closer look at the literature exposes a gap where there is little or no focus on the effects that the COVID-19 pandemic had on depression in Malawi, bar a few studies recently published by Kainja et al. (2022) and M'manga et al. (2023). The utmost need for the study on which this chapter reports was to examine the socioeconomic factors associated with the prevalence of depression in Malawi during COVID-19.

According to the sociological theory of mind, cognitive development starts in the mind; anything affecting the mental health of citizens, thus, has an implicit negative effect on the human economic development of a country as it affects human resources, an essential component of production. The Solow economic growth model illustrates this (Todaro & Smith, 2011). This model was used to study mental health issues in COVID-19. Firstly, the containment measures implemented in Malawi undermined the country's long-term human and economic development. Secondly, the response plans undermined the country's long-term human and economic development. Thirdly, the COVID-19 pandemic jeopardised the achievement of the Sustainable Development Goals (SDGs), particularly SDG 3, which focuses on good health and well-being. As the UN draft discussion paper posits, the diversion of national focus from national priorities towards containing the spread of the pandemic may likely undo the progress made so far on sustainable development, and the countries will witness people falling back into poverty and widening inequalities (Thula et al., 2020; United Nations Development Programme [UNDP], 2020).

In light of the aforementioned, this chapter will contribute knowledge that could play an integral part in realising the Malawi 2063 vision of achieving an inclusively wealthy and self-reliant nation (Government of Malawi, 2020). In the first place, discussions in this chapter will directly affect enabler number one in Vision 2063, namely a mindset change. Some mental health problems, particularly depression, may be overcome by a literal mindset change from negative to positive thinking. Additionally, for an individual to change his or her mindset, he or she needs to be in the right state of mental health. Otherwise, mindset change may lead to mental health issues, such as pathological hatred (xenophobia) and extremism. Vision 2063 has been developed not bearing in mind the adverse effects the pandemic had added on the already existing mental health issues. It may prompt one to rethink the vision with a COVID-19 lens (Government of Malawi, 2020).

The current study looked at the prevalence of depression, coping mechanisms, and the associated socioeconomic factors. Of the participants, 22.7% met the criteria for depression; none had been diagnosed as such by the clinicians (Author, date). These results show that one in five participants presented significant symptoms of depression during the COVID-19 pandemic. The current estimate of 22.7% is slightly lower compared to the one reported by another study conducted at two clinics for non-communicable diseases in Lilongwe on the validity of the Patient Health Questionnaire-8 (PHQ-8) to screen for depression in patients with type 2 diabetes mellitus (Udedi et al., 2019). The investigation reported that 41% of diabetes patients were depressed. However, the estimates of the study by Udedi et al. (2019) are closely related to what has been reported elsewhere in the sub-Saharan region, namely South Africa (32%), Tanzania (30%), Ghana (31.3%), Guinea (34.4%), Tunisia (38%), Uganda (38%), Morocco (33.1%), Ethiopia (39.7%), and

Egypt (32.1%) (see Khan et al., 2019; Mendenhall et al., 2014; Ogunsakin et al., 2021; Teshome et al., 2018).

The current study utilised nationally representative secondary data from the Malawi High-Frequency Phone Survey (HFPS) obtained from the World Bank Group and International Monetary Fund (2021, March 29) and the National Statistical Office (NSO) (2023, March 29). The total sample size comprised 1,584 individuals. Data collection followed the Helsinki 1968 protocol, which anonymises data (World Medical Association, 2014). The data being used do not present respondent metadata that may lead to the identification of who the respondents were.

The variable of interest was depression, measured using the locally validated PHQ-8 questionnaire to identify depression among persons during the COVID-19 pandemic. The eight-item PHQ-8 depression scale is established as a valid diagnostic and severity measure for depressive disorders in large clinical studies (Kroenke et al., 2009). The total score is determined by adding the scores of each of the four items. Scores are rated as normal (0–2), mild (3–5), moderate (6–8), and severe (9–12). The total score ≥ 3 for the first two questions suggests anxiety. The total score ≥ 3 for the last two questions suggests depression. The PHQ-8 is a useful depression measure for population-based studies, and either its diagnostic algorithm or a cut-point > or = 10 can be used for defining current depression (Kroenke et al., 2009).

2.2 COVID-19 Related Depression

Out of 1,584 respondents, the majority (1,254; 79.20%) were male, while 330 (20.80%) were female. A high number, 997 (62.91%) of the respondents, were from rural areas, whereas 587 (37.09%) were from urban areas. Out of 1,584 of these respondents, 677 (42.68%) were from the southern region, 676 (42.62%) were from the central region, and 231 (14.69%) were from the northern region of Malawi.

The prevalence of depression following the analysis of the results for this study stood at 22.39%. Of the 1,584 respondents, 1,005 (63.42%) reported having coping mechanisms for depression, whereas 579 (36.58%) did not have any coping mechanisms for depression. According to the WHO Newsletter published on 2 March 2022, in the first year of the COVID-19 pandemic, the global prevalence of anxiety and depression increased by 25% (World Health Organization, 2021). The brief also highlighted who had been most affected. It summarised the effect of the pandemic on the availability of mental health services, and how this has changed during the pandemic. This estimate by the WHO is not far-fetched from what the current study found.

These findings indicate significant depressive symptoms in one-fifth of participants during the COVID-19 pandemic. The current prevalence estimate (22.7%) is higher than Kauye et al.'s (2014) estimate of 19% and slightly lower than Udedi et al.'s (2019) report of 30.3% in a diabetes mellitus study. Previous studies' settings may account for the relatively lower prevalence, as they were not conducted during the pandemic. Higher depression prevalence in low- and middle-income countries might result from inequalities, healthcare inequities, poor diabetic care, poverty, financial difficulties, and economic stressors (Yekta et al., 2010). However, the current study aligns with findings in the sub-Saharan region (Anderson et al., 2013; Muhia & Nanji, 2021). These results emphasise the urgency of addressing mental health during the COVID-19 pandemic. Mental health policies, clinician training, and access to mental health services are essential (Khan et al., 2019; Mendenhall et al., 2014; Ogunsakin et al., 2021; Teshome et al., 2018).

2.3 Correlates of COVID-19 Related Depression

Of 1,584 respondents, 352 (22.73%) were depressed, and 1,220 (77.61%) were not depressed. Of the respondents, 25% were depressed and selected sales of assets as a way of coping with depression, whereas 22.35% did not select sales of assets as a way of coping with depression. Out of 1,584 respondents, only 18 (75%) were not depressed and selected sales of assets as a way to deal with depression, while 1,202 were not depressed and did not select sales of assets as a coping mechanism for depression. Engaged in additional income-generating activity was selected by 23.08% of the respondents who were depressed, while 22.33% who were depressed did not select it. Of the respondents, 76.92% were not depressed but managed to select coping mechanisms, while 77.67% who were not depressed did not engage themselves in additional income-generating activity. The majority of respondents (1,174; 77.65%) were not depressed and did not receive assistance from friends and family, while 46 (76.66%) respondents still selected receiving assistance from friends and family as a way of coping with depression. Of the respondents, 14 (23.33%) were depressed and selected receiving assistance from friends and family, whereas 338 (22.35%) did not select it. The study's sample size of 1,584 respondents provides a significant representation of the population, allowing for meaningful observations regarding depression. The reported depression rate of 22.73% emphasises the impact of the pandemic on mental health in Malawi. This rate warrants attention from policymakers, healthcare professionals, and society at large (Dale et al., 2021).

Whether depressed or not depressed, 79 (5.03%) selected borrowing from friends and family as a coping mechanism, while 1,493 (94.97%) did not select it. Taking a loan from a financial institution was one way of dealing with depression, and only 1 depressed respondent selected it, whereas 351 (99.72%) did not select it. However, 3 people selected it despite not being depressed, while 1,217 (99.75%) did not select it and were not depressed. Credit purchase was another coping mechanism and was selected by 5 people who were depressed and 12 people who were not depressed, whereas 1,567 (99.68%) people did not select it. The role of social support networks is evident in the choice of coping mechanisms. While a majority of non-depressed respondents did not seek assistance from friends and family, a noteworthy proportion of depressed individuals opted for this form of support (Fang, 2019). This emphasises the importance of strong social connections in managing mental health during the pandemic.

Out of 352 respondents who were depressed, only 1 chose to select "sold harvest in advance" as a coping mechanism, whereas 351 did not select it, and 6 respondents who were not depressed selected "sold harvest in advance" as a coping mechanism. In contrast, 1,214 (77.59%) did not select it and were not depressed. Almost 22.22% of respondents who were depressed selected reducing food consumption as a way of coping, while 22.41% did not select it even if they were depressed. Of the respondents, 77.78% who were not depressed selected to reduce food consumption, whereas 77.59% who were not depressed did not select it. Engaging in additional income-generating activities was chosen as a coping mechanism by a significant proportion of depressed respondents. This indicates the population's resilience and adaptive strategies to combat both financial and emotional challenges. However, the marginal difference between depressed and non-depressed individuals in selecting this option suggests that while financial stability can influence mental well-being, it might not be the sole determinant of depression (Dadson et al., 2018).

Of the respondents who were depressed or not depressed, only 6.30% selected "reduced non-food consumption" and 93.70% did not select it despite being depressed or not depressed. Relying on savings was one way of coping with depression selected by 73 respondents who were depressed, while 279 respondents did not select it even if they were depressed. Of the respondents who were not depressed, 277 managed by relying on savings as a coping mechanism, while 943 respondents who were not depressed did not select it. The study indicates that both depressed and non-depressed individuals considered reducing food consumption as a coping mechanism. This reflects the intricate interplay between economic challenges and mental health (Zhang, 2021). However, the slight variation between the two groups suggests that while economic factors contribute, depression might also be influenced by a range of other factors.

Only 1 depressed respondent depended on assistance from NGOs to deal with depression, while 352 people were depressed but did not select assistance from NGOs. Of the respondents, 1,219 were not depressed and did not select NGO assistance. Only 1 depressed respondent selected taking advance payment from employers as a way of coping, while 352 depressed people did not select it. Of the respondents, only 2 people were not depressed and managed to select "take an advanced payment from employers," whereas 1,218 did not select it. The limited selection of NGO assistance as coping mechanisms by depressed individuals might highlight a lack of awareness, accessibility, or perceived effectiveness of such support systems (McDaid et al., 2008). Addressing these barriers could lead to more holistic strategies for managing depression during crises.

Assistance from the government was specified as a coping mechanism, and 6 depressed respondents selected it, while 346 depressed respondents did not select it. Of the respondents, 18 were not depressed, but they were selected to be assisted by the government, whereas 1,202 respondents who were not depressed did not select assistance from the government. Other people found ways to cope with depression. Of the respondents, 30.23% of those who were depressed selected to find their coping mechanism, whereas 69.77% of respondents who were depressed also selected coping mechanisms for depression. Of the respondents, 22.17% who were depressed did not specify their coping mechanisms, while 77.83% who were not depressed also did not specify their coping mechanisms. The study underscores the diversity of coping mechanisms adopted by respondents. Many depressed individuals opted not to specify their coping mechanisms (Aranda & Lincoln, 2011). This highlights the complex and individualised nature of mental health management.

2.4 The Risk Factors Associated with COVID-19 Related Depression

Among males, the odds of becoming depressed were 17% lower than females. A p-value of 0.212 indicates that the difference is statistically not significant. The findings showed that individuals in the second wealth quintile had 38% higher odds of being depressed compared to the ones in the lowest wealth quintile. The difference is statistically significant, with a p-value of 0.04. Individuals in the middle wealth quintile had 37% higher odds of becoming depressed compared to those in the lowest quintile. However, the p-value of 0.08 shows that the difference was statistically insignificant. The odds of becoming depressed among respondents from the fourth wealth quintile were 16% higher than the lowest. However, the difference was statistically not significant with a p-value of 0.37. The households from the highest wealth quintile reflected 80% higher odds of becoming depressed than those in the lowest wealth quintile. Statistically, the difference was significant with a p-value of 0.01.

The findings of this study are contrary to what (M'manga et al., 2023) found in research conducted in Malawi, where females showed a higher percentage of anxiety symptoms than males. This is also consistent with several studies on gender differences in different anxiety disorders, which indicate that females suffer from anxiety more than males, and are diagnosed with the most anxiety disorders (Asher et al., 2017; Asher & Aderka, 2018; Schneier & Goldmark, 2015). Studies have consistently shown that one of the contributing factors is that males have better resilience to stress than females (see Hou et al., 2020). The findings of the current study are also contrary to the findings by Matandika et al. (2022), who found that the prevalence of mental disorders was higher in men than in women; hence, there is a need for more research to establish and understand the magnitude of the problem of a comparison between men and women when it comes to depression prevalence.

The results also showed that respondents from households with 3 to 4 members had 8% lower odds of becoming depressed compared to those with fewer than 3 members. However, the difference was statistically not significant with a p-value of 0.7. Respondents from households with 5 to 6 members had 17% higher odds of becoming depressed than those with fewer than 3 members. The difference was statistically not significant with a p-value of 0.29. Respondents from households with 7 to 8 members had 10% higher odds of becoming depressed compared to those from households with fewer than 3 members. Statistically, the difference was not significant, with a p-value of 0.6. Respondents from households with more than 9 members had 17% higher odds of becoming depressed than those with fewer than 3 members. However, the difference was statistically not significant, with a p-value of 0.37.

The findings also indicated that households with 3 to 4 members above 18 years of age had equal odds of becoming depressed compared to those with fewer than 3 members. The difference was statistically not significant with a p-value of 0.98. The category reflecting households with 5 to 6 members above 18 years of age, showed 15% lower odds of becoming depressed than those with fewer than 3 members. However, the difference was statistically not significant with a p-value of 0.55. The category of more than 6 members in the household above 18 years of age had 50% higher odds of becoming depressed than the category with fewer than 3 members. However, the difference was statistically not significant with a p-value of 0.5.

A study by Munyenyembe and Chen (2022) showed an inverse gradient in the association between wealth quintile and coping with the depression. In the current study, the assumption was that this result could be an effect of the consequences of the pandemic on family income, since by July 2020, 59.4% of households had seen their income decrease, and 30.1% of the respondents had lost their jobs due to the pandemic (Thula et al., 2020; UNDP, 2020). Public policies to help families economically initially focused on those with the lowest income, with benefits subsequently being extended to the most vulnerable 80% of the population (Langer et al., 2022). In the case of Malawi, the fear of business closures, lockdowns, and loss of employment provided an extrapolation as to why the wealthier were more depressed due to the COVID-19 pandemic, as it meant a loss of income and subsequent loss in livelihood.

Moreover, the findings in a study by Qin et al. (2022) suggest that the socioeconomic gradient in depression among older people may have deteriorated during the initial phase of the pandemic, and this might be explained in part by increased financial hardship, difficulties in accessing services, and reduced social contact. These results align with previous studies, before and during COVID-19 (Lima et al., 2020; Muhia & Nanji, 2021; UNDP, 2020), which found a relationship between social and economic factors and depression. These studies expand on what has been reported in the literature by showing differences in the association between depression and age according to the associated available coping mechanisms (O'Connell et al., 2009; Shah et al., 2020; Shigemura et al., 2020).

From a theoretical perspective, the current study's findings resonate with the stress and coping model, which posits that individuals experience stressors and that their coping mechanisms determine their psychological outcomes (Lazarus & Folkman, 1984). The COVID-19 pandemic has brought significant stressors that may have contributed to the high prevalence of depression observed in the current study. Respondents may have experienced financial stress, job insecurity, social isolation, and fear of contracting the virus (Ye et al., 2020). Coping mechanisms, such as social support, problem-solving, and emotional regulation, may have influenced their psychological outcomes (Fluharty & Fancourt, 2021).

2.5 Conclusion

The COVID-19 pandemic crisis has greatly affected human lives across the world. Uncertainty and quarantine have been affecting people's mental health. Estimations of mental health problems are needed immediately for better planning and management of these concerns at a global level. The current study suggests that participating males (19%) were more likely to be depressed compared to females. Furthermore, in terms of age, the older age group seemed to experience less depression. The effect of wealth status on depression was heterogeneous, indicating no universal relationship exists between wealth and depression. Rather, the association can be influenced by many factors that interact in complex ways. There needs to be a focus on strengthening mental healthcare services to which persons with depression could be connected. It is, therefore, important to explore ways to identify depression during any future pandemic and devise coping mechanisms to assist the citizenry during such times. By examining the prevalence of depression and socioeconomic factors associated with depression in Malawi during the COVID-19 pandemic, this study offers a local mental health perspective. The study found similarities and differences that should be considered in developing mental health programmes in pandemic situations. The high prevalence of depression in Malawi during the COVID-19 pandemic revealed a pressing need to develop programmes and tools that could address mental health from a global perspective in the context of a low- and middle-income country.

References

Anderson, L. M. C., Schierenbeck, I., Strumpher, J., Krantz, G., Topper, K., Backman, G., Ricks, E., & Van Rooyen, D. (2013). Help-seeking behaviour, barriers to care and experiences of care among persons with depression in Eastern Cape, South Africa. *Journal of Affective Disorders, 151*(2), 439–448.

Aranda, M. P., & Lincoln, K. D. (2011). Financial strain, negative interaction, coping styles, and mental health among low-income Latinos. *Race and Social Problems, 3*, 280–297.

Asher, M., & Aderka, I. M. (2018). Gender differences in social anxiety disorder. *Journal of Clinical Psychology, 74*(10), 1730–1741.

Asher, M., Asnaani, A., & Aderka, I. M. (2017). Gender differences in social anxiety disorder: A review. *Clinical Psychology Review, 56*, 1–12.

Banda, G. T., Banda, N., Chadza, A., & Mthunzi, C. (2021). Suicide epidemic in Malawi: What can we do? *The Pan African Medical Journal, 38*(69). https://doi.org/10.11604/pamj.2021.38.69.27843

Barbisch, D., Koenig, K. L., & Shih, F.-Y. (2015). Is there a case for quarantine? Perspectives from SARS to Ebola. *Disaster Medicine and Public Health Preparedness, 9*(5), 547–553.

Chen, J., Farah, N., Dong, R. K., Chen, R. Z., Xu, W., Yin, J., Chen, B. Z., Delios, A. Y., Miller, S., & Wan, X. (2021). Mental health during the Covid-19 crisis in Africa: A systematic review and meta-analysis. *International Journal of Environmental Research and Public Health, 18*(20), 10604.

Chirwa, G. C. (2020). "Who knows more, and why?" Explaining socioeconomic-related inequality in knowledge about HIV in Malawi. *Scientific African, 7*, e00213. https://doi.org/10.1016/j.sciaf.2019.e00213

Chirwa, G. C., Suhrcke, M., & Moreno-Serra, R. (2020). The impact of Ghana's national health insurance on psychological distress. *Applied Health Economics and Health Policy, 18*(2), 249–259.

Dadson, D. A., Annor, F., & Salifu Yendork, J. (2018). The burden of care: Psychosocial experiences and coping strategies among caregivers of persons with mental illness in Ghana. *Issues in Mental Health Nursing, 39*(11), 915–923.

Dale, R., O'Rourke, T., Humer, E., Jesser, A., Plener, P. L., & Pieh, C. (2021). Mental health of apprentices during the COVID-19 pandemic in Austria and the effect of gender, migration background, and work situation. *International Journal of Environmental Research and Public Health, 18*(17), 8933.

DeLuca, J. S., Andorko, N. D., Chibani, D., Jay, S. Y., Rakhshan Rouhakhtar, P. J., Petti, E., Klaunig, M. J., Thompson, E. C., Millman, Z. B., & Connors, K. M. (2020). Telepsychotherapy with youth at clinical high risk for psychosis: Clinical issues and best practices during the COVID-19 pandemic. *Journal of Psychotherapy Integration, 30*(2), 304.

Fang, M. (2019). *Three essays on the relationship between social ties and mental health* [Doctoral dissertation].

Fiorillo, A., & Gorwood, P. (2020). The consequences of the COVID-19 pandemic on mental health and implications for clinical practice. *European Psychiatry, 63*(1), 1–2.

Fluharty, M., & Fancourt, D. (2021). How have people been coping during the COVID-19 pandemic? Patterns and predictors of coping strategies amongst 26,016 UK adults. *BMC Psychology, 9*(1). https://doi.org/10.1186/s40359-021-00603-9

Gordon, M., Patricio, M., Horne, L., Muston, A., Alston, S. R., Pammi, M., Thammasitboon, S., Park, S., Pawlikowska, T., & Rees, E. L. (2020). Developments in medical education in response to the COVID-19 pandemic: A rapid BEME systematic review: BEME Guide No. 63. *Medical Teacher, 42*(11), 1202–1215.

Government of Malawi. (2020). *Malawi 2063*. National Planning Commission.

Gujarati, D. N., Bernier, B., & Bernier, B. (2004). *Econométrie*. De Boeck.

Hou, F., Bi, F., Jiao, R., Luo, D., & Song, K. (2020). Gender differences of depression and anxiety among social media users during the COVID-19 outbreak in China: A cross-sectional study. *BMC Public Health, 20*(1). https://doi.org/10.1186/s12889-020-09738-7

Kainja, J., Ndasauka, Y., Mchenga, M., Kondowe, F., M'manga, C., Maliwichi, L., & Nyamali, S. (2022). Umunthu, Covid-19 and mental health in Malawi. *Heliyon, 8*(11), e11316. https://doi.org/10.1016/j.heliyon.2022.e11316

Kauye, F., Jenkins, R., & Rahman, A. (2014). Training primary health care workers in mental health and its impact on diagnoses of common mental disorders in primary care of a developing country, Malawi: A cluster-randomized controlled trial. *Psychological Medicine, 44*(3), 657–666.

Khan, Z. D., Lutale, J., & Moledina, S. M. (2019, January 15). Prevalence of depression and associated factors among diabetic patients in an outpatient diabetes clinic. *Psychiatry Journal, 2019*, 2083196. https://doi.org/10.1155/2019/2083196. PMID: 30775378; PMCID: PMC6350613.

Kroenke, K., Strine, T. W., Spitzer, R. L., Williams, J. B. W., Berry, J. T., & Mokdad, A. H. (2009). The PHQ-8 as a measure of current depression in the general population. *Journal of Affective Disorders, 114*(1–3), 163–173.

Kutcher, S., Wei, Y., Gilberds, H., Brown, A., Ubuguyu, O., Njau, T., Sabuni, N., Magimba, A., & Perkins, K. (2017). Addressing adolescent depression in Tanzania: Positive primary care workforce outcomes using a training cascade model. *Depression Research and Treatment, 2017*, 9109086. https://doi.org/10.1155/2017/9109086. Epub November 26, 2017. PMID: 29333294; PMCID: PMC5733241.

Langer, Á. I., Crockett, M. A., Bravo-Contreras, M., Carrillo-Naipayan, C., Chaura-Marió, M., Gómez-Curumilla, B., Henríquez-Pacheco, C., Vergara, R. C., Santander, J., & Antúnez, Z. (2022). Social and economic factors associated with subthreshold and major depressive episode in university students during the COVID-19 pandemic. *Frontiers in Public Health, 10*, 893483. https://doi.org/10.3389/fpubh.2022.893483

Lazarus, R. S., & Folkman, S. (1984). *Stress, appraisal, and coping*. Springer.

Lima, C. K. T., De Medeiros Carvalho, P. M., Lima, I. de A. A. S., De Oliveira Nunes, J. V. A., Saraiva, J. S., De Souza, R. I., Da Silva, C. G. L., & Neto, M. L. R. (2020). The emotional impact of Coronavirus 2019-nCoV (new coronavirus disease). *Psychiatry Research, 287*, 112915. https://doi.org/10.1016/j.psychres.2020.112915

Matandika, I., Mategula, D., Kasenda, S., Adeniyi, Y., & Muula, A. (2022). Prevalence and correlates of common mental disorders among children and adolescents in Blantyre-Urban, Malawi. *Malawi Medical Journal, 34*(2), 105–110.

McDaid, D., Knapp, M., & Raja, S. (2008). Barriers in the mind: Promoting an economic case for mental health in low-and middle-income countries. *World Psychiatry, 7*(2), 79.

Mendenhall, E., Norris, S. A., Shidhaye, R., & Prabhakaran, D. (2014). Depression and type 2 diabetes in low-and middle-income countries: A systematic review. *Diabetes Research and Clinical Practice, 103*(2), 276–285.

M'manga, C., Ndasauka, Y., Kainja, J., Kondowe, F., Mchenga, M., Maliwichi, L., & Nyamali, S. (2023). The world is coming to an end! COVID-19, depression, and anxiety among adolescents in Malawi. *Frontiers in Psychiatry, 13*, article 1024793. https://doi.org/10.3389/fpsyt.2022.1024793.

Muhia, J., & Nanji, N. (2021). *Youth mental health in the context of COVID-19 in East and Southern Africa: A desk review* (EQUINET Discussion Paper 122). IWGHSS and TARSC, EQUINET.

Munyenyembe, B., & Chen, Y.-Y. (2022). COVID-19 anxiety-coping strategies of frontline health workers in a low-income country Malawi: A qualitative inquiry. *Journal of Workplace Behavioral Health, 37*(1), 47–67. https://doi.org/10.1080/15555240.2021.2011303

Mweninguwe, R. (2019). Suicide on the rise. *Development & Cooperation Online Magazine*. www.dandc.eu/en/article/people-who-suffer-depression-need-better-care-malawi

National Statistical Office. (2023). *Malawi high frequency phone survey 2020–2023*. https://microdata.worldbank.org/index.php/catalog/3766/related-materials

O'Connell, M. E., Boat, T., & Warner, K. E. (Eds.). (2009). *Preventing mental, emotional, and behavioral disorders among young people: Progress and possibilities*. The National Academies Press.

Ogunsakin, R. E., Olugbara, O. O., Moyo, S., & Israel, C. (2021). Meta-analysis of studies on depression prevalence among diabetes mellitus patients in Africa. *Heliyon*, *7*(5), e07085.

Park, S. C., & Park, Y. C. (2020). Mental health care measures in response to the 2019 novel coronavirus outbreak in Korea. *Psychiatry Investigation*, *17*(2), 85.

Qin, M., Evandrou, M., Falkingham, J., & Vlachantoni, A. (2022). Did the socio-economic gradient in depression in later life deteriorate or weaken during the COVID-19 pandemic? New evidence from England using path analysis. *International Journal of Environmental Research and Public Health*, *19*(11), 6700.

Rowling, L. (2002). School mental health promotion: Perspectives, problems and possibilities. *International Journal of Mental Health Promotion*, *4*(4), 8–13.

Ryff, C. D., & Singer, B. (1998). The contours of positive human health. *Psychological Inquiry*, *9*(1), 1–28.

Schneier, F., & Goldmark, J. (2015). Social anxiety disorder. *Anxiety Disorders and Gender*, 49–67.

Sen, A. (1980). Equality of what? *The Tanner Lecture on Human Values*, *1*, 197–220.

Shah, K., Kamrai, D., Mekala, H., Mann, B., Desai, K., & Patel, R. S. (2020). Focus on mental health during the coronavirus (COVID-19) pandemic: Applying learnings from the past outbreaks. *Cureus*, *12*(3), e7405.

Shigemura, J., Ursano, R. J., Morganstein, J. C., Kurosawa, M., & Benedek, D. M. (2020). Public responses to the novel 2019 Coronavirus (2019-nCoV) in Japan: Mental health consequences and target populations. *Psychiatry and Clinical Neurosciences*, *74*(4), 281–282.

Southern Africa Litigation Centre. (2022, November 10). *Malawi: Man arrested and convicted for attempting to commit suicide.* www.southernafricalitigationcentre.org/2022/11/10/malawi-man-arrested-and-convicted-for-attempting-to-commit-suicide/

Stewart, F. (2014). Against happiness: A critical appraisal of the use of measures of happiness for evaluating progress in development. *Journal of Human Development and Capabilities*, *15*(4), 293–307. https://doi.org/10.1080/19452829.2014.957751

Teshome, H. M., Ayalew, G. D., Shiferaw, F. W., Leshargie, C. T., & Boneya, D. J. (2018, May 23). The prevalence of depression among diabetic patients in Ethiopia: A systematic review and meta-analysis, 2018. *Depression Research and Treatment*, *2018*, 6135460. https://doi.org/10.1155/2018/6135460. PMID: 29951313; PMCID: PMC5989296.

Thula, M., Matola, J. U., Nyasulu, T., & Nyasulu, K. (2020). *Assessment of the impact of COVID-19 on the labor market in Malawi: Final report.* https://malawi.un.org/sites/default/files/2020-09/Assessment%20of%20the%20Impat%20of%20Covid-19%20on%20the%20Labour%20Market%20in%20Malawi_ECAM%20Final%20Report.pdf

Todaro, M. P., & Smith, S. C. (2011). *Economic development.* Pearson.

Udedi, M. (2014). The prevalence of depression among patients and its detection by primary health care workers at Matawale health centre (Zomba). *Malawi Medical Journal*, *26*(2), 34–37.

Udedi, M., Muula, A. S., Stewart, R. C., & Pence, B. W. (2019). The validity of the patient health Questionnaire-8 to screen for depression in patients with type-2 diabetes mellitus in non-communicable diseases clinics in Malawi. *BMC Psychiatry*, *19*(1), 1–7.

United Nations Development Programme. (2020). *Covid 19 pandemic in Malawi: Final report.* www.undp.org/malawi/covid-19-pandemic

World Bank Group, & International Monetary Fund. (2021). *World bank group and international monetary fund support for debt relief under the common framework and beyond* (Policy Papers 022, p. 15). World Bank. https://doi.org/10.5089/9781513576039.007

World Health Organization. (1992). *The ICD-10 classification of mental and behavioural disorders: Clinical descriptions and diagnostic guidelines.* World Health Organization.

World Health Organization. (2004). *Promoting mental health: Concepts, emerging evidence, practice. Summary report.* World Health Organization.

World Health Organization. (2005). *Mental health atlas 2005.* World Health Organization.

World Health Organization. (2008). *The global burden of disease: 2004 update.* World Health Organization.

World Health Organization. (2010). *Mental health and development: Targeting people with mental health conditions as a vulnerable group* (p. 74). World Health Organization.

World Health Organization. (2012). *World suicide prevention day 2012.* www.emro.who.int/media/news/suicide-prevention-day2012.html

World Health Organization. (2021). *Improving health systems and services for mental health: Mental health policy and service guidance package.* World Health Organization.

World Medical Association. (2014). World medical association declaration of Helsinki: Ethical principles for medical research involving human subjects. *The Journal of the American College of Dentists, 81*(3), 14–18.

Xiang, Y.-T., Yang, Y., Li, W., Zhang, L., Zhang, Q., Cheung, T., & Ng, C. H. (2020). Timely mental health care for the 2019 novel Coronavirus outbreak is urgently needed. *The Lancet Psychiatry, 7*(3), 228–229.

Ye, B., Wu, D., Im, H., Liu, M., Wang, X., & Yang, Q. (2020, November). Stressors of COVID-19 and stress consequences: The mediating role of rumination and the moderating role of psychological support. *Children and Youth Services Review, 118*, 105466. https://doi.org/10.1016/j.childyouth.2020.105466. Epub September 25, 2020. PMID: 32994656; PMCID: PMC7515821.

Yekta, Z., Pourali, R., & Yavarian, R. (2010). Behavioural and clinical factors associated with depression among individuals with diabetes. *EMHJ: Eastern Mediterranean Health Journal, 16*(3), 286–291.

Zhang, J. (2021). The bidirectional relationship between body weight and depression across gender: A simultaneous equation approach. *International Journal of Environmental Research and Public Health, 18*(14), 7673.

3 Challenging Notions of Heightened Female Disadvantage During COVID-19

Rachel NyaGondwe Fiedler, Atipatsa Chiwanda Kaminga, Joshua Isaac Kumwenda, Joyce Dainess Mlenga, Rhodian Munyenyembe and Felix Chimera Nyika

3.1 Introduction

Both men and women suffered from psychological distress during the COVID-19 pandemic. Psychological distress is associated with increased mortality (Prior et al., 2016). One of the traditional roles of African women is to care for the sick at home and in hospitals. Statistics have established that, in Africa, fewer women than men have died due to COVID-19 (Frąckowiak-Sochańska, 2021). In Malawi, a case fatality rate analysis indicated that men had an increased risk of COVID-19-related deaths than women (case fatality ratio: 1.58 with 95% CI=1.11–2.22) (see Nyasulu et al., 2021). Globally, the proportion of COVID-19-related deaths for men ranged between 57% and 75% (Frąckowiak-Sochańska, 2021). Gender disaggregated data of infections of men and women during the HIV and AIDS pandemic show that more men contracted the virus than women; for example, the 2010 Malawi figures show that 5.2% of men between the ages of 15 and 24 years old contracted HIV compared to 1.9% of women in the same category (MacIntyre et al., 2013).

A study on women in Southern Malawi found that women, although disempowered, were vital in shaping an effective community response to HIV and AIDS (MacIntyre et al., 2013). Some researchers have shown how the Bible does not promote the oppression of women (see Chifungo, 2014; Chilenje, 2021; Chipeta, 2022). Others have shown how African culture sometimes liberates African women (Chirwa, 2020; Phiri, 1997). These have shown how women occupy leadership positions in African culture and traditional religions. Others have shown how African women have been agents of political transformation (O'Neil et al., 2016).

Some scholars have stated that, during COVID-19, women bore the brunt of the pandemic because of their gender roles (Ndonde & Mukuka, 2021). But what if the fact that more men than women died of COVID-19 in Malawi and globally influences how men and women cope with psychological distress during COVID-19? The primary purpose of this chapter is to report on factors that helped African women in Malawi to suffer less from psychological

DOI: 10.4324/9781003425861-4

distress than men during the COVID-19 pandemic. The chapter builds on the link between women's and men's health against the background of pandemics (Kaunda, 2021; Sibanda et al., 2022). Specifically, the focus is on the psychological health of women and men during pandemics (Frąckowiak-Sochańska, 2021). It extends the academic reflection on how sociological factors help women suffer less psychological stress than men. In this chapter, sociological factors, such as spirituality (Landman, 2007), traditional gender roles (MacIntyre et al., 2013), and lifestyle (Van der Werf et al., 2021) play a role in helping women suffer less psychological distress than men during COVID-19.

3.2 Theoretical and Methodological Considerations

The study employed African feminist theory and grounded theory to consider gender inequalities between men and women in urban churches in Malawi, which put women in an advantaged position in coping with COVID-19 distress. Scholars have argued that religious commitment (Landman, 2007) and improved lifestyle habits (Van der Werf et al., 2021) increased women's resilience against distress. The African feminist theory centres on gender inequalities between men and women in church and society. The theory builds on interdisciplinary feminist theories with multiple constructs (Roberts & Connell, 2016; Fiedler, 2016).

This chapter is based on a study using ethnography and grounded theory, where the study participants were vital sources of information (Stevens, 2017). We collected information through participant observation and intensive conversations with key participants on a one-to-one basis and in focus group discussions. We used virtual participation methods in cases where we could not attend the funeral services due to lockdown regulations by the government.

Since we used participant observation, we had a large group of interviewees. We observed our participants in group meetings, such as at funerals, conferences, church services, and prayer meetings. It was difficult to account for all the participating numbers in these groups. Here we only provide numbers of critical informants with whom we had conversations. We selected these using random, convenient, and purposive sampling. We used purposive sampling to select critical informants based on their information on areas where we could not get clear information through participant observation. We used random sampling in cases where we wanted clarity on issues we had observed and convenient sampling in selecting interviewees whom we could easily reach and those open to having conversations with us. Among these were those who survived bouts of COVID-19 and those close to family members whom COVID-19 had infected.

We chose these three sampling methods because it is congruent with African ways of knowing. Data were processed repeatedly through an iterant method, which included three significant steps: (1) building a thick description of data, (2) reflecting on the data from our different corners of theological and sociological expertise guided by the African feminist theological framework to build thematic blocks that guided the current study, and lastly, (3) subjecting data to another scholar's scrutiny. Our data gained new insights through this iterative method as we repeatedly screened the data we collected over time. We decided to discipline ourselves by focusing on the data we collected and the participants' concepts. This meant we excluded all hearsay and avoided imposing findings from other studies on our data.

Matrilineal and patrilineal ethnic groups characterise Malawi. Malawi has nearly a thousand denominations (Ross & Fiedler, 2020). Our insights into this quest are based on the Christian context of members of selected congregations within Malawian cities. We selected congregations based on the authors' group membership to achieve practical participant observation. The participants were drawn from three congregations of the following churches: mainline, evangelical, and Pentecostal. In this chapter, the term "Pentecostal churches" refers to charismatic churches. This categorisation is based on the local understanding of the churches as *matchalitchi a Pente* (Pentecostal churches).

The names of the churches are withheld for ethical reasons, and churches are only identified by letters, namely A (mainline church), B (evangelical church), and C (Pentecostal church). Quotations by members of these churches are therefore indicated as, for instance (B 2020). In other words, the quotation was from a member of Church B, and the data were collected in 2020. There were 21 key informants, seven from each of the three churches. The fact that there are more references to Congregations B and C does not imply that we included more key informants from these churches. Sources from B and C are quoted more than others depending on the relevance of the information they provided on this chapter's theme. We did not probe deeper, as the information we needed for this chapter had reached saturation (see Creswell, 2003; Longwe, 2016; Ngomezulu & Kalua, 2019).

The study was supported by the Engaging African Realities project of the Nagel Institute of Calvin University and was cleared by the Mzuzu University Research Ethics Committee. We also sought permission from the leaders of the congregations that participated in this study.

3.3 Contribution of Religious Gender Roles

The study found that women were less distressed during COVID-19 because not many were church leaders. Therefore, they were not involved in leadership roles, such as leading the liturgy or visiting and praying for those suffering from COVID-19. On the other hand, we found that men were involved in such leadership roles even though they risked their health and were sometimes infected by COVID-19. Clergy and lay leaders were expected to lead the liturgy and visit the sick and the bereaved. As church leaders, they were considered role models of piety by the church. This means that men had to stand up to the expectations of the church. Leading the burial liturgy at funerals was one of the tasks that the church expected them to fulfil regardless of the dangers attached to this role.

Men were more distressed than women because men as leaders, especially the clergy, were expected to lead by example in receiving COVID-19 vaccinations. As leaders, they were expected to be vaccinated without fear regardless of the threatening theories that came with vaccinations. One such theory was that those vaccinated would turn into animals. If women were not vaccinated, they were not frowned upon because it is traditionally accepted that women demonstrate some weakness. While women were not frowned upon if they rejected vaccines on the basis of fear, it was demeaning for men to do likewise.

During the COVID-19 pandemic, not many women who belong to the church were involved in visiting sick members of the church. During a church service, a leader of the service made the following announcement:

> There is sickness in this family but the pastor and a deacon will visit them on behalf of the church.
>
> (B 2020).

Since women were not pastors, men carried out this function. Like Moses and Esther in the Old Testament and Paul and Lydia in the New Testament (see Fiedler, 2016), these men took up the spiritual role of leaders (see Mafuleka, 2010). At times of sickness or bereavement, men were more in despair than women because Christians looked to the clergy and cooperating leaders to bring hope to those affected by COVID-19. Some church members felt discriminated against when their leaders did not visit them during bereavement (A 2021). Church members who contracted COVID-19 stopped attending churches because of the feeling of being discriminated against by church members (B 2021). Such expectations increased psychological distress among leaders of the church.

Although more women than men are dedicated to the church, most women play support roles in the funeral liturgy (participant observation). Few women in Malawi and beyond are ordained as clergy and are involved in the funeral liturgy (Chilapula, 2023). A large group of lay women leaders are members of church women groups. The names of these groups vary from one church to another. In Nkhoma Synod, it is called *Chigwirizano (Union)* (Phiri, 1997). They usually do not take the coffin to the graveyard. They sing and lead the laying of wreaths at the graveyard after the burial of the deceased. Sometimes these women take the body of their fellow member out of the house for the service (*mwambo*) before the body is taken to the graveyard for burial.

During the COVID-19 pandemic, government regulations were against keeping dead bodies inside the house. The body was transferred from the hospital, where the person died, to the burial place. Hospital personnel and church clergy, with some laymen, were involved in transferring the deceased's body to the graveyard. Clergy were often close to health workers to coordinate with them and their relatives on the burial rituals (A, B, and C 2021).

Lay women leaders involved in administrative roles suffered distress in the course of their work. Such women were those who were involved in serving Holy Communion and managing Sunday cash collections (B 2021). Women leaders who were elders and deacons who served Holy Communion were distressed because they feared contracting COVID-19, as some had become infected and died after serving in this role (A 2021). Although most women attend prayer meetings, men were more distressed than women because they were praying for the sick and often led the prayer meetings (C 2022). This was common among Pentecostal churches. It was common to hear from those clergy and church leaders that they became infected because they were praying for the sick in person.

Ndinatenga COVID-19 chifukwa ife azibusa timanka ndikupempherera anthu (I got COVID-19 infection because we Clergy go and pray for those that area sick).

(C 2022)

When we came back from a night of prayer, I did not feel well. I phoned my friends that also attended the prayer meeting. Everyone was sick.

(C 2021)

In all the churches, men were more distressed than women because of their leadership roles when burying the deceased. Clergy and laymen were leading in burying the dead, coordinating with health workers. Women were mainly involved in leading the laying of wreaths. They were not in touch with health workers. Where people were ill, the clergy and men leaders prayed for the sick, including those infected with COVID-19. However, we did not come across such incidences in Church A. We even found incidences where clergy shunned visiting families that lost a member to COVID-19. Churches B and C were particularly strong on visiting and praying for the sick, believing that solid faith protected them from the virus. Sometimes, they believed faith had even more strength than the vaccinations to protect them. Scholars have argued that religious commitment reduces stress, and leadership is one of the testimonies of one's highest form of religious commitment. It was expected that these people in leadership would be protected against psychological distress, but during COVID-19, leadership positions did not reduce psychological distress. The findings also show that a particular form of religious commitment may bring more psychological distress within one church context than in the other because church leadership functions differ from church to church due to differences in theology and doctrines.

3.4 The Contribution of Traditional Gender Roles

The current study found that women are excluded from traditional leadership roles. Most leaders are male, and men expect to take the leading role during sickness and death. This reduces the distress on women. Women are mothers and carers for the sick. Still, when someone gets sick or dies, men are expected to take a leading role during burial, except in the case of burial of stillborn babies and children that a particular cultural group accords the same burial ritual as stillborn children. Men work with health workers, clergy, and lay leaders to prepare for burying the dead. In this ritual, men are primarily leaders. These are uncles, fathers, or brothers, depending on the cultural context. In a matrilineal society, the maternal uncle is central in these activities. In patrilineal societies, the father, paternal uncle, and brother to the deceased are key leaders during this time (Banda, 2006). Men carry out their leadership roles and risk their lives because society expects them to be strong enough to face danger (Kisembo et al., 1998; Siwila, 2022).

This means that this category of men in the traditional society was more distressed than women because they had to be in conversation with health workers and the church leaders in the processes that led to burying the deceased (A, B, and C 2022). In cities, extended family members sometimes took up this role. During the COVID-19 pandemic, those who took the body from the town to the village were expected to continue with the roles in the village. The village men dug the grave, but they were often told to stay away from the people who came with the dead body from the cities to protect villagers from COVID-19 infection. Health workers reinforced this role. The medical persons often told people not to greet anyone who brought the body and that those who brought the body had to go straight to the car to return to the city (video clip observation). There are traditional women leaders in a matrilineal society, but they are not actively involved in the burial ceremony as chiefs. The traditional role of women to care for the sick bring about less distress for women than for men. Women also did not have to sleep in the hospital to care for those sick from COVID-19. Government COVID-19 regulations did not allow this (A, B, and C 2021).

Some scholars argue that the caring roles of women put women at risk (Ndonde & Mukuka, 2021). This chapter argues that the religious and traditionally ascribed roles of men made men suffer more from psychological distress than women during COVID-19. The chapter concurs with other studies that do not ascribe this reality to biological reasons (Frąckowiak-Sochańska, 2021). Gender inequalities between men and women in church and society influence gender inequalities in distress situations between men and women.

Reconfiguring traditional roles between men and women puts more stress on men than on women. Men in Malawi traditional culture dig graves and bury the dead. This requires that they touch the dead body, which would infect those engaged in this. To avoid this, the government protected men by insisting that health workers bury the dead. But this was not possible when COVID-19 was at its peak. At the time, there were not enough health personnel to bury the dead and care for COVID-19 patients. Men, therefore, buried the dead without the help of medical personnel.

In some instances, people did not believe the person died of COVID-19. In other cases, health workers responsible for burying the dead were chased away by the community (C 2021). This caused men who were not health personnel to bury those who died from COVID-19 just like any dead body. Men consequently suffered more than women because they were unsure whether the person died from COVID.

The expectations of traditional culture restricted men from making decisions that would promote their health during the pandemic. If the death occurred in the matrilineal family context, the maternal uncles and their representatives in the matrilineal context had to coordinate with health workers during funeral services for those who had died of COVID. If the death occurred within the patrilineal context, paternal uncles, fathers, and brothers had to cooperate with health workers in the funeral rituals. If these men abandoned their responsibilities, they would have suffered negative traditionally ascribed consequences. In one instance, the body of the person who had died from COVID-19 only left Blantyre after the uncle of the deceased travelled from Lilongwe to Blantyre (a distance of over 300 km) to arrange the transfer of the body to the village (A 2020). The uncle also died as a result of COVID-19 later. The risk of women in the city conflicting with traditional culture was minimal. Women, therefore, had less psychological distress because they had limited chances of being in contact with dead bodies.

Traditionally, women are supposed to wash the dead bodies of women but also stay close to the dead body in the house where the mourning takes place. But because of COVID-19, women are not allowed to be in the vigil house with the dead body in their midst. The body was transferred from the hospital to the graveyard without much delay. Health officials implemented health-friendly approaches that protected women from being distressed by the possibility of infection. In the village, health officials restricted contact between those who came with the body from town to the graveyard and those at the burial site. Health workers also insisted that those at the burial site sit far from others to avoid contracting COVID-19. Wearing of masks was also enforced (A, B, and C 2021).

3.5 The Contribution of Government Machinery

The study found that women's traditional role of caring for patients was taken away from them through the government's isolation policy for COVID-19 patients. Without this policy, more women than men would have been distressed as they would have been in contact with infected relatives.

> We went to a private clinic because we had hoped that they would treat him as an outpatient but instead, the doctor called for an ambulance without our consent because the private clinic had already established that he was optimistic with COVID-19. Since they did not allow guardians, we could only visit him. Although it was hard emotionally not to see him at the hospital, God protected me from getting COVID-19 infection from my husband. He was discharged and is now recovered.
>
> (B 2020)

The government policy protected women from caring for those who were ill due to COVID-19 in the following ways:

- Guardians such as spouses and close family members were not allowed to take care of a COVID-19 patient in the isolation room. This meant that women could not care for the patients, as is their traditional duty.
- Guardians were allowed to bring food to the hospital, but the patients only got the food through the medical staff. As women traditionally bring food for the patients, this policy prevented women from having direct contact with the patients.
- One was not permitted to be on hospital premises without a mask. The hospitals were fenced, and no one was allowed to enter the gate without a mask.

3.6 Contribution of African Lifestyles

The study found that women had more health-friendly lifestyles than men. Men often travelled to places that were likely to spread COVID-19 infection. These were places such as drinking joints, where men often go to watch soccer or to play chess or related games (B and C 2021). On the other hand, women were perceived to frequent health-friendly places, such as church services and women-only functions, such as bridal showers and village banking meetings, which promote livelihoods of their families and communities. Women also display better health-seeking behaviour than men (A, B, and C). They often go to seek medical treatment even during COVID-19 because they are used to seeking medical treatment for themselves, their relatives, and their families. On the other hand, men often ignore the need for medical treatment. They are also not traditional caregivers of the sick, and this means that they do not frequent hospitals often.

3.7 Contribution of Differences in Theology

The study found that all three churches under study had clergymen and were all involved in funeral liturgies. We found that the main leadership roles that predisposed men to psychological stress were

- leading liturgy at burials of those who died from COVID-19;
- praying for COVID-19 patients;
- providing examples of faith, such as leading in getting vaccinations;
- living a healthy lifestyle; and
- leading in resisting harmful practices that promoted COVID-19 infection.

All three churches provided leadership in burial services. However, we found some differences in leadership practices among the leaders of these churches. Church A was the only one that avoided harmful practices that would endanger clergy and other leaders. These practices included avoiding drinking joints and visiting families that lost someone to COVID-19 and praying for the sick through visitation. On the other hand, Churches B and C prayed for and visited the sick. Some of the leaders – except clergy from Churches B and C – also visited drinking places. The theology of Church A does not allow its members to drink alcohol.

A few previous studies have established that religion has healing properties (see Landman, 2007; Lovinger, 1990). In the context of this study, more women than men attended prayer meetings, church women groups were much larger than men's groups, and there were more women than men in the churches. These aspects combined confirm that more women than men take religion seriously, and this, in turn, helps women to cope better with stress than men. However, this chapter argued that cumulative effects (see Lindgren et al., 2013) made leaders of congregation B and C more predisposed to the virus than leaders of church A because the latter congregations had more avenues of exposure to the virus than church A due to differences in theologies.

3.8 Conclusion

This chapter has shown that women beat the odds because of sociological factors, especially friendly lifestyles such as religious life and belonging to support groups which helped women relieve psychological distress better than men. Augmenting this fact, the government had social protection measures favouring women, such as restricting care for COVID-19 patients to health workers. This finding suggests that there is a need to have social protection measures that will help men to relieve stress during crises such as COVID-19. Since religious and traditional leadership roles are key stresses to men, churches, the government, and other actors implementing programmes to curb mental stress should balance their programmes and include social protection programmes that will help women and men during crises such as pandemics.

References

Adogame, A. (2021). *Indigeneity in African religions: Oza worldviews, cosmologies and religious cultures.* Bloomsbury Academic.

Banda, R. N. [Fiedler]. (2006). *Women of Bible and culture: Baptist convention women in Southern Malawi.* Kachere.

Chifungo, P. F. (2014). *Women in the CCAP Nkhoma Synod: A practical theological study of their leadership roles* [Doctoral dissertation, Stellenbosch University].

Chilapula, M. K. (2023). *Towards inclusion: Experiences of women clergy in the Church of Central Africa Presbyterian (CCAP) Blantyre Synod* [Doctoral dissertation, Mzuzu University].

Chilenje, L. (2021). *Paul's gender theology and the ordained women's ministry in the CCAP in Zambia.* Mzuni Press.

Chipeta, S. (2022). *Paul and women: An examination of selected Pauline texts in relation to the role of women in the seventh-day adventist Church in Malawi* [Doctoral dissertation, Mzuzu University].

Chirwa, F. (2020). *Mission in progress: The developing role of women in the church. An SDA perspective from Malawi.* Mzuni Press.

Creswell, J. W. (2003). *Research design: Qualitative, quantitative and mixed method approaches.* Sage.

Fiedler, R. N. (2016). *The history of the circle of concerned African women theologians, 1989–2007.* Mzuni Press.

Foresti, M. (2016). *Women on the move: Migration, gender equality and the 2030 agenda for sustainable development.* Overseas Development Institute.

Frąckowiak-Sochańska, M. (2021). Men and social trauma of Covid-19 pandemic: The maladaptiveness of toxic masculinity. *Society Register, 5*(1), 73–94. http://doi.org/10.14746/sr.2021.5.1.04

Kanyongolo, N., & Malunga, B. (2016). Legal empowerment: Laws promoting women's participation in politics. In I. Amundsen & H. Kayuni (Eds.), *Women in politics in Malawi* (pp. 23–31). CMI.

Kaunda, C. J. (2021). *Religion, gender and wellbeing in Africa.* Lexington Books.

Kisembo, B., Magesa, L., & Shorter, A. (1998). *African Christian marriage.* Pauline Publications Africa.

Landman, C. (2007). *Doing narrative counselling in the context of township spirituali-ties* [Doctoral dissertation, UNISA].

Lindgren, T., Schell, E., Phiri, J., Fiedler, R., & Chakanza, J. L. (2013). A response to Edzi (AIDS): Malawi faith-based organizations' impact on HIV prevention and care. *Journal of the Association of Nurses in AIDS Care, 24*(3), 227–241. https://doi.org/:10.1016/j.jana.2012.05.004

Longwe, H. (2016). *Academic research and writing in theology and religious studies.* Mzuni Press.

Lovinger, R. (1990). *Religion and counselling: The psychological impact of religious beliefs.* Continuum.

MacIntyre, L. M., Rankin, S., Pinderhughes, H., Waters, C., Schell, E., Fiedler, R. N. (2013). Socially disempowered women as key to addressing change in Malawi: How do they do it? *Health Care for Women International, 34*(2), 103–121. https://doi.org/10.1080/07399332.2011.630116

Mafuleka, F. (2010). *Leadership lessons from the story of Jethro's visit to Mosses (Exodus 18:13–24)* [MA Module: Theology and Religious Studies, Mzuzu University].

Media Observation. (2021). *Video clip of a funeral in Kasungu.* Media Observation.

Nadar, S. (2009). Her stories and her-theologies: Charting feminist theologies in Africa. *Studia Historiae Ecclesiasticae.*

Ndonde, B., & Mukuka, B. N. M. (2021). Covid-19 and violence against women and children in Zambia: A gendered perspective. In C. J. Kaunda (Ed.), *Religion, gender and wellbeing in Africa* (pp. 49–62). Lexington Books.

Ngomezulu, V., & Kalua, F. A. (2019). *A companion to academic writing.* Mzuni Press.

Nyasulu, J. C. Y., Munthali, R. J., Nyondo-Mipando, A. L., Pandya, H., Nyirenda, L., Nyasulu, P. S., & Manda, S. (2021). COVID-19 pandemic in Malawi: Did public sociopolitical events gatherings contribute to its first-wave local transmission? *International Journal of Infectious Diseases, 106,* 269–275. https://doi.org/10.1016/j.ijid.2021.03.055

O'Neil, T., Kanyongolo, N., & Wales, J. (2016). *Women and power: Representation and influence in Malawi's parliament.* Oversees Development Institute.

Phiri, I. A. (1997). *Women, presbyterianism and patriarchy: Religious experience of Chewa women in Central Malawi.* CLAIM-Kachere.

Prior, A., Fenger-Grøn, M., Larsen, K. K., Larsen, F. B., Robinson, K. M., Nielsen, M. G., Christensen, K. S., Mercer, S. W., & Vestergaard, M. (2016). The association between perceived stress and mortality among people with multimorbidity: A prospective population-based cohort study. *American Journal of Epidemiology, 184*(3), 199–210. https://doi.org/10.1093/aje/kwv324

Roberts, C., & Connell, R. (2016). Feminist theory and the global South. *Feminist Theory, 17*(2), 135–140. https://doi.org/10.1177/17464700116645874.

Ross, K. R., & Fiedler, K. (2020). *A Malawi church history 1860–2020.* Mzuni Press.

Sibanda, F., Muyambo, T., & Chitando, E. (Eds.). (2022). *Religion and the COVID-19 pandemic in Southern Africa.* Routledge.

Siwila, L. C. (2022). Masculinity and empire in religion and public life: Social construction of a "real man" in Zambia. In L. C. Siwila, S. Mukuka, & N. Mwale (Eds.), *Gender and empire in religion and public space* (pp. 33–54). Mzuni Press.

Stevens, B. A. (2017). Grounded theology? A call for a community of practice. *Practical Theology, 10,* 201–206. https://doi.org/10.1080/17560773X.2017.1308485

Van der Werf, E. T., Busch, M., Jong, M. C., & Hoenders, H. J. C. (2021). Lifestyle changes during the first wave of the COVID-19 pandemic: A cross-sectional survey in the Netherlands. *BMC Public Health, 21,* article 1226.

4 COVID-19 Crisis Communication, Infodemics, and Psychological Distress Among Sub-Saharan African Youth

Pascal Newbourne Mwale

4.1 Introduction

The COVID-19 pandemic comprised a source of complex psychological stress (Su et al., 2021). Globally, many people reported symptoms of stress, anxiety, depressive disorders leading to insomnia, eating disorders, suicide ideation, suicide, increased substance abuse, worsening chronic conditions, and overdose deaths during the pandemic (Panchal et al., 2021; Xu & Liu, 2021). According to Albuquerque and Santos (2021), children are at a higher risk of mental health effects, given their limited capacity to understand their surroundings, their inability to cope with stressors, such as parents' short illness and sudden death, and to control their environments. Research has demonstrated that COVID-19-related rates of depression and anxiety were prevalent among children and adolescents (see Wang et al., 2022; Ma et al., 2021). Victims of the coronavirus left behind many grieving children and grandchildren, with European family rates of 2.2 children and 4.1 grandchildren for each person who dies. Evidence points to the societal failure to address the needs of grieving children proactively and continuously, which may result in poor mental and physical health (Albuquerque & Santos, 2021). It is estimated that globally, 5 to 10% of children and adolescents who have suffered the loss of loved ones developed clinically significant psychiatric difficulties (Albuquerque & Santos, 2021).

This chapter reflects on the plight of sub-Saharan African (SSA) youth vis-à-vis the COVID-19 pandemic. The chapter reports on the effects of the COVID-19 infodemic on the SSA youth. The study's rationale was that the SSA youth is one of the most neglected, marginalised, and high-risk groups regarding public health interventions during the COVID-19 pandemic. No public health intervention was specifically tailor-made for the SSA youth. Therefore, this chapter argues that since the SSA youth had been neglected and marginalised as public health interventions focused on adults only, the youth suffered psychological stress, leading to idleness, leading to teenage and unplanned pregnancies, and early marriages.

The chapter is structured as follows: section 1 is the introduction. Section 1.1 looks at COVID-19, e-learning as an educational intervention to

DOI: 10.4324/9781003425861-5

sustain teaching and learning for the youth during the pandemic and general mental health issues among the youth. Section 1.2 discusses crisis communication in relation to the COVID-19 infodemic and how the latter negatively affected mental health. Section 1.3 reviews the extant literature on the COVID-19 infodemic in relation to legacy media[1] and social media. Section 1.4 reflects on the SSA youth and COVID-19 aftershocks, most especially psychological stress leading to idleness and alcohol and drug abuse, leading to teenage and unplanned pregnancies and early marriages. Section 1.4.1 deploys the reconstructed version of the Ubuntu thought system to reflect further on the plight of the SSA youth, subsequently suggesting an ethical framework for handling the ongoing COVID-19 pandemic and similar pandemics in the future. The section aims to appreciate how African philosophy could reflect on the COVID-19 infodemic and psychological stress debate.

4.2 COVID-19, E-learning, and Mental Health among the Youth

Mental health can be defined as a state of well-being in which the individual realises his or her own abilities, can cope with the everyday stresses of life, can work productively and fruitfully, and is able to contribute to his or her own community (Su et al., 2021, p. 1). For Golberstein et al. (2020, p. 819), e-learning refers to home-based distance-learning models in the United States of America. Due to COVID-19, educational institutions were closed. E-learning was introduced as a remedial measure to continue with teaching and learning at all levels while the learners and students were at home. Golberstein et al. (2020) remind us that, globally, the first school closures began by mid-March 2020. Closure of educational institutions substantially disrupted the lives of learners and students and their families and might have had consequences for child health. Golberstein et al. (2020, p. 819) summarise the main points further:

> Children and adolescents are generally healthy and do not require much healthcare outside regular check-ups and immunisations. However, mental healthcare is very much important for children and adolescents. Most mental health disorders begin in childhood, making it essential that mental health needs are identified early and treated during this sensitive time in child development. If [left] untreated, mental health problems can lead to many negative health and social outcomes. Economic downturns are associated with increased mental health problems for youth that may be affected by the ways that economic downturns affect adult unemployment, adult mental health, and child maltreatment.

The quotation cited earlier argues that the COVID-19 pandemic had great potential to exacerbate existing mental health disorders, such as stress, depression, and anxiety among children, adolescents and not only the US youth but also globally, SSA youth included. Golberstein et al. (2020, p. 819) bemoan closures of educational institutions and argue, "educators, administrators and policy makers must minimise the disruptions that [educational institutions'] closures . . . have on academic development."

According to a United Kingdom (UK) Foreign Commonwealth Development Office (FCDO)-supported project report, Africans have been killed by both COVID-19 and mental illnesses since the outbreak of COVID-19 in December 2019. COVID-19 has aggravated mental health disorders on the African continent to an unimaginable extent.

The effects of the COVID-19 pandemic in Africa have been far-reaching and disproportionate. For the recovery from COVID-19 to be sustainable, the high prevalence of mental health cases should be addressed urgently. Societies, especially those individuals that are most marginalised, continue to suffer severe psychological distress, anxiety disorders, post-traumatic stress disorders, and depression.

> In [2020], there [was] increased co-morbidity of mental illness and disorders and COVID-19 in Africa. [Pandemic] disease experience, physical distancing, [self-isolation or quarantine], stigma, discrimination, and job loss are some of the ways that COVID-19 . . . stimulated the surge of mental health disorders in Africa.
> (Foreign Commonwealth Development Office, UK, 2020, p. 2)

In the quotation, the implication is that during the COVID-19 pandemic, there were two dangerous mass killers: COVID-19 and mental illness. Media attention, especially social media, was focused on the former. No wonder there is little to no, if not very scanty, information on the deaths resulting from psychological stress, anxiety disorders, depression, and other mental illnesses during the COVID-19 pandemic. Given the high levels of poverty and youth unemployment, psychological stress and anxiety are the norm of the day in Africa. During the pandemic in Malawi, for example, the police reported on a monthly basis hundreds of alarmingly unprecedented figures of persons who had committed suicide or had attempted suicide due to income and/ or job loss (The Southern Africa Litigation Centre, 2022). Shame, stigma, and discrimination were also common in Malawi, for example. The author's two eldest children, a young man and a young woman, unfortunately became infected by the deadly coronavirus. They shunned the entire family for several weeks and remained in self-isolation very long after they had been healed of COVID-19. They said they were too ashamed to tell their family. The feeling of shame can be identified as a mental health disorder. During the COVID-19 pandemic, shame went hand in hand with stigma and discrimination because in a good number of cases, the persons who had the feeling of shame actually ended up being stigmatised and discriminated against by their own relatives, families, friends, and colleagues when it was discovered COVID-19 infected them. Stigma and discrimination can be seen as enhancers or stimulants of shame; they most often lead to or cause mental illness.

4.3 Crisis Communication, COVID-19 Infodemic, and Mental Health

Crisis communication is "the collection, processing and dissemination of information required to address a crisis" (Su et al., 2021, p. 2). Crisis communication tends to degenerate into infodemic (Su et al., 2021), increasing the risk of mental health problems, such as stress, distress, anxiety, and depression. For example, exposure to infodemic reduces vaccination intention, leading to vaccine hesitancy due to stress, anxiety, confusion, pressure, and low motivation (Kim & Tandoc, 2022; Loomba et al., 2021). Infodemic makes it hard for people to find trustworthy information for sound health decision-making (Xu & Liu, 2021). Crisis communication is indispensable during global pandemics, such as COVID-19, in dispelling fears and uncertainty and in unifying individuals worldwide in a concerted global fight against health threats (Xu & Liu, 2021). Mounting research shows two things: first, seemingly endless newsfeeds related to COVID-19 infection and death rates that increased the risk of mental health problems (see Xu & Liu, 2021). Second, media reports that include infodemic regarding the influence of COVID-19 on mental health may be a source of adverse psychological effects on individuals (Xu & Liu, 2021).

Owing partly to insufficient crisis communication practices, media and news organisations across the globe have played minimal roles in battling the COVID-19 infodemic (see Xu & Liu, 2021). Common refrains include but are not limited to QAnon conspiracies,[2] the "Chinese Virus" (see Xu & Liu, 2021), and the use of disinfectants as cure (see Xu & Liu, 2021). These narratives are false and dishonest (See Xu & Liu, 2021). Infodemic can potentially deteriorate mental health (see Xu & Liu, 2021). Infodemic fuelled by a kaleidoscopic range of misinformation can be dangerous (see Elbarazi et al., 2022; Gisondi et al., 2022; Su et al., 2021). Su et al. (2021) claim that there is a lack of research on improving crisis communication across news media organisation channels. In their article, they identified ways that legacy media reports on COVID-19 and the way social media-based infodemic can result in mental health concerns. They suggest possible crisis communication solutions to address these mental health concerns. These solutions comprise e-Health (Su et al., 2021). In their envisaged e-Health promotion, global media try to forge a fact-based, person-centred, and collaborative response to COVID-19 reporting (Su et al., 2021, p. 1). According to Su et al. (2021), the scope and severity of the pandemic further fuelled a global mental health crisis, especially among underserved populations, such as older adults, healthcare professionals, and women.

The rapid pace at which COVID-19 spread and its unprecedented transmissibility, causing it to spread fast and far in a short period were rare among other pandemics (Su et al., 2021, p. 1). Together with consequent spikes, variants of the virus, and quick death caused a range of psychological and physical issues in individuals across the globe, including among SSA youth (Su et al., 2021, p. 1). The authors go on arguing that, triggered by a global health crisis, mental health issues could have severe health consequences on personal and population health, ranging from stress to distress, anxiety, depression, and suicidal ideation or complete suicide. They also argue, "COVID-19 has been a source of complex, multifaceted stress for many" (Su et al., 2021, p. 1). This was due to fears and uncertainty associated with the coronavirus, together with the stress and anxiety following on lockdowns and social distancing mandates. All these have exacerbated mental health issues to varying degrees across the globe, sub-Saharan Africa included.

In summary of the foregoing, COVID-19 has diminished the mental health and well-being of individuals. COVID-19 has also severely limited people's access to mental health services due to the rationing of medical services during the pandemic, leading to an instigated restructuring and repurposing across mental health institutions dealing with the pandemic. Well-intentioned public health measures, such as lockdowns and social distancing, have further reduced access to mental health services, leaving people with little to no access to onsite assistance. The unending barrage (or the disproportionate media attention to COVID-19) of news from legacy media outlets and social media platforms has further complicated the situation, as COVID-19 infodemic gave little or no consideration to how pandemic-related media coverage might affect people's mental health. Misinformation and disinformation surrounding COVID-19 include references to the "Wuhan Virus," the "China Virus," the "Chinese Virus," and using disinfectants as cure. (Mwale et al., 2023) Misinformation in particular has affected individuals' mental and physical health and well-being (see Elbarazi et al., 2022; Gisondi et al., 2022; Leung et al., 2022; Su et al., 2021, p. 2). Little to no research has explored ways to mitigate the mental health consequences of COVID-19 media coverage.

According to Su et al. (2021), crisis communication could address complex, multifaceted issues that erupt in society. It could also mitigate negative effects of adverse events like pandemics. Su et al. (2021) identified areas where legacy media reports on COVID-19 and social media-fuelled infodemic could harm people's mental health. This outlined potential crisis communication solutions that media and news organisations could adopt to alleviate the mental health consequences of COVID-19 media coverage. In other words, Su et al. (2021)'s article explained the effect of legacy media coverage of COVID-19 on people's mental health (Su et al., 2021).

According to Su et al. (2021), during the COVID-19 pandemic, the public witnessed three forms of news media coverage, balanced, fact-based and truth-oriented reporting, biased and misleading reporting, and false and dishonest reporting.

Further, the adverse effects of biased and misleading COVID-19 coverage on personal and population health and well-being could have been more pronounced (See Leung et al., 2021, 2022). Right-wing-leaning legacy media outlets often issued biased and misleading news as well as false and dishonest reports on COVID-19, which could have facilitated the spread of misinformation on the virus (Su et al., 2021, p. 3). For example, in 2020, at the peak of the pandemic, misinformation was neither challenged nor fact-checked before being distributed by legacy media to reach the public. This effectively exposed especially the American media public to common or widely known misinformation, such as miracle cures, or the Democratic Party hoax, which could have resulted in substantial personal mental health issues and economic concerns (see Leung et al., 2021, 2022).

Importantly, fear and panic generated by COVID-19-related misinformation might have had a long-lasting effect on the media public's mental health that will outlive COVID-19 media cycles (Leung et al., 2021, 2022).

During the pandemic, false and dishonest COVID-19 media coverage manifested through the prevalence of common or widely known mass media narratives referring to the "Wuhan Virus," the "Chinese Virus," and the "China Virus," which suggests that some legacy media outlets were capable of producing sensational news (Mwale et al., 2023). Directly associating a group, a nation, and an entire race to a virus inevitably evoked or triggered substantial mental health concerns in those targeted by racism or xenophobia. In general, fake news eroded public trust in official public health information on the COVID-19 pandemic (Egelhofer & Lecheler, 2019; Leung et al., 2021, 2022; Su et al., 2021, p. 3).

4.4 COVID-19 Infodemic, Legacy Media, and Social Media

Infodemic involves the purposeful spread of misinformation and disinformation via the media, particularly on social media platforms. Infodemic can detract from efforts by health officials and experts by fuelling public fear, panic, uncertainty, and mistrust, all of which could have grave mental health as well as personal and economic consequences (Elbarazi et al., 2022; Gisondi et al., 2022; Su et al., 2021). Bearing in mind the infodemics as discussed earlier, crisis communication amid COVID-19 was indispensable at the time of the global pandemic in dispelling fear and uncertainty and by unifying citizens in a concerted fight against disease. Crisis communication promotes sound health decision-making; hence, it is pro-e-Health[3] (Su et al., 2021). Crisis communication is usually adopted as an emergency communication strategy during a crisis. For Su et al. (2021), a crisis can arise in one of three ways:

- First, a crisis can be seen as an unprecedented event with widespread personal and economic consequences, for example, the COVID-19 pandemic.
- Second, it can be a communication crisis that could put off and prevent stakeholders from working towards a solution, for example, COVID-19 infodemic.
- Third, it can be a potential trust crisis either already present or in development partially due to the first two crises, for example, public trust crisis (Su et al., 2021).

4.5 SSA Youth and COVID-19 Aftershocks

According to Rukasha (2021), the effects of COVID-19 on children appeared to have been largely invisible and/or minimised or underestimated. Moreover, for Rukasha, African leaders have largely ignored the effects of COVID-19 on children in favour of more pressing issues, such as food security, adult COVID-19, economic turmoil, internal political wars, and internecine or inter-tribal conflict. However, in Africa, where half of the population is under 18 (Rukasha, 2021), the direct and indirect effects of COVID-19 need to be carefully examined because they (the children) represent the present and future of Africa's youthful population. By "direct effects" of COVID-19, Rukasha is probably referring to a UK Foreign Commonwealth Development Office (FCDO)-supported project that defines the direct effects of COVID-19 as including death or near-death experience in the family as a result of hospitalisation and/or illness, self-isolation or quarantine, anxiety about reported deaths, or about those at a great risk, such as healthcare workers. Stigmatisation and social discrimination of survivors in the family were also prevalent (FCDO, 2020, p. 2).

By "indirect effects," Rukasha (2021), again, refers to the FCDO-supported project report, which defined these as the result of containment measures taken by African governments in response to the COVID-19 pandemic. These included indefinite closure of educational institutions for all levels; strict border controls; screening and vaccination; mandatory wearing of face masks in banks, markets, shops and other public facilities; drastic reduction of hours of business for places of entertainment, such as bottle stores, bars, pubs, and clubs; and banning of assemblies, such as religious gatherings, weddings, and engagements (Rukasha, 2021).

Rukasha's (2021) study focused on South Africa because, in her opinion, the "rainbow nation" was the hardest hit country in Africa by COVID-19. She critically examined the effects of COVID-19 on children on three fronts: economy, education, and health. Although she looked at the effect of COVID-19 on children only, her study is still relevant because children and adolescents are considered generally as belonging to the youth. For Aborode et al. (2020, p. 4), in 2020, students were at home following the indefinite closure of tertiary educational institutions in sub-Saharan Africa (SSA), which included Nigeria, the base of their study. Many SSA governments had to shut down their educational institutions ranging from kindergarten to university, momentarily to curb the unprecedented rapid spread of COVID-19 to the rest of the country as well as to neighbouring countries. Numerous tertiary educational institutions had to organise a variety of e-learning interventions to assist students and to ensure that learning continues uninterrupted so that the academic calendar was not disrupted due to the COVID-19 pandemic. Aborode et al. (2020) argue that a synchronised effort was required for all tertiary education stakeholders to search for alternative models for the e-learning solution.

Namukasa (2021) conducted an undergraduate study at Makerere University to look into factors that contributed to teenage pregnancy during

COVID-19 in the Bugiri municipal council of Uganda. Her findings highlighted that the outbreak of the COVID-19 pandemic was largely responsible for the dramatic and unprecedented increase in the numbers of teenage pregnancy in Bugiri, which registered 60 teenage pregnancies. This was compounded by the harsh economic conditions, including youth and adult unemployment, anxiety and depression, a lack of access to family planning services, as well as idleness (Namukasa, 2021, p. 1).

Still in Uganda, in its latest country strategy (2021), World Vision International (WVI) (World Vision Uganda) focused on the psychosocial and economic effect of the COVID-19 pandemic on children and emerging humanitarian needs. In its area of operation, which comprises 46 districts, WVI found that 25% of teenagers between the ages 15 and 19 fell pregnant during the COVID-19 pandemic lockdown (27% for rural areas while for urban areas it was slightly lower, at 19%) (World Vision International Uganda, 2022, p. 4). World Vision International Uganda (2022) reports thus:

> Across Uganda, eight out of ten citizens (79%) said the lockdown had increased cases of teenage pregnancy and sexual violence . . . After the first lockdown, teenage pregnancies rose by 28% with the Ministry of Education reporting that over 90,000 girls under 18 fell pregnant during the [COVID-19] period when they were not attending school, and this included more than 9,000 underage girls . . . Another worrying (and related) trend has been an increase in child marriage . . . In most cases, child marriage is the outcome of teenage pregnancies and sexual abuse.
> (World Vision International Uganda, 2022, p. 6)

The previous quotation testifies to the calamity into which COVID-19 has plunged children and the youth in Uganda. The pre-pandemic rate of child or early marriage was 12% in Uganda, but during the COVID-19 pandemic in 2021 alone, it skyrocketed to 46%, an unprecedented rate of child or early marriages being hastily contracted among, and for, teenagers. For World Vision International Uganda (2022), both child marriages and teenage pregnancies are associated with shame, stigma, and mental health issues that sometimes lead to suicidal tendencies (World Vision International Uganda, 2022, p. 6). World Vision International Uganda (2022) also reported that, before 2021, more than 298,127 teenagers visited public health facilities for their first antenatal care in 2020 during the COVID-19 lockdown in Uganda. Teenage pregnancies unimaginably and unexpectedly escalated amidst COVID-19, adversely affecting underage girls aged between 10 and 17 (World Vision International Uganda, 2022, p. 6).

World Vision International (2020c) also looked at other countries than Uganda in sub-Saharan Africa in terms of how COVID-19 has adversely affected children and adolescents and the youth in general. The affected sub-Saharan African countries include but are not limited to Ghana, Malawi, and Kenya. In the aforementioned region of sub-Saharan Africa, teenage pregnancy kept about a million girls from returning to school, according to World Vision International estimates for 2020. World Vision International (2020c) went further to report that school closures during crises could lead to increases in teenage pregnancy by as much as 65%, as was the case before COVID-19. This is the case because girls end up spending more time with men and boys than they would had they been in school, leading to the greater likelihood of engaging in risky sexual behaviour, and an increased risk of sexual violence and exploitation (World Vision International, 2020c).

The SSA region has the highest rate of adolescent pregnancy in the world (World Vision International, 2020c). More alarmingly, in 2018, before the outbreak of the COVID-19 pandemic, the estimated global adolescent birth rate stood at 42 births per 1,000 girls aged between 15 and 19; the adolescent birth rate for the SSA region stood at 101 births per 1,000 girls aged between 15 and 19 during the same period. This was more than double the global adolescent birth rate of 1.5 births per 1,000 girls of the same age range (WHO, 2023). Compared with South Asia, 26% of women aged from 20 to 24 in sub-Saharan Africa report giving birth for the first time before the age of 18; the estimate in South Asia is only 11% (World Vision International, 2020c). Let us look closely at what happened in some countries during the COVID-19 pandemic, especially in Ghana, Malawi, and Kenya (World Vision International, 2020c).

During COVID-19, the Krachi West Area Programme in Ghana experienced an almost nine-fold rise in teenage pregnancy. In that one area, 51 children were reported to have fallen pregnant between March and May 2020. According to WVI, the majority of these 51 pregnancies occurred as a result of the lockdown instituted by the Ghanaian government as a preventive measure to stop the infection and spread of COVID-19 (World Vision International Ghana, 2020b, p. 12).

According to World Vision International (2020c), the Malawian government shut its schools, colleges, and universities in March 2020 after being threatened greatly by the rising infections and the rapid pace of the spread of the COVID-19 pandemic. World Vision International (2020c) reported several hundreds of thousands of teenage pregnancies across Malawi, with Phalombe district topping the list. The report narrated that cases of child marriages and teenage pregnancies are not new in Phalombe "but [had] become more common since schools closed due to the COVID-19 pandemic" (World Vision International Malawi, 2020d, p. 15). More worrisome, psychosocially speaking, the report went on to narrate that children out of school and pregnant or children caught up in early marriages had "no hope for the future" even after undergoing intensive counselling by the WVI Child Protection counsellors (World Vision International Malawi, 2020d, p. 15). The Malawian government policy does not exclude or ban girls who fall pregnant from attending school. Only a one-year suspension is imposed on those girls who are found pregnant in schools. This is unlike Togo, Equatorial Guinea, and Tanzanian that have exclusionary laws and policies for girls who, unfortunately, fall pregnant while at school (World Vision International Malawi, 2020d, pp. 15–16).

According to World Vision International Kenya (2020c) (the Kenyan Chapter), Kenya registered an unusually high rise in the number of teenage pregnancies in 2020 due to the COVID-19 pandemic lockdown. In 2020, Machakos County alone registered about 4,000 teenage pregnancies of school-going girls in that district only. This is an extremely alarming figure without having to learn what the normal estimate was pre-pandemic. World Vision International (2020) sums up its SSA regional report thus:

> Many teenage pregnancies relate to lack of education on sexual and reproductive health. In the home, children may receive little or no guidance on sexuality, or [if any at all], it may be based on stereotypical gender roles and social expectations. Meanwhile in schools, many African governments have failed to implement comprehensive, scientifically-accurate, age-appropriate sexual and reproductive health education . . . Countries across Sub-Saharan Africa have the world's youngest median age of first intercourse. Many children and adolescents lack understanding of relationships, consent, sexually transmitted infections, healthy timing and spacing of pregnancies or family planning.
>
> (World Vision International, 2020, p. 6)

No wonder teenage pregnancies are rampant in times of idleness when they are out of school. World Vision International (2020) estimates that one million teenage girls fell pregnant during the COVID-19 lockdowns in the SSA region alone. SSA girls know little to nothing about pregnancy, ovulation, menstruation, and safe timing for having sex (or safe sex), and this mass ignorance explains the SSA youth's highly risky sexual behaviour (Rukasha, 2021). The ministries of education of many SSA governments are similarly ill-equipped in terms of sex and/or sexuality education curriculum-wise: the ill-prepared, if not shy, teachers do not know how to teach sexuality and reproduction in schools (Rukasha, 2021).

Worse, almost no SSA parents openly discuss sexuality with their children. Consequently, SSA youth must source information on sexuality and reproduction from peers ignorant of such intimate and intricate matters (Panchal et al., 2021). Worse still, contraception (for example, the male or female condom) for protection against STIs (sexually transmitted infections) and unplanned pregnancies is either unknown or out of reach and/or inaccessible financially, or if available, it is not much used by the youth let alone by older men and women in the SSA region (Panchal et al., 2021). The same goes for family planning methods, which are virtually unknown among the SSA youth. When it comes to negotiating sex, SSA youth behave and operate as if the girls need not give their consent before sexual intercourse and as if they have no options but to have unprotected sex with their sexual partners (both boys and men) (Panchal et al., 2021). Because abortion is illegal in most SSA countries, the scenario of backstreet abortion is common for the few girls who consider abortion as an option when the responsible boys and men deny their pregnancies (Panchal et al., 2021).

SSA youth are among high-risk groups predisposed to poor mental health outcomes during pandemics (Panchal et al., 2021). Following the indefinite closure of all educational institutions, there was a surge in teenage and adolescent pregnancies and early marriages in Malawi and the rest of sub-Saharan Africa. Sub-Saharan African youth were affected psychologically by the COVID-19 infodemic. They were bombarded with excessive information on the subject of COVID-19 due to the dissemination of both balanced, fact-based, and truth-oriented news stories on COVID-19 and biased and misleading as well as false and dishonest news stories – in short, misinformation and disinformation (Panchal et al., 2021). The same cannot be said about the SSA youth's access to sexual and reproductive health information and services. Sexual and reproductive health information and services were, and remain, inaccessible to most school-going children and adolescents in the SSA region (Panchal et al., 2021). During the pandemic, the COVID-19 infodemic in the SSA region ran parallel with youth mass ignorance about sexual and reproductive e-health, where e-health refers to online health knowledge, information, and services (Panchal et al., 2021).

4.6 COVID-19 Infodemic and Psychological Stress among SSA Youth

This section draws on the reconstructed Ubuntu thought system (Kayange & Mwale, forthcoming) to propose an ethical intervention tailor-made for the SSA youth in the ongoing COVID-19 pandemic. Moreover, it generally suggests an ethical framework of virtues required for global public health crises, such as COVID-19. What is Ubuntu? Kayange and Mwale (forthcoming) describe thus:

> The notion ubuntu is a Nguni term which is translated by different terms such as humanity and humanness (Gade, 2011). It is a common term in the sub-Saharan context, which refers to different terms in various languages such as "*umunthu*" in ciChewa and Huhnu in Shona. Ubuntu in the philosophical community is often summarised in the following aphorisms, (a) "a person is a person through others" (Tutu, 1999), and "To be a human being is to affirm one's humanity by recognizing the humanity of others and, on that basis establish humane relations with them" (Ramose, 2002). In both aphorisms, the central concept is the community, which guarantees personhood in Tutu's citation and "being human" in Ramose's. These dictums of ubuntu are amenable to different philosophical interpretations, for instance the ontological perspective and the ethical perspective.
>
> (Kayange & Mwale, forthcoming)

The inference that can be drawn from the previous quotation is that Ubuntu is humanness and humaneness. To be human and humane, one exists communally and cooperatively, not singularly and solitarily. The community defines a human being as a person. It is a different question whether such a communal human being – the person – has autonomy, freedoms, and rights, beholden to the community as they are (Kayange & Mwale, forthcoming).

The alarming and unprecedented high increases in teenage and adolescent pregnancies across the SSA region during the COVID-19 pandemic are symptomatic of and testimonial to the lack of the reconstructed Ubuntu, which recognises and upholds individual critical thinking and moral decision-making. Had the SSA youth been inducted into reconstructed Ubuntu, they would have practised self-regarding virtues of self-control and temperance, self-esteem, self, responsibility, foresight, and wisdom – thereby avoiding engaging in unsafe or unprotected sex, or they would have wisely avoided pre-marital sex altogether.

4.7 Conclusion

Owing to COVID-19 pandemic-related stress and infodemic, SSA youth were generally unable to sift and utilise useful information for sound health decision-making. They demonstrated unmitigated ignorance about sexual and reproductive health knowledge, information, and services; hence, the one million teenage and adolescent pregnancies the WVI estimated in 2020 for the SSA region alone. The SSA youth did not practise e-health, despite their social media savvy. This book chapter aimed to depict at least two things. First, it intended to demonstrate how COVID-19 pandemic-related infodemic has affected the youth, leading to psychological stress. This, in turn, has led to their idleness – the high price of which are the one million teenage and adolescent pregnancies that World Vision International estimated for the SSA region in 2020. Malawi, Ghana, Mozambique, Kenya, and Uganda had their fair share of such alarming and unprecedented high increases in teenage and adolescent pregnancies during the COVID-19 pandemic in 2020 and 2021. Idleness, a mental health issue among the SSA youth due to the indefinite closure of all educational institutions at the outbreak of the COVID-19 pandemic, was a recipe for disaster, for it wreaked social havoc in SSA society. Second, the chapter deployed the reconstructed Ubuntu thought system to reflect critically on the role of African philosophy on the debate on COVID-19 infodemic and psychological stress.

Notes

1 **Legacy media** are mass media or mainstream or traditional media that include but are not limited to print news media, television, and radio (see Diel, 2017).
2 **QAnon** is a conspiracy theory contending, among other things, that COVID-19 is a conspiracy orchestrated by powerful actors and aimed at repressing civil liberties (Chan et al., 2021).
3 Pro-e-Health means innovations intended to promote e-health, where e-health itself stands for emerging technologies in internet medicine or telemedicine (Wicks et al., 2014).

References

Aborode, A., Anifowoshe, O., Ayodele, I. T., Iretiayo, R. A., & David, O. O. (2020). *Impact of COVID-19 on education in sub-Saharan Africa.* EDTechHub. https:// docs.edtechhub.org

Albuquerque, S., & Santos, A. R. (2021). "In the same storm, but not in the same boat": Children grief during the COVID-19 pandemic. *Frontiers in Psychiatry, 15,* 1–4. https://doi.org/10.3389/fpsyt.2021.638866

Chan, H. F., Rizio, S. M., Skali, A., & Torgler, B. (2021). Early COVID-19 government communication is associated with reduced interest in the QAnon conspiracy theory. *Frontiers in Psychiatry, 12,* 1–12.

Diel, S. (2017). New media, legacy media and misperceptions regarding sourcing. *KOME: An International Journal of Pure Communication Inquiry, 5*(1), 104–120.

Egelhofer, J. L., & Lecheler, S. (2019). Fake news as a two-dimensional phenomenon: A framework and research agenda. *Annals of the International Communication Association, 43*(2), 97–116.

Elbarazi, I., Saddik, B., Grivna, M., Aziz, F., Elsoris, D., Stip, E., & Bandak, E. (2022). The impact of the COVID-19 "infodemic" on well-being: A cross-sectional study. *Journal of Multidisciplinary Healthcare, 15,* 289–307. https://doi.org.10.2147/ JMDH.S346930

FCDO. (2020). *Mental health and COVID-19 recovery in Africa: Policy options for Africa. Policy brief.* Foreign Commonwealth Development Office.

Gade, C. B. N. (2011). The historical development of the written discourses on *Ubuntu. South African Journal of Philosophy, 30*(3). Published Online on January 1, 2011.

Gisondi, M. A., Barber, R., Faust, J. S., Raja, A., Strehlow, M. C., Westafer, L. M., & Gottlieb, M. (2022). A deadly infodemic: Social media and the power of COVID-19 misinformation. *Journal of Medical Internet Research, 24*(2), e35552. https://doi. org/10.2196/35552

Golberstein, E., Wen, H., & Miller, B. F. (2020). Corona virus 2019 (COVID-19) and mental health for children and adolescents. *JAMA Paediatrics, 174*(9), 819–820. https://doi.org/10.1001/jamapediatrics.2020.1456

Kayange, G. M., & Mwale, P. N. (forthcoming). African condition of agro-epistemicide: Reintroducing the ubuntu framework. In M. Ramose, P. Chaminuka, Y. Ebabu, B. Boogaard, D. Ludwig, & S. Diop (Eds.), *African philosophy and the politics of food systems.* Springer.

Kim, H. K., & Tandoc, E. C., Jr. (2022). Consequences of online misinformationon COVID-19: Two potential pathways and disparity by eHealth Literacy. *Frontiers in Psychology, 13,* 1–11. https://doi.org/10.3389/fpsyg.2022.783909

Leung, J., Schoultz, M., Chiu, V., Bonsaksen, T., Ruffolo, M., Thygesen, H., Price, D., & Geirdal, A. Ø. (2021, January). *Concerns over the spread of misinformation and fake news on social media – challenges amid the Coronavirus pandemic* (pp. 1–6). The 3rd International Electronic Conference on Environmental Research and Public Health. Conference Paper, MDPI AG, Basel. https://doi.org/10.3390/ECERPH-3-09078

Leung, J., Schoultz, M., Chiu, V., Bonsaksen, T., Ruffolo, M., Thygesen, H., Price, D., & Geirdal, A. Ø. (2022). Concerns over the spread of misinformation and fake news on social media: Challenges amid the coronavirus pandemic. *Journal of Multidisciplinary Healthcare, 15,* 289–307. https://doi.org/10.3390/ECERPH-3-09078

Loomba, S., De Figueiredo, A., Piatek, S. J., De Graaf, K., & Larson, H. J. (2021). Measuring the impact of COVID-19 vaccine misinformation on vaccination intent in the UK and USA. *Nature Human Behaviour, 5,* 337–348. https://doi. org/10.1038/s41562-021-01056-1

Ma, L., Mazidi, M., Li, K., Li, Y., Chen, S., Kirwan, R., Zhou, H., Yan, N., Rahman, A., Wang, W., & Wang, Y. (2021). Prevalence of mental health problems among children and adolescents during the COVID-19 pandemic: A systematic review and meta-analysis. *Journal of Affective Disorders, 293*, 78–89.

Mwale, P. N., Tamani, B., & Chisi-Kasunda, T. (2023). Politics and media: The Covid-19 pandemic and its discursive public. *Journal of Humanities, 31*, 43–72. https://dx.doi.org/10.4314/jh.v31i1.3

Namukasa, S. (2021). *Factors that contribute to teenage pregnancy during COVID-19 in Uganda: A study of Bugiri municipal council in Bugiri district* [BA dissertation, Makerere University].

Panchal, U., De Pablo, G. S., Franco, M., Moreno, C., Parellada, M., Arango, C., & Fusar-Poli, P. (2021). The impact of COVID-19 lockdown on child and adolescent mental health: Systematic review. *European Child and Adolescent Psychiatry, 32*, 1151–1177. https://doi.org/10.1007/s00787-021-01856-w

Ramose, M. B. (2002). The philosophy of ubuntu and ubuntu as a philosophy. In P. H. Coetzee & A. P. J. Roux (Eds.), *Philosophy from Africa: A text with readings* (pp. 230–237). Oxford University Press.

Rukasha, I. (2021). COVID-19 and sub-Saharan African children: Direct and indirect impacts. *Commonwealth Youth and Development, 19*(2), 20. https://doi.org/10.25159/2663-6549/11048

Su, Z., McDonnell, D., Wen, J., Kozak, M., Abbas, J., Segalo, S., Li, X., Ahmad, J., Cheshmehzangi, A., Cai, Y., Yang, L., & Xiang, Y. (2021). Mental health consequences of COVID-19 media coverage: The need for effective crisis communication practices. *Global Health, 17*(4), 1–8. https://doi.org/10.1186/s12992-020-00654-4

Tutu, D. (1999). The theology of liberation in Africa. In *Philosophy of religion: The big questions* (pp. 257–262). Blackwell Publishers.

Wang, S., Chen, L., Ran, H., Che, Y., Fang, D., Sun, H., Peng, J., Liang, X., & Xiao, Y. (2022). Depression and anxiety among children and adolescents pre and post COVID-19: A comparative meta-analysis. *Frontiers in Psychiatry, 13*, 1–10. https://doi.org/10.3389/fpsyt.2022.917552

Wicks, P., Stamford, J., Grootenhuis, M. A., Haverman, L., & Ahmed, S. (2014). Innovations in e-health. *Quality of Life Research, 23*, 195–203.

World Health Organization. (2023). www.who.int›newsroom›factsheets›detail

World Vision International. (2020a). *Annual report, Ghana.* www.wvi.org/publications/annual-report/ghana/world-vision-ghana-annual-report-2020

World Vision International. (2020b). *COVID-19 aftershocks: Access denied. Teenage pregnancy threatens to prevent a million girls across sub-Saharan Africa from returning to school.* www.wvi.org/sites/default/files/2020-08-21-%20Aftershocks%20%Education%20Final_3.pdf

World Vision International. (2020c). *Annual report, Kenya.* World Vision Kenya 2020 Annual Report. www.wvi.org/publications/annual-report/kenya/world-vision-kenya-annual-report-2020

World Vision International. (2020d). *Waking our wonder, annual report, Malawi. Waking our wonder: World vision Malawi annual report 2020.* World Vision International.

World Vision International. (2022). *Child protection and the COVID-19 response in Uganda.* www.wvi.org/sites/default/files/2022-02/Uganda_Case%Study_Final.pdf

Xu, J., & Liu, C. (2021). Infodemic vs. pandemic factors associated to public anxiety in the early stage of the COVID-19 outbreak: A cross-sectional study in China. *Public Health, 9*, 1–10. https://doi.org/10.3389/fpubh.2021.723648

5 Academic Staff Coping Responses to COVID-19 Disruptions in Universities

Peter J. O. Aloka and Mary Ooko

5.1 Introduction

Coronavirus disease (COVID-19) emerged as a significant pandemic with effects globally. According to the World Health Organization (WHO) (2020a), statistics revealed a global infection of 12,322,393 cases and 556,335 reported deaths because of the disease. COVID-19 led to the abrupt closure of universities, upending students' in-person learning and living conditions. The pandemic is thus associated with psychological distress among academic staff and other global university workers (Cao et al., 2020) due to health-related fears, uncertainty, and downstream academic consequences. During the outbreak and months into the pandemic, most university academic staff reported a high prevalence of stress among them. A study by the World Health Organization (2020b) reiterated that the effect of the COVID-19 pandemic on mental and psychological well-being has increased because of fear, worry and anxiety related to the virus outbreak. Son et al. (2020) reiterate that during the same period, depression increased from 22% to 26% and anxiety from 11% to 15% among university staff in the United States. Moreover, Rodríguez-Rey et al. (2020) study found that most working people in Spain experienced moderate to severe psychological effects, some showed mild to severe anxiety levels, and more than half reported depressive symptoms.

In addition, Serrano-Ripoll et al. (2020) reported pooled prevalence estimates of 40% for acute stress disorder, 30% for anxiety, 28% for burnout, 24% for depression, and 13% for post-traumatic stress disorder (PTSD) among academic staff at universities. The increased incidences of stress and depressive symptoms among workers could be attributed to high workloads, unattainable performance evaluation processes, the competitive environment in academia and contract employment, a sudden demand to adjust to online teaching, ambiguous boundaries between work and home and social disconnection from students, additional administrative duties, and limited organisational support (Poalses & Bezuidenhout, 2018). In addition, Van Niekerk and Van Gent (2021) state that academic staff at universities thus experienced psychological distress, including fear, worry, and anxiety during the disease. Moreover, Araújo et al. (2020) argue that this increased depression and anxiety among

DOI: 10.4324/9781003425861-6

academic staff members in higher education worldwide. Reports before the pandemic showed an escalation in the poor mental health of university staff members in the United Kingdom due to work environment conditions and challenges (Van Niekerk & Van Gent, 2021).

From an African continent perspective, studies also found that the pandemic significantly affected universities. For example, Rono and Waithera's (2021) study in Kenya reported that most universities experienced challenges in adapting quickly to the effects of the pandemic due to significant challenges to infrastructure, digital fluency of their staff members and students, having appropriate devices, Internet connectivity, and, in many cases, adequate power supply. According to Makiyi (2021), the pandemic affected the learning institutions in Malawi, and the government responded by introducing online and radio lessons. At that time, however, only 5% of Malawians had access to information and communication technology (ICT) facilities, and 45% of the households had radios. Araújo et al. (2020) also reported that increased depression and anxiety were found among staff members in higher education. In Kenya, Odhiambo (2020) noted that the Ministry of Education recognised that the universities had significant numbers of older people, senior professors, deans, principals, and vice-chancellors. They adopted an approach where the older staff and those with underlying health problems were the first members asked to conduct most of their duties from home.

In addition, Mkumbo (2014) reported a high prevalence of stress among higher education academic staff. Moreover, a study by Sahu (2020) also acknowledged that university staff members' main concern was a shift from the usual face-to-face teaching to an online work mode. In Nigeria, Ogunode (2020) found that the COVID-19 pandemic had led to suspending the academic calendar of higher institutions. Adeoye et al. (2020) also reported that the rapid spread of COVID-19 forced the Nigerian government to shut down schools, and schools were directed to adopt an online learning system, which most universities in Nigeria were not used to before the pandemic. In the South African context, Wangenge-Ouma and Kupe (2020) argue that due to the COVID-19 pandemic, universities in South Africa faced an uncertain future, as dwindling funds in the sector are challenging. Van Niekerk and Van Gent (2021) found that during the pandemic, university academic staff experienced uncertainty and instability coupled with fatigue, characterised by new realities and new fears and consequently demanded an adjustment to the work context. Atibuni (2019) argues that during the COVID-19 pandemic, academic staff generally had to cope with stressful conditions to be effective in their various roles and responsibilities. During the COVID-19 pandemic, work at academic institutions was even more stressful than usual because it involved shifts to a complete online learning mode.

Based on the research in the introduction section, the COVID-19 pandemic placed academic staff at African universities at an increased risk of high stress, panic, anxiety, depression, burnout, and obsessive behaviours. In response to the pandemic, universities had to unexpectedly shift their teaching modes from traditional lectures to online teaching with very little time to prepare. This negatively affected the mental health and well-being of university academic staff because of the increased demand for information communication and technology in classrooms due to changes in the teaching mode. Psychological stress is a risk factor in terms of poor mental and physical health outcomes, and academic staff at universities are prone to suffer long-term effects of psychological distress if this is not well addressed. However, very little literature is available on the coping mechanisms adopted in response to psychological distress by academic staff in African universities. Therefore, this chapter provides a conceptual review of coping strategies for psychological distress among academic staff in African universities during the COVID-19 pandemic.

5.2 Coping Mechanisms to Psychological Distress

Coping has been described as a response intended to diminish the physical, emotional, and psychological burdens related to stressful life events and daily disturbances (Snyder, 1999). Synder further argues that the ability to manage stressors created in difficult situations entails constantly changing cognitive, behavioural, and emotional efforts. Appraisal of risks and available coping resources result in the inclination to see complicated situations as challenges rather than threats (Chemers et al., 2001). Coping strategies play a critical role in shaping the meaning and impact of stressful life events. These strategies are used to restore the balance that has been displaced, and are the responses a person displays to a stressful event or situation, which can be adaptive or maladaptive (Carver, 1997). The next section 5.2.1 that follows presents literature which indicates that academic staff in African universities adopted both adaptive and maladaptive coping mechanisms during the COVID-19 pandemic period in an effort to manage psychological distress experienced. This section 1.2.1 discusses literature that was reviewed and which reflected coping mechanisms as adopted by academic staff in African universities and as seen from both perspectives (i.e., adaptive and maladaptive coping strategies).

5.2.1 Adaptive Coping Strategies

According to Du Plessis and Martins (2019), adaptive strategies are positively associated with affect modulation and physiological and psychological health and well-being. Folayan et al. (2017) reiterate that adaptive coping strategies are those that traditionally benefit or positively affect the lives of those who use them. Individuals who utilised adaptive coping strategies are thus able to modulate felt emotions so that their perception of the stressor or coping success to psychological distress, which affects them, is changed. The adaptive coping strategies include cognitive coping, active coping, social support coping, leisure coping, and religious coping strategies. The available literature on the adaptive coping strategies is presented in the following subsections.

Cognitive Coping Strategy

A cognitive coping strategy is based on a mental process of how the individual appraises the situation (Carver, 1997). A cognitive strategy refers to the processes of acquiring knowledge and understanding through thought and experiences to manage the intake of emotion arousing stimuli (Carver, 1997). Previous studies (see Hagan et al., 2022; El-Monshed et al., 2022) at selected African universities found that there were instances when academic staff adopted cognitive coping strategies in an attempt to manage psychological distress during the COVID-19 pandemic period. For example, in Egypt, a study by El-Monshed et al. (2022) found that academic staff had the ability to rationalise or justify their inactive lifestyles and adapted effectively in terms of social distancing measures, hence, being less frustrated by the restrictive measures during the pandemic. Another study in Ghana by Hagan et al. (2022) found that in the case of active coping, the result could be explained from the view that awareness of COVID-19 inherently lent itself to the adoption of active coping mechanisms. In a study done in Egypt, Shehata et al. (2021) found that coping strategies, such as anxiety management, was significantly correlated with anxiety and depression.

Active Coping Strategy

According to Rothmann et al. (2011), active coping strategies are either behavioural or psychological responses designed to change the nature of the stressors themselves or the way one thinks about them. The reviewed studies in this section indicates that some academic staff in certain African universities adopted this active coping strategy. For example, based on a study done in Ghana, Frimpong et al. (2022) reported that university staff adopted active coping strategies to manage the effects of the COVID-19 pandemic. Hagan et al. (2022), also doing research in Ghana, indicate that university lecturers embraced the use of functional management strategies, such as active coping mechanisms, for the duration of the pandemic. In South Africa, Du Plessis (2020) revealed that academics mostly adopted adaptive coping strategies, such as cognitive coping, social support coping, and vacation time, to modulate their emotions so that their perceptions of the stressors during the COVID-19 pandemic could be altered. Rawat and Choudhary's (2020) study found that staff at universities adopted proactive approaches, stayed connected with the universe, reflected and connected with their selves, focused on their health, and managed their time. Another study in North Africa by Chaabane et al. (2021) reported that staff at universities utilised strategies within the problem-focused mechanism, such as active coping, which in turn included specific strategies, namely "problem understanding and solving" and "seeking support" (pp. 136). In this context, these include active coping, planning, restraint coping, seeking social support for instrumental reasons, and suppression of competing activities.

Social Support Coping Strategy

Social support coping strategy is the perceived support that individuals receive from their social support network, such as the family members, friends, and colleagues at work or personal relationships (Rothmann et al., 2011). Previous literature (see Sehularo et al., 2021; Chirombe et al., 2020) indicated that academic staff in African universities adopted social support as a coping strategy during the COVID-19 pandemic. A study by Mokogwu (2022) reported that staff at Nigerian universities utilised strategies such as sharing jokes with friends and families, keeping themselves busy around their homes, and engaging in exercises in an effort to cope with the effects of the pandemic. Sehularo et al.'s (2021) study in South Africa found that staff adopted social support as a coping mechanism during the COVID-19 pandemic, such as support from the spouse, relatives, friends, co-workers and the community. The members of the community provided support to each other to cope with the effects of the pandemic. In addition, Chirombe et al.'s (2020) study reported that staff at universities adopted social support in the form of social media to communicate with friends and colleagues at work to cope with the pandemic. In Egypt, Hafez and Salah El-Din (2021) also noted that academic staff at universities utilised social media as a coping strategy during lockdown through socialisation with family and friends on different social media platforms. Moreover, the study found that academic staff at public and private universities in Egypt used social support in the form of socialising with friends using audio and/or video tools. In Nigeria, Ojewale (2022) noted that staff at universities adopted social support strategies, such as use of social media – WhatsApp, status challenges, and/or Instagram – as they interacted with colleagues in an effort to cope with the pandemic.

In a related study in Nigeria, Isah et al. (2020) observed that using social media was a very common coping strategy among staff and students at universities during the COVID-19 pandemic period. Isah et al. (2020) further argue that social support was associated with reduced cortisol response to stress and better immunity, and it was the most vital psychosocial protective resource. In addition, emotionally satisfying social bonds reduce the effects of stress and, hopefully, the negative impact stress might have on health. Likewise, Son et al. (2020) show that the coping mechanisms of students and staff due to stress and anxiety caused by the pandemic comprised seeking support from others or helping themselves by adopting negative or positive methods. Yu et al. (2020) indicate that social support was one of the preferred coping mechanisms for academic staff at universities during the pandemic. Cao et al. (2020) also report that various forms of concrete or tangible social support were adopted by staff at universities in an effort to cope with the psychological distress caused by the pandemic. Taylor (2015) agrees that social support is the most vital psychosocial protective resource, as emotionally satisfying social bonds reduce the effects caused by stress and its bad effects on health.

In South Africa, Hardman et al. (2022) found that collective responsibility emerged, which circumvented official and apathetic forms of leadership, which disregarded involvement in decisions and were thus unable to contend with the social complexity of crisis management. These apathetic forms of leadership remained one-dimensional in their focus on productive output and forms of capital accumulation, which paid no heed to human need. Goldman and Bell (2022) also reported that staff members at university adopted the use of positive reinterpretation, use of instrumental social support, active coping, suppression of competing activities, and planning to cope with the distresses associated the negative effects of the pandemic.

Emotional Coping Strategy

Emotional coping strategy is the subjective, psychological, and physiological expression of and reaction to stressful encounters that are considered taxing or exceeding an individual's coping resources. According to Sinha (2013), emotion-focused coping refers to the management of an individual's emotional distress coupled with the stressful event rather than the cause of the stress. Sinha further argues that emotion-focused coping involves self-reflection, and the goal is to facilitate expression and process emotions to reappraise an unchangeable stressor (Stanton et al., 2000). Folkman and Moskowitz (2004) argue that emotions are integral to the coping process, as this strategy first regulates negative emotions that may interfere with instrumental forms of coping. Folkman and Moskowitz further contend that within this coping strategy, two mechanisms, namely emotional expression and processing, are always adopted. Previous research indicates that some university staff adopted this strategy to manage stressful conditions. For example, in Egypt, a study by Elkayal et al. (2022) found that the methods of adaptation used by most academic staff at universities relied on emotional-focused coping to manage stressful conditions during the COVID-19 pandemic. A study by Shen and Slater (2021) further found that most academics employed positive coping styles to deal with occupational stress during the COVID-19 outbreak, including emotional support. Du Plessis (2020) revealed that South African academics mostly adopted adaptive emotional-focused coping strategies to modulate the felt emotions so that their perceptions of the stressor were altered. In a related study, Hagenauer and Volet (2014) indicated that being aware of the effectiveness of emotion sharing, staff at universities expressed their positive and negative emotions with family members and departmental colleagues. However, they believed there were not many opportunities to share and discuss negative emotions and their triggers due to the lonely nature of university teaching profession.

Finally, a study done in North Africa by Chaabane et al. (2021) reported that academic staff at universities adopted emotional-focused mechanisms, positive reinforcement and growth strategy, which includes "staying optimistic" and "wishful thinking" to manage stress and its effects experienced during the pandemic period. Therefore, it is concluded that emotion-focused coping is used to manage all forms of emotional distress, including feeling of depression, anxiety, frustration, and anger.

Leisure Coping Strategy

Leisure coping strategy refers to physical activities that individuals voluntarily engage in to regulate heightened emotions in response to environmental demands, and this includes passive leisure, active leisure, social leisure activities, and vacation time. Previous researches (see Mohammed et al., 2021; Gulam, 2016) indicate that staff in higher education institutions also adopted leisure as a coping strategy to psychological stress during the pandemic period. For example, in Egypt, Mohammed et al. (2021) observed that most staff at universities resorted to engaging in other relaxing and meaningful activities, such as reading or listening to news stories mainly on social media, which helped them cope with the stress. Other strategies included staying busy at home doing activities to keep their minds away from COVID-19, getting enough rest, finding spare time during work or between shifts, and eating regular meals. Gulam (2016) also asserts that exercise not only improves one's body image but also helps to improve one's mood and reduces stress. It further improves one's ability to cope with stress in an event of lockdown or stress associated with being incapacitated to live one's normal life. Gulam (2016) further observed that most university staff turned to sleeping during the lockdown as a coping mechanism. In addition, Schuch et al. (2020) noted that leisure activities, such as exercise, yoga, watching movies, and singing, could be used in the treatment of depression and stress. In Zimbabwe, Ngwenya (2021) noticed that the majority of staff managed stress by engaging in relaxation activities, trying to remain aware of the job expectations management had, avoiding being overzealous when duties were being allocated, moving away from a stressful situation, avoiding being pessimistic when confronted with a challenging situation, and sharing their stressful situation with management. Finally, Shamsuddin (2022) reported that leisure can be versatile, and it can adapted to be utilised as a coping tool in various settings and populations.

Religious Coping Strategy

Religious coping strategy is one of the ways of understanding and dealing with negative life events. This strategy is related to the sacred and includes organisational and non-organisational religious activities (Zahid, 2020). Religion seeks to provide meaning to life, particularly in times of calamity, and members of the Islam and other faiths rely on divine intervention in times of crisis (Zahid, 2020). Zahid further argues that Muslims capitalise on their belief, religiosity, and spirituality to cope with life problems and stressors. Sehularo et al. (2021), doing research in South Africa, reported that some staff at universities adopted faith-based practices as a strategy during the COVID-19 pandemic. Similarly, a study by Achour et al. (2021) also noted that staff at higher education institutions depended on faith-based practices, such as prayer, meditation, and spending time with family. A study by Attia et al. (2022) reported that staff at Egyptian universities resorted to prayer to relieve their stress. In their study in Egypt, Bhat et al. (2020) found that the staff at universities adopted religious activities and social work as coping mechanisms during the pandemic. Yawe's (2022) study in Uganda reported that staff at universities resorted to religious coping strategies in an effort to manage the stressful experiences during the pandemic. A Malawian study by Baluwa et al. (2021) reported that religion was one of the coping strategies to alleviate fears in relation to contracting the COVID-19 virus in clinical practice. Similarly, Ozcan et al. (2021) suggest a faith-based and spiritual approach helped university staff to feel grounded, calm, resilient, and present in difficult environments.

5.2.2 Maladaptive Coping Strategies

The term "maladaptive coping strategies" refers to methods that often lead to adverse consequences, including mental health challenges (Javed & Parveen, 2021). Maladaptive coping strategies are only effective in reducing symptoms in the short term, as they tend to increase dysfunction by maintaining and strengthening the disorder (Javed & Parveen, 2021). The reviewed literature in the section indicates that the most common maladaptive coping strategies adopted by academic staff at universities in their response to the pandemic and stressful events were avoidant coping strategy, expressive suppression coping strategy, rumination coping strategy, and alcohol and substance abuse. These maladaptive coping strategies are discussed in the subsection that follows.

Avoidant Coping Strategy

An avoidant coping strategy is an individual's cognitive and behavioural attempt to avoid or escape from dealing with a situation, person, emotion, thought, or entity that causes harm (Hayes et al., 1994). Avoidance coping comprises an attempt to reject or deny that the stressor occurred, to quit any attempts to change the stressor or to engage in tasks not associated with the stressor. An avoidant coping strategy is an activity individuals engage to alter the form and frequency of any adverse experience and distress (Hayes et al., 1994). Avoidant coping is a form of maladaptive coping and was found to be the strongest predictor of adverse well-being outcomes (Gibbons et al., 2011). Previous research indicated that during the COVID-19 pandemic, most staff at higher education institutions adopted avoidant coping strategies to manage their psychological stress. For example, Ojilong et al. (2022) reported that some university staff opted to avoid news, events, or situations that added to their stress or that they thought increased their risk of contracting or transmitting COVID-19. Moreover, Rodino et al. (2018) noted that avoidant coping strategies were significantly positively associated with stress. Li et al. (2018) argue that avoidance is an escapist response to stressful circumstances and that this is regarded as maladjustment in stressful situations rather than flexible adaptation. Kubo et al. (2020) observed that most university staff adopted avoidant coping strategies during the pandemic. Du Plessis (2020) found that negative relationships were observed between avoidant coping on the one hand and coping success on the other among academic staff. Academics who adopted maladaptive coping strategies could not change the adverse experiences or events that elicited emotions and continued to experience distress (Du Plessis, 2020).

Engelbrecht et al. (2021) similarly reported that avoidant coping styles, including self-distraction, denial, venting, substance use, behavioural disengagement, and self-blame, were adopted by university staff to manage psychological distress during the pandemic. Engelbrecht further argues that individuals opt for dysfunctional coping strategies when faced with an uncontrollable event, such as the COVID-19 pandemic. When calamity occurs, the focus is on coping with the problem and not dealing with emotions. Moreover, a study in Nigeria by Oyin et al. (2022) found that some of the avoidant coping responses among the university staff were that they gave up trying to deal with the COVID-19 pandemic. Baluwa et al. (2021) assert that staff at Malawian universities were using avoidance coping strategies to cope with stress during the COVID-19 pandemic due to fear of contracting the coronavirus while in clinical practice. Sehularo et al. (2021) observed that nurses and doctors at a South African university hospital adopted avoidance strategies during the COVID-19 pandemic. Moreover, Okechukwu et al. (2022) found that some university lecturers adopted avoidance as a coping mechanism when dealing with stressful experiences during the pandemic.

Expressive Suppression Coping Strategy

Expressive suppression as a coping strategy is the conscious suppression of emotions (Taylor & Heimberg, 2018). This coping strategy has been adopted by few individuals in handling stressful situations because it does not allow them to express themselves. Taylor and Heimberg (2018) define thought as a conscious cognitive avoidance strategy that individuals adopt when actively attempting to suppress unwanted thoughts or feelings. A study by Mahoney et al. (2011), for example, found genuine expression of negative emotions, faking positive emotions, and suppressing negative emotions to predict greater emotional exhaustion. In contrast, genuine expressions of positive emotions, faking negative emotions, and suppressing positive emotions predicted lower emotional exhaustion. Taylor and Heimberg (2018) argue that individuals who use expressive suppression frequently report receiving less social and emotional support from their peers than those who use other coping strategies.

Hong et al. (2018) observed that expressive suppression – which heightens the intensity of the negative emotion felt and dampens the experience of positive emotion – may negatively affect mental health in the long term. García-Batista et al. (2021) agree that contextual contingencies demand immediate responses and may not allow health personnel to use cognitive re-evaluation strategies, leaning towards emotion suppression. This study by García-Batista is still relevant to the university environment because the health personnel are in the same age category as the academic staff at universities. Finally, Mariani et al. (2021) found that the prevalence and persistence of predominantly negative feelings – without the presence of positive emotions to balance the emotional baseline – could induce a significant risk of psychopathology when facing future stressful events. The imbalanced evaluation of the environment, therefore, increases the perception of risk and the negative evaluation of the strength of the individual.

Rumination Coping Strategy

Rumination as a coping strategy is a method of responding to distress that involves a repetitive and passive focus on the causes, symptoms, and consequences of distress (Shen & Slater, 2021). Few previous studies indicate that university staff utilised rumination as a coping mechanism during times of crisis (see Shen & Slater, 2021). In a related study in South Africa, Du Plessis (2020) noted negative relationships between avoidant coping and rumination coping strategy. Taylor (2015) also argues that academic staff adopted negative coping mechanisms, such as blaming themselves for everything, crying easily, losing appetite, worrying excessively about various things, thinking that everything requires considerable effort, somatic symptoms (such as headache), and bearing with the consequences of having difficulty sleeping. Holman et al. (2020) noticed that a rumination coping mechanism adopted by staff was likely a unique and salient risk factor for poor sleep quality. Moreover, Ye et al. (2022) argue that rumination was a mechanism by which COVID-19 stressors were linked with poor sleep quality. This was positively associated with poor sleep quality among academic staff at universities

Alcohol and Substance Abuse

Previous studies (Shen & Slater, 2021; Patterson et al., 2021) that are presented in this section indicate that some academic staff at universities resorted to alcohol and substance abuse to manage psychological stress and its effects during the pandemic period. Such abuse is regarded as a maladaptive coping strategy because it does not help the sufferers to manage the psychological stress effectively but only temporarily makes them feel comfortable about the problem that they have encountered. For example, in their study, Shen and Slater (2021) found that most academics had a low risk of alcohol dependence and few academics had an increasing risk of alcohol dependence during the pandemic period.

Patterson et al. (2021) observed that the COVID-19 pandemic introduced a significant set of stressors into the lives of many university staff, a population that was already at high risk of developing mental health and substance use disorders. Patterson et al. (2021) further noted that coping with problematic substance use, stressors associated with COVID-19, and overall trends in substance use, more problematic substance use could be expected among academic staff at universities. Gritsenko et al. (2020) noticed that the most commonly reported reasons for increasing alcohol consumption among university staff were the lack of a regular schedule and increased boredom and stress. The university staff who reported increased alcohol use displayed greater fear, loneliness, and depression compared to those who did not increase substance use.

Niba et al. (2022) found that some university staff and even students indulged in smoking, drinking alcohol, taking drugs, and gambling for the first time, while others did this more often than before. Similarly, Attia et al. (2022) found that academic staff adopted smoking as a coping mechanism to handle stressful conditions. The study by Attia et al. further attributed adopting this coping strategy to the fact that some people smoke as self-medication to ease feelings of stress. Moreover, because nicotine creates immediate and temporary relaxation, people falsely think smoking reduces stress and anxiety (Attia et al., 2022). Similarly, Priyadarshini et al. (2015) found that academics adopted negative coping styles, such as drinking alcohol.

5.3 Conclusion

This chapter concludes that some academic staff at African universities adopted adaptive coping strategies to alleviate the psychological distress they experienced during the pandemic. The chapter has argued that the changing emotional factors were positive under stress related to the COVID-19 pandemic, indicating that individual balancing can be achieved through positive affect. However, it is essential to note that during the pandemic, academic staff often learned to cope with the university's unique circumstances without formal training. The chapter further argued that maladaptive coping strategies are less effective in helping an individual to cope with distress because such strategies only provide temporary relief. Still, they tend to increase dysfunction by maintaining and strengthening the distress.

This chapter has highlighted the importance of safeguarding the mental health of academic staff at universities to ensure students' well-being and high-quality teaching. African universities should therefore continue to develop mental well-being support programmes for academic and administrative staff to enable them to cope with the after-effects of the pandemic. The universities should develop wellness centres to assess the well-being of staff, as this would assist in identifying those at risk of maladaptive coping strategies. Moreover, the chapter recommends that universities adopt role-modelling strategies in which staff who utilised adaptive coping strategies during the pandemic would mentor those struggling to cope with stressful events.

References

Achour, M., Souici, D., & Bensaid, B. (2021). Coping with anxiety during the COVID-19 pandemic: A case study of academics in the Muslim world. *Journal of Religious Health, 60,* 4579–4599. https://doi.org/10.1007/s10943-021-01422-3

Adeoye, I. A., Adanikin, A. F., & Adanikin, A. (2020). COVID-19 and e-learning: Nigeria tertiary education system experience. *International Journal of Research and Innovation in Applied Science, 5*(5), 28–30.

Araújo, F. J. O., De Lima, L. S. A., Cidade, P. I. M., Nobre, C. B., & Neto, M. L. R. (2020). Impact of SarsCov-2 and its reverberation in global higher education and mental health. *Psychiatry Research, 288,* 112977–112978. https://doi.org/10.1016/j.psychres.2020.112977

Atibuni, D. Z. (2019). Roles, stress and coping mechanisms among middle-level academic leaders in multi-campus universities in Africa. *Journal of Higher Education in Africa, 17*(1–2), 95–124.

Attia, M., Ibrahim, F. A., Elsady, M. A., Khorkhash, M. K., Rizk, M. A., Shah, J., & Amer, S. A. (2022). Cognitive, emotional, physical, and behavioral stress-related symptoms and coping strategies among university students during the third wave of COVID-19 pandemic. *Frontiers in Psychiatry, 13,* 1–20. https://doi.org/10.3389/fpsyt.2022.933981

Baluwa, M. A., Konyani, A., Chipeta, M. C., Munthali, G., Mhango, L., Chimbe, E., Lungu, F., & Mpasa, F. (2021). Coping with fears of Covid-19 pandemic among nursing students during clinical practice: Malawi's perspective. *Advances in Medical Education and Practice, 12,* 1389–1396. https://doi.org/10.2147/AMEP.S337783

Bhat, B. A., Khan, S., Manzoor, S., Niyaz, A., Tak, H. J., Anees, S. M., Gull, S., & Ahmad, I. (2020). A study on impact of COVID-19 lockdown on psychological health, economy and social life of people in Kashmir. *International Journal of Science and Healthcare Research, 5*(2), 36–46.

Cao, W., Fang, Z., Hou, G., Han, M., Xu, X., Dong, J., & Zheng, J. (2020). The psychological impact of the COVID-19 epidemic on college students in China. *Psychiatry Research, 287,* 112934–112938. https://doi.org/10.1016/j.psychres.2020.112934

Carver, C. S. (1997). You want to measure coping but your protocol's too long: Consider the brief COPE. *International Journal of Behavioral Medicine, 4,* 92–100.

Chaabane, S., Chaabna, K., & Bhagat, S. (2021). Perceived stress, stressors, and coping strategies among nursing students in the Middle East and North Africa: An overview of systematic reviews. *Systematic Review, 10,* 136–145. https://doi.org/10.1186/s13643-021-01691-9

Chemers, M. M., Hu, L. T., & Garcia, B. F. (2001). Academic self-efficacy and first year college student performance and adjustment. *Journal of Educational Psychology, 93*(1), 55–67.

Chirombe, T., Benza, S., Munetsi, E., & Zirima, H. (2020). Coping mechanisms adopted by people during the COVID-19 lockdown in Zimbabwe. *Business Excellence and Management, 10*(1), 33–45.

Du Plessis, M. (2020). Model of coping with occupational stress of academics in a South African higher education institution. *SA Journal of Industrial Psychology, 46*(1), 1–11. https://dx.doi.org/10.4102/sajip.v46i0.1714

Du Plessis, M., & Martins, N. (2019). Developing a measurement instrument for coping with occupational stress in academia. *South African Journal of Industrial Psychology*, *45*, 1–13. https://doi.org/10.4102/sajip.v45i0.1653

Elkayal, M. M., Shahin, M. A. H., & Hussien, R. M. (2022). Psychological distress related to the emerging COVID-19 pandemic and coping strategies among general population in Egypt. *Journal of the Egyptian Public Health Association*, *97*(3), 1–12. https://doi.org/10.1186/s42506-021-00100-2

El-Monshed, A. H., Loutfy, A. S., Moustafa, T., Ahmed, S., Mohamed, A., Soliman, A., Mahmoud, S., & Zoromba, M. (2022). Satisfaction with life and psychological distress during the COVID-19 pandemic: An Egyptian online cross-sectional study. *African Journal of Primary Health Care & Family Medicine*, *14*(1), 1–6. https://dx.doi.org/10.4102/phcfm.v14i1.2896

Engelbrecht, M. C., Heunis, J. C., & Kigozi, N. G. (2021). Post-traumatic stress and coping strategies of South African nurses during the second wave of the COVID-19 pandemic. *International Journal of Environmental Research and Public Health*, *18*(15), 7919–7933. https://doi.org/10.3390/ijerph18157919

Folayan, M. O., Cáceres, C. F., Sam-Agudu, N. A., Odetoyinbo, M., Stockman, J. K., & Harrison, A. (2017). Psychological stressors and coping strategies used by adolescents living with and not living with HIV infection in Nigeria. *AIDS Behaviour*, *21*(9), 2736–2745. https://doi.org/10.1007/s10461-016-1534-3

Folkman, S., & Moskowitz, J. (2004). Coping: Pitfalls and promise. *Annual Review of Psychology*, *55*(1), 745–774.

Frimpong, J. B., Agormedah, E. K., Srem-Sai, M., Quansah, F., & Hagan, J. E., Jr. (2022). Examining risk perception and coping strategies of senior high school teachers in Ghana: Does COVID-19-related knowledge matter? *COVID*, *2*(5), 660–673. https://doi.org/10.3390/covid2050050

García-Batista, Z. E., Guerra-Peña, K., Nouri, K. V., Marte, M. I., Garrido, L. E., & Cantisano-Guzmán, L. M. (2021). COVID-19 pandemic and health worker stress: The mediating effect of emotional regulation. *PLOS One*, *16*(11), e0259013. https://doi.org/10.1371/journal.pone.0259013

Gibbons, C., Dempster, M., & Moutray, M. (2011). Stress, coping and satisfaction in nursing students. *Journal of Advanced Nursing*, *67*(3), 621–632.

Goldman, J. A., & Bell, S. C. (2022). Student and faculty coping and impacts on academic success in response to COVID-19. *Journal of Interdisciplinary Studies in Education*, *11*(1), 74–91.

Gritsenko, V., Skugarevsky, O., Konstantinov, V., Khamenka, N., Marinova, T., Reznik, A., & Isralowitz, R. (2020). COVID 19 fear, stress, anxiety, and substance use among Russian and Belarusian university students. *International Journal of Mental Health and Addiction*, *19*, 2362–2368. https://doi.org/10.1007/s11469-020-00330-z

Gulam, A. (2016). Need, importance and benefits of exercise in daily life. *International Journal of Physical Education, Sports and Health*, *3*(2), 127–130.

Hafez, O., & Salah El-Din, Y. (2021). Egyptian educators' online teaching challenges and coping strategies during COVID-19. *Arab World English Journal*, *12*(4), 279–301. https://dx.doi.org/10.24093/awej/vol12no4.19

Hagan, J. E., Jr., Quansah, F. A., Kwesi, A. E., Medina, S. J. B., & Schack, T. (2022). Linking COVID-19-related awareness and anxiety as determinants of coping strategies' utilization among senior high school teachers in Cape Coast Metropolis, Ghana. *Social Sciences, MDPI*, *11*(3), 1–15. https://doi.org/10.3390/socsci11030137

Hagenauer, G., & Volet, S. E. (2014). "I don't hide my feelings, even though I try to": Insight into teacher educator emotion display. *Australian Educational Researcher*, *41*, 261–281. https://doi.org/10.1007/s13384-013-0129-5

Hardman, J., Shankar, K., Crick, T., McGaughey, F., Watermeyer, R., Ratnadeep Suri, V., Knight, C., & Chung, R. (2022). "Does anyone even notice us?" Covid-19's impact on academics' well-being in a developing country. *South African Journal of Higher Education*, *36*(1), 1–19. https://dx.doi.org/10.20853/36-1-4844

Hayes, S. C., Jacobson, N. S., Follette, V. M., & Dougher, M. J. (Eds.). (1994). *Acceptance and change: Content and context in psychotherapy*. Context Press.

Holman, E. A., Thompson, R. R., Garfin, D. R., & Silver, R. C. (2020). The unfolding COVID-19 pandemic: A probability-based, nationally representative study of mental health in the United States. *Science Advances*, *6*, eabd5390. https://doi.org/10.1126/sciadv.abd5390

Hong, F., Tarullo, A. R., Mercurio, A., Liu, S., Cai, Q., & Malleymorrison, K. (2018). Childhood maltreatment and perceived stress in young adults: The role of emotion regulation strategies, self-efficacy, and resilience. *Child Abuse Neglect*, *86*, 136–146.

Isah, A., Oyine, A. D., Abba, A., Ogbonna, C. P., Okpara, M. E., Sadiq, A., Uchenna, I. N., Ogochukwu, A., & Nworu, C. (2020). Impact of the COVID-19 national lockdown on pharmacy students' productivity and their coping strategies in a developing country: An online survey in Nigerian universities. *Pharmacy Education*, *20*(2), 249–259. https://doi.org/10.46542/pe.2020.202.249259

Javed, S., & Parveen, H. (2021). Adaptive coping strategies used by people during Coronavirus. *Journal of Educational Health Promotion*, *10*, 122–134. https://doi.org/10.4103/jehp.jehp_522_20

Kubo, T., Sugawara, D., & Masuyama, A. (2020). The effect of ego-resiliency and COVID-19-related stress on mental health among the Japanese population. *Personality and Individual Differences*, *175*, a110702. https://doi.org/10.1016/j.paid.2021.110702

Li, M. H., Eschenauer, R., & Persaud, V. (2018). Between avoidance and problem solving: Resilience, self-efficacy, and social support seeking. *Journal of Counseling & Development*, *96*(2), 132–143.

Mahoney, K. T., Buboltz, W. C., Buckner, J. E., & Doverspike, D. (2011). Emotional labor in American professors. *Journal of Occupational Health Psychology*, *16*, 406–423. https://doi.org/10.1037/a0025099

Makiyi, P. (2021). Striking a balance between prevention of COVID-19 and the promotion of child and adolescent mental health: A case study of long closure of schools in Malawi. *Malawi Medical Journal*, *33*(4), 297–299. https://doi.org/10.4314/mmj.v33i4.11

Mariani, R., Renzi, A., Di Monte, C., Petrovska, E., & Di Trani, M. (2021). The impact of the COVID-19 pandemic on primary emotional systems and emotional regulation. *International Journal of Environmental Research and Public Health*, *18*, 5742–5758. https://doi.org/10.3390/ijerph18115742

Mkumbo, K. (2014). Prevalence of and factors associated with work stress in academia in Tanzania. *International Journal of Higher Education*, *3*(1), 1–11.

Mohammed, R. S., Salem, M. R., Mahmoud, A. T., El Sabbahy, L., & El-Jaafary, S. I. (2021). Stress coping strategies among critical care medicine physicians during COVID-19 pandemic in Egypt: A qualitative study. *Open Access Macedonian Journal of Medical Sciences*, *9*(E), 283–288. https://doi.org/10.3889/oamjms.2021.5934

Mokogwu, N. (2022). Psychological challenges and coping strategies of quarantined healthcare workers exposed to confirmed COVID-19 cases in a tertiary hospital in Edo state. *The Journal of the Pan African Thoracic Society*, *3*, 71–77.

Ngwenya, V. C. (2021). Recognising stressors and managing stress in Bulawayo Metropolitan Province primary schools. *South African Journal of Human Resource Management, 19*, a1549. https://doi.org/10.4102/sajhrm.v19i0.1549

Niba, R. N., Akwah, E. A., Musisi, J., Awanchiri, K., Babirye, R., & Emalieu, D. (2022). Perceived risks of COVID-19, attitudes towards preventive guidelines and impact of the lockdown on students in Uganda: A cross-sectional study. *PLOS One, 17*(4), e0266249. https://doi.org/10.1371/journal.pone.0266249

Odhiambo, W. (2020, July 16). COVID-19: Managing the risk to older university staff members. *University World News: Africa Edition.* www.universityworldnews.com/post.php?story=20200716062706283

Ogunode, N. J. (2020). Investigation into the impact of COVID-19 pandemic on higher institutions in FCT, Abuja, Nigeria. *Journal of Social Science, Education and Humanities, 1*(1), 8–16.

Ojewale, L. Y. (2022). *Psychological state, family functioning and coping strategies among students of the University of Ibadan, Nigeria, during the COVID-19 lockdown.* Springer. https://doi.org/10.1101/2020.07.09.20149997

Ojilong, D., Kanyike, A. M., Nakawuki, A. W., Lutwama, D. M, Nakanwagi, D., & Nekaka, R. (2022). Anxiety and coping strategies during the Covid-19 pandemic among students at a multi-campus university in Uganda. *Research Square, 3*, 1–23. https://doi.org/10.21203/rs.3.rs-1446865/v1

Okechukwu, F. O., Ogba, K. T. U., Nwufo, J. I., Ogba, M. O., Onyekachi, B. N., Nwanosike, C. I., & Onyishi, A. B. (2022). Academic stress and suicidal ideation: Moderating roles of coping style and resilience. *BMC Psychiatry, 22*(1), 546–555. https://doi.org/10.1186/s12888-022-04063-2

Oyin, O. G., Adaramola, O. M., Oluwanisola, T., Olu-Festus, D. M., Toluwanimi, E. O., Uche-Orji, C. I., Oluseun, P. O., & Oluwakemi, O. O. (2022). Coping strategies of Nigerian medical students during the COVID-19 pandemic. *Ghana Medical Journal, 56*(1), 15–22. http://dx.doi.org/10.4314/gmj.v56i1.3

Ozcan, O., Hoelterhoff, M., & Wylie, E. (2021). Faith and spirituality as psychological coping mechanism among female aid workers: A qualitative study. *International Journal of Humanitarian Action, 6*, 15–27. https://doi.org/10.1186/s41018-021-00100-z

Patterson, Z. R., Gabrys, R. L., Prowse, R. K., Abizaid, A. B., Hellemans, K. G. C., & McQuaid, R. J. (2021). The influence of COVID-19 on stress, substance use, and mental health among postsecondary students. *Emerging Adulthood, 9*(5), 516–530. https://doi.org/10.1177/21676968211014080

Poalses, J., & Bezuidenhout, A. (2018). Mental health in higher education: A comparative stress risk assessment at an open distance learning university in South Africa. *The International Review of Research in Open and Distributed Learning, 19*(2), 169–191. https://doi.org/10.19173/irrodl.v19i2.3391

Priyadarshini, C., Ponnam, A., & Banerjee, P. (2015). Role stress and coping among business school professors: A phenomenological study. *Qualitative Report, 20*(12), 2050–2066.

Rawat, N. S., & Choudhary, K. C. (2020). Coping strategies with stress and anxiety of tri-pillar of the education system in COVID-19 pandemic period. *SSRN Electronic Journal, 2020.* https://doi.org/10.2139/ssrn.3596912

Rodino, I. S., Gignac, G. E., & Sanders, K. A. (2018). Stress has a direct and indirect effect on eating pathology in infertile women: Avoidant coping style as a mediator. *Reproductive Biomedicine & Society Online, 5*, 110–118. https://doi.org/10.1016/j.rbms.2018.03.002

Rodríguez-Rey, R., Garrido-Hernansaiz, H., & Bueno-Guerra, N. (2020). Working in the times of COVID-19. Psychological impact of the pandemic in frontline workers in Spain. *International Journal of Environmental Research and Public Health*, *17*(21), 8149–8172. https://doi.org/10.3390/ijerph17218149

Rono, R. C., & Waithera, K. L. (2021). The mental and psychosocial impact of COVID-19 pandemic on university faculty and students. *Alliance for African Partnership Perspectives*, *1*, 73–81.

Rothmann, S., Jorgensen, L., & Hill, C. (2011). Coping and work engagement in selected South African organisations. *SA Journal of Industrial Psychology*, *37*(1), 1–11. https://doi.org/10.4102/sajip.v37i1.962

Ruisoto, P., Vaca, S. L., López-Goñi, J. J., Cacho, R., & Fernández-Suárez, I. (2017). Gender differences in problematic alcohol consumption in university professors. *International Journal of Environmental Research and Public Health*, *14*(9), 1069–1080. https://doi.org/10.3390/ijerph14091069.

Sahu, P. (2020). Closure of universities due to coronavirus disease 2019 (COVID-19): Impact on education and mental health of students and academic staff. *Cureus*, *12*(4), e7541. https://doi.org/10.7759/cureus.7541

Schuch, F. B., Bulzing, R. A., Meyer, J., Vancampfort, D., Firth, J., & Stubbs, B. (2020). Associations of moderate to vigorous physical activity and sedentary behavior with depressive and anxiety symptoms in self-isolating people during the COVID-19 pandemic: A cross-sectional survey in Brazil. *Psychiatry Research*, *1*, 292–309.

Sehularo, L. A., Molato, B. J., Mokgaola, I. O., & Gause, G. (2021). Coping strategies used by nurses during the COVID-19 pandemic: A narrative literature review. *Health SA Gesondheid*, *26*, 1–8. https://dx.doi.org/10.4102/hsag.v26i0.1652

Serrano-Ripoll, M. J., Meneses-Echavez, J. F., Ricci-Cabello, I., Fraile-Navarro, D., Fiol-deRoque, M. A., Pastor-Moreno, G., Castro, A., Ruiz-Pérez, I., Zamanillo Campos, R., & Gonçalves-Bradley, D. C. (2020). Impact of viral epidemic outbreaks on mental health of healthcare workers: A rapid systematic review and meta-analysis. *Journal of Affective Disorders*, *277*, 347–357. https://doi.org/10.1016/j.jad.2020.08.034

Shamsuddin, S. (2022). *Leisure as a coping mechanism: The relationship between leisure and stress*. Poster presented at the International Research Conference for Graduate Students, San Marcos, TX.

Shehata, G. A., Gabra, R., Eltellawy, S., Elsayed, M., Gaber, D. E., & Elshabrawy, H. A. (2021). Assessment of anxiety, depression, attitude, and coping strategies of the Egyptian population during the COVID-19 pandemic. *Journal of Clinical Medicine*, *10*(17), 3989–3899. https://doi.org/10.3390/jcm10173989

Shen, P., & Slater, P. (2021). The effect of occupational stress and coping strategies on mental health and emotional well-being among university academic staff during the COVID-19 outbreak. *International Education Studies*, *14*(3), 82–95. https://doi.org/10.5539/ies.v14n3p82

Sinha, R. (2013). The clinical neurobiology of drug craving. *Current Opinion in Neurobiology*, *23*(4), 649–654.

Snyder, C. R. (1999). *Coping: The psychology of what works*. Oxford University Press.

Son, C., Hegde, S., Smith, A., Wang, X., & Sasangohar, F. (2020). Effects of COVID-19 on college students' mental health in the United States: Interview survey study. *Journal of Medical Internet Research*, *22*, e21279. https://doi.org/10.2196/21279

Stanton, A. L., Kirk, S. B., Cameron, C. L., & Danoff-Burg, S. (2000). Coping through emotional approach: Scale construction and validation. *Journal of Personality and Social Psychology, 78*(6), 1150–1169.

Taylor, D. M., & Heimberg, R. G. (2018). Emotion regulation in social anxiety and depression: A systematic review of expressive suppression and cognitive reappraisal. *Clinical Psychology Review, 65,* 17–42.

Taylor, S. E. (2015). *Health psychology.* McGraw-Hill.

Van Niekerk, R. L., & Van Gent, M. M. (2021). Mental health and well-being of university staff during the coronavirus disease 2019 levels 4 and 5 lockdowns in an Eastern Cape university, South Africa. *South African Journal of Psychiatry, 27*(4), a1589. https://doi.org/10.4102/sajpsychiatry.v27i0.1589

Wangenge-Ouma, G., & Kupe, T. (2020). *Uncertain times: Re-imagining universities for new, sustainable futures.* USAf. www.usaf.ac.za/wp-content/uploads/2020/09/Uncertain-Times-Paper.pdf

World Health Organization. (2020a). *Mental health and psychosocial considerations during the COVID-19 outbreak.* www.who.int/docs/default-source/coronaviruse/mental-health-considerations.pdf

World Health Organization. (2020b). *Coronavirus disease (COVID-2019) situation reports.* www.who.int/emergencies/diseases/novel-coronavirus-2019/situation-reports

Yawe, M. J. (2022). Managing burnout among teaching staff at private universities in Uganda: A case study. *International Journal of Educational Development in Africa, 7*(1), 33–46. https://doi.org/10.25159/2312-3540/10233

Ye, B., Wu, D., & Wang, P. (2022). COVID-19 stressors and poor sleep quality: The mediating role of rumination and the moderating role of emotion regulation strategies. *International Journal of Behavioral Medicine, 29,* 416–425. https://doi.org/10.1007/s12529-021-10026-w

Yu, H., Li, M., Li, Z., Xiang, W., Yuan, Y., & Liu, Y. (2020). Coping style, social support and psychological distress in the general Chinese population in the early stages of the COVID-19 epidemic. *BMC Psychiatry, 20,* 426–438. https://doi.org/10.1186/s12888-020-02826-3

Zahid, M. A. (2020, April 11). COVID-19: An Islamic prescription. *The Muslim Vibe.* https://themuslimvibe.com/faith-islam/COVID-19-an-islamic-prescription

6 Experiences of Media Workers During the COVID-19 Crisis

Tendai Makaripe and Lazarus Sauti

6.1 Introduction

The emergence of the COVID-19 pandemic had socioeconomic and political ramifications on people's lives. Most, if not all, enterprises within and across the world lost considerable planned revenue while jobs and lives were also lost (Cepel et al., 2020). The media sector was not spared from the consequences of the pandemic. Several studies have been conducted on the nexus between the pandemic and the journalism sector. Chibuwe and colleagues (2022) investigated newsroom disruptions and opportunities in times of crisis and focused on examining Southern African media during the COVID-19 crisis. In their study, Ncube and Mare (2022) focused on fake news and multiple regimes of truth during the COVID-19 pandemic in Zimbabwe. Mututwa and Mare (2022) analysed the mediation of the COVID-19 pandemic by mainstream and peripheral content creators in Zimbabwe. For Matsilele et al. (2022), the need to understand how news operations, newsroom cultures, news gathering, and news dissemination practices were affected by the COVID-19 pandemic formed the basis of their investigation. However, there appears to be a dearth of literature regarding the psychological effects of COVID-19 on journalists in Zimbabwe and other countries worldwide.

There is little coverage of how media practitioners, especially news reporters, editors, and sub-editors dealt with mental health issues, such as anxiety, depression, event-specific distress, and a decline in psychological well-being during the pandemic. Against this backdrop, this chapter seeks to bridge this gap by analysing how Zimbabwean journalists dealt with anxiety issues during the COVID-19 pandemic. This chapter starts by contextualising the effect of COVID-19 on journalistic practice and the profession. The chapter then discusses the theoretical framework, methodology, findings, and discussions.

6.2 The Effect of COVID-19 on Journalistic Practice and the Profession

Pneumonia-like cases first appeared in China in December 2019, and the coronavirus, known as severe acute respiratory syndrome coronavirus 2

DOI: 10.4324/9781003425861-7

(SARS-CoV-2) (also known as COVID-19), was later shown to be responsible (Laguna et al., 2020). This disease was and is still spread mainly through contact with infected people, respiratory droplets from symptomatic individuals, and/or contact with contaminated objects and surfaces. The media has been crucial in informing and educating the public about COVID-19, which has affected people around the globe. Casero-Ripollés (2020) argues that during a global crisis such as the COVID-19 pandemic, the media provide data, information, and ideas that can directly contribute to citizens' potential for self-protection and safety. True to this, the media were central in mediating the COVID-19 pandemic from the start of the disease up to now. Data from the Pew Research Center (2020) reveal that most citizens in the United States relied on websites, newspapers, cable and free-to-air television, and social media platforms to get information about the COVID-19 pandemic. In Spain, Ruiz de Gauna (2020) found that most people also relied on television, digital press, the Internet and social media networks, and printed media to learn about COVID-19.

Even though the media played a crucial role in informing and educating people in the United States, Spain, and other countries worldwide, journalists were exposed to the virus. Media houses also grappled and struggled to stay afloat due to the devastating consequences of the COVID-19 pandemic. The working conditions for journalists were negatively affected by media companies' lack of financial revenue owing to COVID-19. For instance, major newspapers in Spain, such as *Prisa, Vocento, Prensa Ibérica, Unedisa, Godó, Henneo*, and *Joly* reduced their working hours and the wages of their staff reporters by between 11% and 50% over a period of three to six months (Ministerio de Trabajo y Economia Social, 2020). This has directly influenced the creation of journalistic content, which fell 14.2% overall during the first stage of the health emergency in Spain.

Daniels (2020) affirms that the COVID-19 pandemic-induced crisis in the media caused roughly 50% of formally hired South African journalists to lose their jobs between March 2020 and December 2020. The effect was also felt in Zimbabwe where various social domains, such as education, sports, entertainment, and the media were severely affected (Matsilele, 2021; Nhamo et al., 2020). News publishers halted the printing and delivery of newspapers in response to the forced changes brought about by the pandemic in the political economy, slashing pay and firing journalists, and declaring bankruptcy (Matsilele et al., 2022). While COVID-19 had a positive effect on journalism, as evidenced by increased news consumption and the promotion of new formats and information products, such as infographics or newsletters, it also had devastating effects, as it contributed to the deterioration of the working conditions of journalists, the reinforcement of political control mechanisms over the media, and the rise in disinformation.

Because of restrictive measures imposed by the government of Zimbabwe to flatten the COVID-19 curve, some news stations used simulcasting while others alternated between working from home and employing digital media technology. This was a double-edged sword for journalists. On the one hand, it restrained journalists as they lost their jobs. On the other hand, it helped journalists and newsrooms to adapt and develop digital techniques and practices (Mungwari et al., 2022). Matsilele et al. (2022) observe that journalists in Zimbabwe, Botswana, and South Africa also experienced traumatic events, such as COVID-19-related illness, fatalities, and job losses when media houses reduced their operations to stop the spreading of the virus.

The scholars add that despite the difficult working conditions, journalists had to complete their assignments timeously. Their standard function is to disseminate essential information to the public, which is crucial during a public health emergency, such as the COVID-19 epidemic. Since news organisations typically form part of a communication ecology, it is reasonable to assume that during the COVID-19 pandemic, journalists and news organisations were engaged in that ecosystem (Perreault, 2020). While juggling their struggles during the crisis, journalists acted as a resource for others inside the news and/or information ecology. Perreault and Perreault (2021) posit that during COVID-19, journalists discursively positioned themselves in a responsible but exposed position within the media ecology – not just due to the pandemic but also from environmental factors that long preceded it. During the pandemic, journalists had difficulties reporting and working to counteract these factors, environmental and otherwise, while attempting to stop spreading false information.

6.3 The Sociology of News Production

In his articulation of the sociology of news production theory, Schudson (2003, pp. 5–6) argues, "the vast majority of daily news in newspapers or on television comes from planned, intentional events, press releases, press conferences, and schedule interviews." Schudson argues that this means that news is primarily the result of the interaction between journalists and sources. Supporting this, Belair-Gagnon and Revers (2018) assert that the news production process is routinised. They explain that journalists make news following a set of professional values and organisational routines and structures, which they hardly articulate. In the sociology of news production, journalists interact with sources daily.

As mentioned before, the communication ecology is still influenced by the formal, professional, informal, and personal methods used by journalists (Christians et al., 2010; Lewis, 2020). Given what they believe their audience requires, journalists develop their roles and carry them out accordingly. For instance, studies have shown that a journalist takes on

- the role of a storyteller when covering dangerous situations;
- an enrichment role when striving to provide full services to a particular community; and
- the role of a disseminator when attempting to uphold objectivity in a fragile cultural area (Perreault et al., 2020).

To Christians et al. (2010), journalists also play a facilitative role by monitoring or observing the environment in search of relevant information about events, conditions, trends, and threats and by carrying out the role in response to a perceived need for collaboration. The scholars add that the facilitative function is based on the idea that journalists have a social responsibility to help the public make decisions in times of need.

The COVID-19 pandemic and its prevention protocols, such as national shutdowns, prevented journalists in Zimbabwe and other parts of the world from fulfilling their roles. It also disrupted the physical interaction of journalists and their news sources. In their limited interactions, journalists were exposed to the virus. This justifies the applicability of the sociology of news production theory in this chapter. We argue that the COVID-19 pandemic disrupted news-gathering practices and routines, straining some journalists. The disruption resulted in job losses, increased workload, stress, and depression.

The study employed semi-structured interviews with purposively selected editors, sub-editors, and journalists from purposively selected newsrooms. Specifically, we conducted five telephonic interviews from print and online publications: *The Sunday Mail, H-Metro,* and *263Chat.* The justification for interviewing five participants is that, in qualitative research, meaning is more important than numbers. Having few respondents in qualitative research can be important for several reasons. One reason is that it allows for an in-depth exploration of the experiences, perspectives, and attitudes of each participant. This could lead to a richer understanding of the phenomenon being studied and provides valuable insights that would be missed with larger sample size.

The intention of interviewing five participants – three males and two females – was to gather information on the effect of the COVID-19 pandemic on the psychological well-being of journalists in Zimbabwe. The following questions were asked: (1) How can you describe your state of mind as a practising journalist during COVID-19? (2) Do you think your media house and other stakeholders did enough to protect journalists from COVID-19 in their line of work? And (3) From your experiences, which intervention methods can be implemented to curb the psychological impact of pandemics among journalists? To analyse the data, we employed thematic analysis. This method identifies, analyses, and reports patterns (themes) within data (see Braun & Clarke, 2006). Thematic analysis organises and describes data in rich detail. Through thematic analysis, commonly recurring themes are drawn from the data (Braun & Clarke, 2006). The scholars contend that thematic analysis is a familiar method of analysing interview data, especially from in-depth and semi-structured interviews.

6.4 Psychological Effect of COVID-19 on Zimbabwean Journalists

This section focuses on the psychological outcomes COVID-19 had on journalists in Zimbabwe. Findings from the interviews with participants showed that COVID-19 negatively affected them, their work, and their social relations.

For instance, P1 from *The Sunday Mail* said the COVID-19 pandemic negatively affected her work, social relations, and economic life. She added that fear developed just from hearing how COVID-19 had affected China and how the virus was spreading to other countries. As a result, there was much fear of leaving home and meeting colleagues at work, especially after the disease began spreading in the workplaces. Please note that all quotations are reproduced verbatim and unedited.

> This caused anxiety because I feared contracting the virus and taking it back to my family, including my unborn and then newly born child.
>
> (P1, *The Sunday Mail*)

P1 further said her anxiety worsened when she saw her colleagues dying because of COVID-19. She said,

> It was heart-breaking that workmates we had soldiered within the industry were lost overnight, some we spoke often on the phone, and some we worked side by side. Those statistics became so real as the pandemic hit home. So, it was so draining. It also then made me fear to execute my duties because there was that fear that maybe I'm next. Journalism thrives on networking, interactions, and fieldwork – so COVID-19 disrupted this and we couldn't be doing that anymore. Because of that, coming up with stories, apart from those linked to COVID-19 became difficult.
>
> (P1, *The Sunday Mail*)

Additionally, P1 said government-induced measures, such as lockdowns, enabled her to work from home and talk to sources on the phone. She explained,

> It was also good that even the sources preferred using online platforms to do interviews so getting a positive response for stories was possible. There was also lots of spiritual and soul searching just to keep the faith and keep going because it was such a difficult time.
>
> (P1, *The Sunday Mail*)

The second respondent (P2 from *H-Metro*) said in the initial stages of COVID-19, it was very scary; it was difficult to have a stable mind as COVID-19 was raging. He stated,

> I was put on the frontline team at my workplace. So, from the onset of COVID-19, my mind was shaky but settled with time. COVID was killing and it was not easy to relax. But I later on managed to cool and following the vaccinations, I relaxed.
>
> (P2, *H-Metro*)

P2 also said fellow journalists succumbing to COVID-19 affected him, since there is a saying in journalism, namely "no story is worth dying for."

> I felt so affected when the country lost Zororo Makamba. It traumatised me that COVID-19 meant business. Emotionally, I felt sorry for the journalists who lost their lives in the line of duty.

He added that the possibility of infecting his family with COVID-19 also caused him significant fear:

> Imagine going for a story at a local hospital and going back to meet the family. To be honest, COVID-19 was deadly and it was not easy to work and come alive. So, each time I go for a story I would make sure, I play it safe. The fear was of infecting the next person.
>
> (P2, *H-Metro*)

Another participant from *H-Metro* (P3) asserted that the COVID-19 pandemic adversely affected his mind. As a sports reporter, he explained that it was a difficult experience considering there were few sports activities; hence, pressure from the editors increased on him to come up with sports stories. He added,

> It was traumatising because I had to come up with stories from little to no activity. At the same time, where sports were being conducted, going there was a risk that my family members did not want me to take. At the same time, I had to go there because that is my source of income.

P4 from *263Chat*, an online publication, said the COVID-19 pandemic affected his state of mind as a practising journalist in Zimbabwe. He stated that COVID-19 not only triggered fear and uncertainty; the pandemic turned his life upside down. He said fear was everywhere, and he even contemplated taking a break from the noble profession considering the way he succumbed to the virus. P4 went further to explain:

> It was a tough experience which up to now has not been easy to grasp considering that in our line of work, we mix and mingle with a lot of people.

The same sentiments were shared by a radio producer (P5), who was working for Radio Zimbabwe at the time – a state-owned and controlled radio station. She said the pandemic stressed her as it had brought her life to a standstill. She explained,

> I was stressed. Some of my colleagues lost their jobs because of the pandemic. Media houses were forced to downsize because of several reasons. This burdened me and as such I experienced anxiety and tension.

The same participant said the COVID-19 pandemic forced newsrooms to embrace digital media technologies. She added that even though these new media technologies improved journalistic practices, some journalists lacked the skills required to use them effectively and to work safely from home.

Evidence from all the participants in the current study revealed that the COVID-19 pandemic had left a lasting impression on the journalism profession and the lives of media practitioners. The pandemic affected their way of life, their social structures, and their economic lives. All participants said they were stressed because of the pandemic, and this strained their relationships with family members. The pandemic thus caused psychological distress among journalists in Zimbabwe. These findings tally with the global study by the International Federation of Journalists on the effects of the COVID-19 pandemic on field journalists (Arab Trade Union Confederation, 2020). The participants were 1 308 journalists from 77 nations. In terms of their coverage of the COVID-19 outbreak, three out of four journalists experienced workplace limitations from government agencies, disruptions of their movements, or intimidation (Arab Trade Union Confederation, 2020). According to two-thirds of the respondents (872), the pandemic also resulted in wage reductions, job losses, the cancellation of production contracts, and a worsening of their financial circumstances.

These findings have significant implications for the quality of news produced. The sociology of news production posits that news is not merely a reflection of reality but a social construct influenced by a variety of societal and professional factors (Tuchman, 1978). The stress and anxiety caused by the pandemic could therefore have altered journalists' perspectives, potentially leading to biased or imbalanced reporting.

The stress, anxiety, and financial insecurity experienced by journalists, as identified in the study, could all interfere with their ability to select, interpret, and present news impartially. Consequently, the societal distress brought on by the pandemic might unintentionally have biased news construction, possibly skewing the depiction of events and issues. Furthermore, the economic pressures induced by the pandemic could have compelled news outlets and journalists to prioritise profitability and survival, potentially leading to sensationalism, a reduction in investigative journalism, and an overreliance on press releases or other easily accessible sources (Singh, 2020). Such practices, driven by economic imperatives, may compromise journalistic integrity and the diversity of news content, reinforcing the influence of power structures on news production (Bourdieu, 1998).

The strain on familial relationships and the reported psychological distress among journalists could also have played a role in news production. These personal challenges might potentially have influenced journalists' news framing, story selection, and interpretation of events, introducing an element of subjectivity (see Shoemaker & Reese, 1996). Ultimately, the findings provide a potent illustration of the intricate relationship between societal conditions – in this case, a global pandemic – and the news production process, as underscored by the sociology of news production theory.

6.5 Support from Media Houses and Other Stakeholders

On the issue of support from media houses and other stakeholders, all the participants said their newsrooms and other stakeholders supported them during the COVID-19 pandemic. P1 had this to say:

> Our media house, the Ministry of Information and Broadcasting Services, the Zimbabwe Union of Journalists, and the Nyaradzo Group supported us. These organisations provided us with protective gear.
>
> (P1, *H-Metro* insert)

P2 argued that, from the onset, COVID-19 was a hard blow for almost everyone, as the virus came unexpectedly. Over the months, as the pandemic continued to run its course, media houses were able to handle it better. He explained,

> The virus caught many people unaware. Had it not been the intervention of the international community, including the World Health Organization it could have been a disaster. But with time, our employers and other stakeholders like the Ministry of Information and Broadcasting Services, Ministry of Health and Child Care, and the Media Institute of Southern Africa-Zimbabwean Chapter began to manage the situation. If you noticed, many people died in the inception of COVID-19 but later on lives were saved. Journalists were given some protective clothing at a later stage but it was not enough to curtail the spread of the virus. So, journalists were not safe just like the health workers.
>
> (P2, *H-Metro*)

To P3, although media houses and other institutions tried to save journalists from COVID-19, most journalists across the country lacked the protective gear they needed for fieldwork. P3 added that some journalists were beaten by police officers and soldiers during their fieldwork.

> Despite the efforts made by media houses and other institutions to ensure the safety of journalists during the pandemic, the reality is that many journalists across the country lacked the necessary protective gear for fieldwork. This, coupled with incidents of police brutality towards journalists, has made it even more difficult for them to carry out their work effectively and safely.

Based on the research findings, it can be concluded that during the pandemic, most newsrooms tried to safeguard their journalists from being infected with COVID-19. They were supported by organisations such as the Ministry of Information and Broadcasting Services, the Ministry of Health and Child Care, the Zimbabwe Union of Journalists (ZUJ), MISA-Zimbabwe, and the Nyaradzo Group. However, most journalists in the country lacked protective gear. Law enforcement agents abused some in the course of their work because they were perceived to be violating lockdown regulations, even when they were performing their duties as essential service providers. These findings are thus in sync with findings by the Arab Trade Union Confederation (2020), which revealed that several journalists in Jordan, Iraq, and Egypt who covered the COVID-19 pandemic and its economic and social effects not only lacked protective gear but were beaten and also subjected to judicial warrants or arrested.

These findings significantly reflect the structural and situational constraints journalists in Zimbabwe faced during the COVID-19 pandemic, providing a real-world application of the sociology of news production theory. This theoretical framework emphasises that news is a social construct shaped by institutional, professional, and societal dynamics (Tuchman, 1978). For instance, a lack of protective gear presented a direct physical risk to journalists, potentially impinging on their ability and willingness to cover stories, particularly those requiring direct contact or proximity to potentially infected people. As McQuail (1994) posits, the physical conditions in which journalists work can considerably affect the news they produce.

Meanwhile, abuse by law enforcement agents suggests institutional pressure that could negatively affect the news-gathering process. It signifies an environment of fear and intimidation that could induce journalists' self-censorship or reluctance to cover specific stories (Shoemaker & Reese, 1996). This situation echoes Bourdieu's (1998) argument that power structures could significantly influence news production. As identified in the current study, these circumstances undoubtedly contribute to a stressful working environment that could adversely affect journalists' mental health. Psychological distress, in turn, could influence journalists' framing of events and story selection, adding a subjective element to news production (see Shoemaker & Reese, 1996). Consequently, these implications reinforce the central tenet of the sociology of news production theory: news is a social construct influenced by many societal, institutional, and professional factors.

6.6 Curbing the Psychological Impact of Pandemics among Journalists

This section focuses on the recommended intervention methods that media houses could implement to curb the psychological impact of pandemics on journalists in Zimbabwe. Interviewed participants recommended several solutions. For instance, P1 believed that media houses should organise counselling sessions with psychologists to assist journalists in understanding what they are facing as frontline workers and how to deal with it. She added that media houses and relevant authorities should ensure journalists have adequate financial and material resources to cushion them against anxiety and other psychological impacts.

P2 stated that one of the most viable solutions to mitigating the psychological impact of pandemics among journalists should be based on workshops where health experts would be invited to share some key information about understanding the psychological impact of journalism. Experts could help journalists understand the potential psychological impact of their work, including the risk of developing conditions such as post-traumatic stress disorder (PTSD), depression, and anxiety. Additionally, experts could help journalists recognise the signs of burnout, such as feeling emotionally and physically exhausted, losing interest in their work, and experiencing a decline in performance. He argues that psychologists should be part and parcel of the workshops to share with journalists. Above all, P2 believed "journalists need money and money helps to calm down the mind."

To P3, media houses, the Ministry of Health and Child Care, the Ministry of Information and Broadcasting Services, the Zimbabwe Union of Journalists, the Young Journalists Association of Zimbabwe (YOJA), the Media Alliance, and other players in the civic society sector should accommodate journalists during pandemics to avoid inconveniences from family members who would be exposed to diseases as well. Journalists have a social responsibility to mediate crises and should be empowered to fulfil that obligation without fear. These sentiments were also shared by participants 4 and 5, respectively.

The current findings indicate that the journalists in the study recognised the importance of their and public safety amid a pandemic. The suggestion of counselling sessions and workshops implied that they understood the importance of education and support in navigating the challenges of covering a health crisis.

The implications of these findings are both theoretical and empirical. From a theoretical perspective, the study highlighted the role of journalists as key stakeholders in the communication and media sector and underscored the importance of their safety and well-being. The suggestion of counselling sessions and workshops highlighted the need for ongoing education and support for journalists, which could help them navigate their profession's challenges.

Empirically, the findings suggest that media organisations and their partners should prioritise the safety and well-being of journalists and provide them with adequate resources to fulfil their roles as information providers and public educators during health crises. This could include the provision of personal protective equipment, training in health and safety protocols, and ongoing support and education.

In terms of the sociology of news production theory, the findings suggest that journalists are not passive recipients of news, but active agents who shape the production and dissemination of news. The suggestion of counselling sessions and workshops also indicates that journalists are aware of their role in shaping public perceptions of health crises, and are willing to take proactive steps to ensure that they are equipped with the necessary knowledge and resources to fulfil this role.

Overall, the findings suggest that journalists have an essential role in informing, educating, and protecting the public during health crises, such as COVID-19. However, they must be supported and equipped with the necessary resources to fulfil this role effectively. The study highlighted the importance of ongoing education and support for journalists. It underscored the need for media organisations and their partners to prioritise the safety and well-being of journalists in the face of health crises.

6.7 Conclusion

As evidenced in this chapter, the COVID-19 pandemic was challenging for Zimbabwean journalists. It had such a severe effect on media personalities that it considerably influenced how they operated. Like many countries in the world, Zimbabwe introduced various restrictive measures to deal with the pandemic, and these measures altered how journalists operated. Some journalists were forced to adopt new technologies with little to no training, reporting without a newsroom, and conducting online interviews, and – those with families – had to learn how to do journalism. At the same time, children were being homeschooled in the adjacent room (Hoak, 2021). All these factors conspired to put a fresh and dynamic strain on the media, as the reporters themselves fell victim to the pandemic they were reporting. Zimbabwean journalists covering the COVID-19 pandemic while adhering to the same social constraints imposed on the general public found themselves on completely unfamiliar ground, as industry press pieces show (Hoak, 2021; King, 2020).

Our main conclusion is that the COVID-19 pandemic has a lasting impact on the journalism profession and the lives of media practitioners in Zimbabwe. The pandemic affected their way of life, their social structures, and their economic lives. Journalists were stressed because of the pandemic, which strained their relationships with family members. The pandemic also caused anxiety and other related psychological misery among journalists in Zimbabwe. Participants reported that most newsrooms in Zimbabwe tried their best to protect their reporters from COVID-19. They were supported by organisations such as the Ministry of Information and Broadcasting Services, the Ministry of Health and Child Care, the Zimbabwe Union of Journalists (ZUJ), MISA-Zimbabwe, and the Nyaradzo Group. However, most journalists in the country lacked protective gear as alluded to by the participants.

Additionally, some journalists were abused by law enforcement agents during the course of their work. These anomalies should be corrected if journalists are to fulfil their social obligations of educating people about political, social, and economic crises. This means that media organisations and other relevant stakeholders should ensure journalists' safety during their work. No journalist should die or be harmed for carrying out his or her duty. The current study highlighted journalists' challenges while reporting political, social, and economic crises and the need to ensure their safety and protection. This aligns with the sociology of news production theory, which examines how social, cultural, and economic factors influence news production, distribution, and consumption. The theory also emphasises the role of journalists and media organisations in shaping public opinion and promoting social change. In this case, the safety of journalists is crucial for them to fulfil their social obligations of educating people about crises, which is a key aspect of the sociology of news production theory.

References

Arab Trade Union Confederation. (2020). *Effects of the Covid-19 pandemic on journalists and the media sector in the Arab world and the Middle East.* Arab Trade Union.

Belair-Gagnon, V., & Revers, M. (2018). The sociology of journalism. In T. P. Vos (Ed.), *Journalism: Handbook of communication science* (pp. 257–280). De Gruyter.

Bourdieu, P. (1998). *Practical reason: On the theory of action.* Stanford University Press.

Braun, V., & Clarke, V. (2006). Using thematic analysis in psychology. *Qualitative Research in Psychology, 3*(2), 77–101.

Casero-Ripollés, A. (2020). Impact of COVID-19 on the media system: Communicative and democratic consequences of news consumption during the outbreak. *El Profesional de la Información, 29*(2), e290223.

Casero-Ripollés, A. (2021). *The impact of Covid-19 on journalism: A set of transformations in five domains.* Artigos Temáticos.

Cepel, M., Gavurova, B., Dvorsky, J., & Belas, J. (2020). The impact of the Covid-19 crisis on the perception of business risk in the SME segment. *Journal of International Studies, 13*(3), 248–263. https://doi.org/10.14254/2071-8330.2020/13-3/16

Chibuwe, A., Munoriyarwa, A., Motsaathebe, G., Chiumbu, S., & Lesitaokana, W. (2022). Newsroom disruptions and opportunities in times of crisis: Analysing southern African media during the COVID-19 crisis. *African Journalism Studies, 43*(2), 53–70.

Christians, C. G., Glasser, T., McQuail, D., Nordenstreng, K., & White, R. A. (2010). *Normative theories of the media: Journalism in democratic societies.* University of Illinois Press.

Daniels, G. (2020, September 28). Job losses in journalism not good news for democracy. *Sowetan Live.* www.sowetanlive.co.za/opinion/2020-09-28-job-losses-in-journalism-not-good-news-for-democracy/

Guest, G., Bunce, A., & Johnson, L. (2006). How many interviews are enough? An experiment with data saturation and variability. *Field Methods, 18*(1), 59–82.

Hoak, G. (2021). Covering COVID: Journalists' stress and perceived organizational support while reporting on the pandemic. *Journalism & Mass Communication Quarterly, 98*(3), 854–874.

Jaguga, F., & Kwobah, E. (2020). Mental health response to the COVID-19 pandemic in Kenya: A review. *International Journal of Mental Health Systems, 14*(1), 1–6. https://doi.org/10.1186/s13033-020-00400-8.

Katz, E. (1989). Journalists as scientists. *American Behavioural Scientist, 33*(2), 238–246. https:// doi.org/10.1177/0002764289033002022.

King, M. S. (2020, April 1). Freelancers, unemployment and the Coronavirus aid, relief and economic security act. *Quill.* www.quillmag.com/2020/04/01/freelancers-unemployment-and-the-coronavirus-aid-relief-and-economic-security-act/

Laguna, L., Fiszman, S., Puerta, P., Chaya, C., & Tárrega, A. (2020). The impact of Covid-19 lockdown on food priorities: Results from a preliminary study using social media and an online survey with Spanish consumers. *Food Quality and Preference*, *86*(104028), 1–9.

Lewis, S. C. (2020). The objects and objectives of journalism research during the coronavirus pandemic and beyond. *Digital Journalism*, *8*(5), 681–689. https://doi. org/abs/10.1080/21670811.2020.1773292

MacNaughtan, H. (2020). Japan, the Olympics, and the COVID-19 pandemic. *East Asia Forum*, 1–4.

Matsilele, T. (2021). The implications of COVID-19 on institutions of higher learning: A case of Zimbabwe and South Africa. *Education in Africa: Perspectives, Opportunities and Challenges*, *1*(1), 93–115.

Matsilele, T., Tshuma, L., & Msimanga, M. (2022). Reconstruction and adaptation in times of a contagious crisis: A case of African newsrooms' response to the Covid-19 pandemic. *Journal of Communication Inquiry*, *46*(3), 268–288.

McManus, J. (1994). *Market-driven journalism: Let the citizen beware?* Sage.

McQuail, D. (1994). *Mass communication theory: An introduction*. Sage.

Ministerio de Trabajo y Economía Social. (2020, October). *Impacto del Covid-19 sobre las estadísticas del Ministerio de Trabajo y Economía Social*. www.mites. gob.es/ficheros/ministerio/estadisticas/documentos/Nota_impacto_COVID_Octubre-2020.pdf

Mungwari, T., Mapuranga, S., & Kembo, S. (2022). Reorganisation of news production in Zimbabwe during COVID-19. *International Journal of Advanced Mass Communication and Journalism*, *3*(1), 8–15.

Mututwa, W. T., & Mare, A. (2022). Competing or complimentary actors in the journalistic field? An analysis of the mediation of the COVID-19 pandemic by mainstream and peripheral content creators in Zimbabwe. *African Journalism Studies*, *42*(4), 1–17, 82–98.

Ncube, L., & Mare, A. (2022). "Fake news" and multiple regimes of "truth" during the COVID-19 pandemic in Zimbabwe. *African Journalism Studies*, *43*(2), 71–89.

Nhamo, G., Dube, K., & Chikodzi, D. (Eds.). (2020). *Counting the cost of COVID-19 on the global tourism industry*. Springer.

Perreault, G., & Bell, T. R. (2020). Towards a "digital" sports journalism: Field theory, changing boundaries and evolving technologies. *Communication & Sport*, *10*(3). Advance online publication. https://doi.org/10.1177/2167479520979958.

Perreault, G., Johnson, B., & Klein, L. (2020). Covering hate: Field theory and journalistic role conception in reporting on white nationalist rallies. *Journalism Practice*, *16*(3), 1–17. https://doi.org/10.1080/17512786.2020.1835525

Perreault, M. F. (2020, August 9). *Journalism beyond the command post* [Paper presentation]. Association of Education in Journalism and Mass Communication Annual Conference, San Francisco, CA.

Perreault, M. F., & Perreault, G. P. (2021). Journalists on COVID-19 journalism: Communication ecology of pandemic reporting. *American Behavioral Scientist*, *65*(7), 976–991. https://doi.org/10.1177/0002764221992813

Pew Research Center. (2020, March 18). *U.S. public sees multiple threats from the coronavirus – and concerns are growing*. www.pewresearch.org/politics/wp-content/uploads/sites/4/2020/03/PP_2020.03.18_Coronavirus_Final-1.pdf

Ruiz de Gauna, P. (2020, March 20). ¿Cómo impacta la crisis del coronavirus en los hábitos de consumo y en los medios? *Marketing Directo.* www.marketingdirecto.com/anunciantes-general/medios/como-impacta-la-crisis-del-coronavirus-en-los-habitos-de-consumo-y-en-los-medios

Schudson, M. (2003). *The sociology of news.* W. W. Norton.

Shoemaker, P. J., & Reese, S. D. (1996). *Mediating the message: Theories of influences on mass media content.* Longman.

Singh, B. (2020). Media in the time of COVID-19. *Economic and Political Weekly (Engage), 55*(16), 1–7.

Tuchman, G. (1978). *Making news: A study in the construction of reality.* Free Press.

Vanderstoep, S. W., & Johnston, D. D. (2009). *Research methods for everyday life: Blending qualitative and quantitative approaches.* Jossey-Bass.

Verpoorten, M. (2005). The death toll of the Rwandan genocide: A detailed analysis for Gikongoro Province. *Population, 60*(4), 331–367.

Villani, L., Pastorino, R., Molinari, E., Anelli, F., Ricciardi, W., Graffigna, G., & Boccia, S. (2021). Impact of the COVID-19 pandemic on psychological well-being of students in an Italian university: A web-based cross-sectional survey. *Globalization and Health, 17*(1), 1–14. https://doi.org/10.1186/s12992-021-00680-w

Part 2

Setting the COVID-19 Narrative

7 Unintended Mental Health Consequences of Media Framing During COVID-19

Wellman Kondowe, Flemmings Fishani Ngwira, and Drinney Labanna

7.1 Introduction

The emergence of a pandemic triggers a considerable threat to physical and mental health and social, political, and economic stability worldwide. Because of the uncertainty they bring, pandemics can harm mental health. Depression and anxiety will likely emerge due to fear of infection and death, worry about one's health, and financial constraints due to the pandemic (Stainback et al., 2020). Severe mental health consequences of COVID-19 were evident worldwide (Bueno-Notivol et al., 2021).

The coronavirus pandemic (COVID-19) was not an exception, as it caused a considerable impact globally (Ogbodo et al., 2020; Su et al., 2021). The World Health Organization (WHO) declared the COVID-19 outbreak a pandemic on 12 March 2020 (WHO, 2020). Africa reported its first COVID-19 case on 14 February 2020 (Aljazeera, 2020). In Malawi, COVID-19 was declared a national disaster on 20 March 2020 (Mzumara et al., 2021), and the country registered its first case on 2 April 2020 (Nyasulu et al., 2021).

Research shows that fear of contagion, suffering and death, social isolation, infodemics, and the economic repercussions associated with COVID-19 present a risk to mental health globally (Garfin et al., 2020). According to the WHO (2004), mental health is a state of well-being in which the individual realises his or her abilities, can cope with the everyday stresses of life, can work productively and fruitfully, and can contribute to his or her community. During COVID-19, mental health issues had adverse health consequences on personal health, ranging from depression and anxiety to suicidal ideation or complete suicide (Wang et al., 2020). In October 2020, for instance, Japan registered more COVID-19-related suicide deaths (2,153) than COVID-19 itself (2,087) (Su et al., 2021). In the same year, Malawi also registered a rise in suicide cases linked to COVID-19. The country recorded a 57% increase in suicide deaths during the pandemic (Banda et al., 2021; Voice of America [VOA], 2020).

Because of the fear and uncertainty associated with pandemics, people feel frightened, confused, and susceptible during crises (Reynolds & Seeger, 2005), and tend to be more attentive to information about the disease (Ophir

DOI: 10.4324/9781003425861-9

et al., 2021). Consequently, during pandemics, the public seeks timely and accurate information about the disease to minimise its effects. Specifically, during these crises, people seek to learn about risk information, including potential threats and actions they could take to minimise the risks (Reynolds & Seeger, 2005). Studies have reported that people tend not to look for such reliable health information through the official channels of communication of health organisations; they often obtain their health information via mass and social media, which often quote or direct people to news articles from the mainstream media (Djerf-Pierre & Shehata, 2017). This suggests that as the only reliable and ubiquitous source of information, mass media play a vital role in times of a public health crisis.

Mass media can influence public opinion and decision-making (Msughter & Phillips, 2020). Whenever there is a public health crisis, such as COVID-19, the flow of health information in the mainstream media becomes overwhelming. This calls for extra care in using language on mass media when communicating the pandemic to the public, as language can either escalate or dowse the tension caused by the pandemic (Ogbodo et al., 2020). This postulates that it is not only what is said that is significant in communicating information but also the way the information is expressed. Research on media effects shows that, in times of pandemics, effective crisis communication is vital in dispelling fears, uncertainties, and panic and unifying citizens in a collective fight against the disease (Wu et al., 2020). It is paramount that during public health crises, media organisations disseminate health information that is balanced, fact-based, and truth-oriented to avoid creating unnecessary panic in the people. Regrettably, research has documented that while crisis and risk communication recommends providing the public with reliable information about potential threats and actions to be taken to mitigate the risks, through the process of media framing, media coverage of pandemics has often been inadequate, biased, and misleading (Motta et al., 2020).

Media framing refers to how the media organise and present information to the public on specific issues, giving them particular context to influence the interpretation of how the public views reality (Msughter & Phillips, 2020). To frame could mean selecting some aspects of reality to make the media more prominent in communicating a text. Through framing, the media therefore make an issue salient and direct the attention of the audience at specific issues and ideas (Caicedo-Moreno et al., 2022). Some notable media framing during pandemics include the coverage of the crisis, the containment of the disease, and the social, economic, and political implications of the outbreak (Ophir et al., 2021; Stainback et al., 2020). In terms of frame tone, journalists choose either to slant their media coverage towards a positive, negative, or neutral tone. During pandemics, as already established, framing may amplify certain aspects of the disease, leaving out other equally important aspects. Regarding frame tone, research shows that most journalists slant media coverage towards the negative rather than the positive tone (Greenslade, 2015).

Specifically, focusing on COVID-19 media coverage, media framing was of particular importance. In a study by Su et al. (2021) at the onset of COVID-19, right-leaning media outlets in the United States often issued biased and misleading reports about COVID-19. Media reports that are biased and misleading may be a source of adverse psychological effects on individuals (Olagoke et al., 2020). During COVID-19, Malawi registered an increased number of cases of COVID-19-related anxiety (Chorwe-Sungani, 2021) and COVID-19-related suicide (Banda et al., 2021; VOA, 2020), but to our knowledge, no attempt has been made to investigate the role media framing had on fuelling the destructive power of the pandemic at the time. To address this research gap, the current chapter aims to identify critical areas, where Malawian main media reports on COVID-19 could have harmed public mental health. While previous media framing studies (see Msughter & Phillips, 2020; Ogbodo et al., 2020) on pandemics primarily relied on deductive, theory-driven approaches in identifying media frames, our study adopted an inductive approach, letting the media frames emerge from the data. On frame tones, the study used a deductive, theory-driven approach.

This chapter, therefore, reports on the framing of COVID-19 by analysing newspaper headlines in Malawi. A headline is the most important cue to activate certain concepts in the reader's mind (Liu et al., 2019). Headlines are also used to convince people to pay attention to the story that follows (Bowles & Borden, 2000). Consequently, journalists use it to influence people's perception on an issue. Media framing researchers consequently often identify and measure frames in news headlines (Bleich et al., 2015). Moreover, in this digital era, many people only read headlines; very few go beyond it (Gabielkov et al., 2016). Overall, examining media frames through newspaper headlines provides the most direct hint of the potential effect of the news coverage.

The current study systematically collected data from two print media outlets in Malawi: Nation Publication Limited (NPL) and Blantyre Newspapers Limited (BNL). The two were chosen based on their nationwide circulation. Samples from NPL comprised *Weekend Nation, The Nation* and *Nation on Sunday* newspapers. Samples from BNL were *The Weekend Times, Malawi News, Daily Times,* and *Sunday Times.* We believe that coverage in these media institutions (i.e., NPL and BNL) provided an appropriate context for understanding the framing of COVID-19, the tone of the frames, and their implications on public mental health.

We collected data from newspaper articles published between 1 March 2020 and 29 February 2021, making it a year. This period was critical for media coverage of the pandemic to prepare for the measures to handle it. The study employed content analysis to identify the most significant COVID-19-related issues in the headlines published by the NPL and BNL media outlets during the early COVID-19 outbreaks in Malawi. To establish frame categories and frame tones, the study on which this chapter is based used a hybrid approach in identifying patterns, creating codes, and arranging codes into overarching themes. The approach incorporates deductive, top-down, theoretical, inductive, bottom-up, and data-driven processes. We employed the inductive, data-driven process to identify media frames; therefore, we did not have the priori codes when identifying patterns. However, for frame tone identification, we used the deductive, theoretical process. This shows that, for frame tone identification, we used the priori codes, namely, cheerful tones – frames that indicated a favourable point of view to COVID-19; negative tones – frames that indicated an unfavourable point of view to COVID-19; and neutral tones – frames that indicated neither favourable nor unfavourable points of view to COVID-19 (see Msughter & Phillips, 2020).

7.2 Media Frames of COVID-19 Coverage in Malawi

Results regarding media frames show four main ways the print media in Malawi framed the information related to COVID-19.

Human Interest

Human interest was the main frame used by the print media when covering COVID-19, with 76 headlines accounting for 37% of the entire headlines analysed. This frame demonstrates how journalists gave an emotional angle to the issue's presentation. Journalists used emotional appeals, categorised as negative or positive, as a sub-frame of the human interest frame. The negative human interest sub-frame was significantly higher in frequency (67 of 76) than the positive sub-frame focused on headlines, which essentially presented the negative effect of the pandemic on human beings. For instance, the headline H1: "Poorer people left behind as rich nations hoard COVID-19 vaccine" (2020) triggers panic, hopelessness, and anger of being poor among poor nations. The understanding here is that people living in poverty cannot afford to develop or procure COVID-19 vaccine, as rich countries secretly keep guard to their vaccines. Despite being used less, the positive human interest sub-scale focused on bringing hope and relief to the people who are already affected by the pandemic. Headlines, such as H2: "Corona relief" (2020), and H3: "COVID test kits arrive today" (Pasungwi, 2020b), gave hope to people that something was happening to cushion the effect of the pandemic on their health.

Containment

The second dominant frame most media outlets employed during the COVID-19 print media coverage was the containment frame, reflected in 51 (24.9%) of the headlines analysed. This frame encompassed all headlines – those that displayed efforts and behaviours towards the containment of the disease and those that demonstrated failure to contain the disease. The frame, therefore, comprised two sub-themes, namely control and failure. The control sub-frame consisting of 41 out of 51 containment headlines, concentrated on headlines that focused on reporting the efforts and capacity of the country – through the Ministry of Health and other non-governmental organisations – to handle the crisis. For instance, headline H4: "Mutharika declares state of disaster over coronavirus" (Chikoko, 2020) suggests the government's commitment to disburse state aid to supplement locally available resources in alleviating the suffering and loss. The failure sub-frame focused on headlines that unveiled the failure by the country to handle the crisis. Consider the following headlines:

- H5: "No COVID-19 test centre in the North" (2020); and
- H6: "Mangochi DHO [District Health Officer] in need of COVID-19 materials" (2020).

The dominance of the control sub-frame pointed to the effort made by the country to contain the crisis by bringing hope to the people.

Economic Consequences

This was the third dominant frame journalists in Malawi employed in the media coverage of COVID-19, with 32 headlines (16.6%) of all headlines analysed in this chapter. In this frame, coders found that certain headlines were written to make the economic consequences of COVID-19 on individuals, organisations, or the country seem relevant. The coding process for this frame inductively yielded three sub-frames, namely the loss, gain, and solution sub-frames. The loss sub-frame, the most frequently used among the three (24 of 32), focused on headlines that largely presented the economic negative effect of the pandemic. For instance, in the headline, H7: "Coronavirus pushing millions to starvation" (2020), COVID-19 is presented as forcing millions of Malawians into poverty. By using the words "pushing" and "millions," every Malawian reading the headline is compelled to put him- or herself among the alleged millions that became poor due to the pandemic. On a positive note, although to a minor extent (5 of 32), some headlines framed the COVID-19-related economic consequences positively, suggesting some economic benefits of the pandemic. For instance, the headline H8: "CAF gives FAM K225M COVID-19 package" (Chinoko, 2020) points in that direction. Some headlines further emphasised the solutions to curb the pandemic's negative consequences. Headlines, such as H9: "Applying Shell planning to COVID-19" (Mtumbuka, 2020), are a case in point.

Politicisation

The politicisation frame emphasised headlines that reported issues from a political perspective. This is where, on the one hand, critics blamed the government for not doing enough, and on the other, the government defended their actions towards the fight against the pandemic. During the coding process, two sub-frames emerged: blame and defence. The blame sub-frame, which was more frequently used (23 of 27), focused on headlines that essentially presented attacks from government critics for not doing enough, let alone embezzling funds meant to cushion the impact the disease had brought to the country. The headline H10, "Akatamuka ndi coronavirus" (2020), which means "they have become rich with COVID-19" insinuates that they (most likely referring to government officials) have misappropriated COVID-19 funds, which were meant for the masses. Regarding the defence sub-frame, headlines such as H11: "Chakwera [the State President] denies COVID-19 laxity" (Phuka, 2021) emphasised defence from the government side in terms of accusations levelled against them that they were not doing enough.

Scholarly evidence points out that the emergence of pandemics, such as COVID-19, threatens human life – mentally, physically, socially, politically, and economically (Stainback et al., 2020). Due to this profound threat to life, people tend to seek timely and accurate information about a pandemic and its risk factors to minimise the potential effects of the disease on their life. Under such circumstances, research shows that people usually use mass media for such information (see Djerf-Pierre & Shehata, 2017). This postulates that during public health crises, the flow of timely and accurate information is vital for people to make sense of the risk information and actions they could take to minimise the risks. Literature documents that accurate, credible, and reliable media coverage about outbreaks helps avoid potential mental health issues, dispelling people's fear and uncertainty about the disease, and improving compliance with preventive measures (Liu et al., 2020; Su et al., 2021).

During the critical period when people in Malawi were keen to seek accurate and reliable information about the pandemic, media coverage on COVID-19 was largely biased and misleading. Our results are in line with other studies on COVID-19 media coverage elsewhere. For instance, Motta et al. (2020) found that right-leaning media outlets in the United States often issued biased and misleading reports on COVID-19. As earlier mentioned, a newspaper headline such as H1: "Poorer people left behind as rich nations hoard COVID-19 vaccine" (2020) was not only misleading but also brought no hope for poor nations, such as Malawi, to afford a vaccine, which is essential to overcome the pandemic. However, on 5 March 2021, Malawi received its first shipment of 360,000 doses of COVID-19 vaccine (WHO, 2021). While COVID-19 had already been a source of multifaceted stress for many people (Su et al., 2021), headlines with misleading frames might have triggered fear and panic to people, and together with the pandemic-related threat, this might have exacerbated mental health issues in the country.

Media coverage of COVID-19 in Malawi was inadequate despite an emphasis on the need for timely and accurate information, especially during the initial stages of the pandemic (Ophir et al., 2021). Media frames in Malawi mainly focused on social, economic, and political issues. It should be noted that this was the time when the country was experiencing political unrest due to the February 2020 ruling for a rerun of presidential elections in July 2020 due to the irregularities observed in the May 2019 general elections (see Nyasulu et al., 2021). Consequently, they hardly balanced the coverage by emphasising required behaviours to mitigate contagion risks. Similarly, Ophir (2018) found that during pandemics, the media tend to focus on the social frame, emphasising the effect of the pandemic on social, political, and economic issues and ignoring the crucial component of individual response to reduce the risks. Such emphasis on reporting may increase mental health issues. In their study, Ophir et al. (2021) found that in Italian media, the social frame, which emphasised the social and economic consequences of COVID-19, was associated with increased morbidity. These findings suggest that the mere emphasis on one or two frames at the expense of other equally essential frames, such as containment, yielded detrimental effects on mental health. The balance in framing is important in promoting mental health.

7.3 Frame Tones of COVID-19 Coverage

The study identified three media frame tones frequently used during COVID-19 print media coverage.

Negative Tone

A negative tone was the most dominant frame tone used by the print media on COVID-19 coverage. Under this frame tone, newspaper headlines expressed unfavourable and non-sympathetic perspectives on COVID-19. Out of the 205 headlines, 129 (63%) were framed negatively. This suggests that most journalists slant their COVID-19 media coverage towards a negative tone. Except for the containment media frame, all frames established in this chapter had a higher percentage of negative tone than positive and/or neutral tones. Headlines such as H12: "COVID-19 worsens" (2020) (which fell under the human interest frame) and H13: "COVID-19 bites" (Pasungwi, 2020a) under the economic frame, drew people's attention towards the adverse, hostile, and non-sympathetic nature of COVID-19.

Positive Tone

Despite the negative tone being the most dominant frame, some newspaper headlines employed a positive frame tone displaying perspectives that were favourable and generally sympathetic to COVID-19. This frame was apparent in 55 headlines, which accounted for 26.8% of all the headlines analysed in this study. Of all the media frames identified in this study, the containment frame had the highest number of cheerful frame tones (41). Headlines such as H14: "Nipping coronavirus in the bud" (2020), and H15: "Together we can win the war against COVID-19" (2020) gave people hope and a belief that COVID-19 could be defeated. Such headlines probably did not cause panic or fear; hence, they were categorised with a positive frame tone.

Neutral Tone

Although on a lower scale, some newspaper headlines employed a neutral frame tone during COVID-19 media coverage. This frame comprised newspaper headlines that did not appear to discuss COVID-19 either positively or negatively. This was the frame tone used least of all, consisting of 21 headlines (which accounted for 10.2% of all the headlines analysed). Instances of such headlines were H16: "Former presidents speak on COVID-19" (Kachere, 2020), and H17: "How are major religions respond to COVID-19?" (2020). These headlines did not show whether the sentiments of former presidents or the responses from major religions were positive or negative towards the pandemic.

Findings show that a negative tone was the one most dominantly used by the print media during COVID-19 coverage. Except for the containment media frame, all five media frames had a higher percentage of a negative tone than a positive and/or a neutral tone. Greenslade (2015) also notes that most journalists slant their media coverage towards the negative rather than the positive tone. On COVID-19 media coverage in Nigeria, Msughter and Phillips (2020) equally found a negative tone to be the most dominant of the three tones. Negative media coverage could cause adverse psychological effects in individuals. Research on media effects shows that negative media coverage of pandemics may lead to severe mental health issues among media consumers (Olagoke et al., 2020). Negatively framed news may accentuate public fear and panic, eventually leading to adverse mental health consequences. While negative news has detrimental effects on mental health, positively framed news may enhance mental health and facilitate support for preventive measures (Caicedo-Moreno et al., 2022).

7.4 Language Use in COVID-19 Coverage

Regarding language use, it was found that the media outlets used two languages: Chichewa, the language of wider communication, and English, the official language of Malawi. The coding process for language use revealed that English was the most dominant language used by the print media on COVID-19 coverage. Of the 205 headlines, 195 (95.1%) were written in English. This heavy use of a foreign language in public media, and later the only language used to report on a critical public health problem, such as COVID-19, might have acted as a barrier to the majority of Malawians who cannot comfortably read and understand the foreign language, considering the literacy level of 62.14% of people above 15 years of age (World Bank, 2022).

This shows that English was highly favoured in communicating COVID-19 issues to the public. Studies have shown that not all segments of society understand their official languages (Lha, 2020). In Kenya, for instance, despite English being their official language, people understood texts translated into

Kiswahili better than English source (see O'Brien & Cadwell, 2018). In Malawi, the situation is similar. Certainly, with a literacy level of 62.14% for people above 15 (World Bank, 2022), not everyone would understand texts in English. Accurate media coverage of COVID-19 should reach everyone, including the indigenous people, irrespective of their educational levels. Yet, findings from the current study show that COVID-19 information was not often available in the language indigenous people in Malawi understood. Such a language choice defeats people's need to be informed, prepared, and responsive to the pandemic. Instead, the foreign language further fuels misconceptions that could considerably increase the risk of mental health problems.

7.5 Conclusion

This chapter has demonstrated that media coverage is critical during a public health crisis, such as the COVID-19 pandemic. The public should be equipped with accurate, credible, and reliable health information to make informed decisions towards their health protection. Since newspaper headlines are used to convince people to pay attention to the entire story, choosing words is important in crafting headlines that do not send exaggerated, inaccurate, and/ or misleading information about the pandemic.

The excessive use of the human-interest frame, which emphasised the negative effects of the pandemic on human beings, might have given rise to severe mental health issues among information consumers. The overemphasis on social and economic consequences of the pandemic might have augmented perceptions of threats to health and economic security and could have created amplified distress in people. The tendency to divert readers' attention from COVID-19 to mere politics and ethnics put public responses towards the pandemic at risk. Overusing negative frame tones in news headlines might accentuate people's fear and panic, eventually leading to adverse mental health consequences. The responsibility to achieve accurate, credible, and reliable media coverage – especially during a pandemic – rests in the hands of the media organisations to ensure that news that would amplify people's distress would be avoided.

The results of this study should be understood in the light of some limitations. First, this study relied on newspaper headlines without looking at the entire story, which might have been framed differently from the headlines as headlines are typically used to lure readers into reading the entire article. Further research must concentrate on the headlines and the rest of the article, even though research indicates that reading the entire article may not correct the headline misdirection (see Liu et al., 2019). Second, the current study relied on the headlines of the published newspapers without investigating responses to such media messages from the members of the public themselves. Further research should extend the investigation to the public to address this gap.

References

Aljazeera. (2020, February). Egypt confirms coronavirus case, the first in Africa. *Aljazeera*. www.aljazeera.com/news/2020/2/14/egypt-confirms-coronavirus-case-the-first-in-africa

Banda, G. T., Banda, N., Chadza, A., & Mthunzi, C. (2021). Suicide epidemic in Malawi: What can we do? *Pan African Medical Journal, 38*(69).

Bleich, E., Stonebraker, H., Nisar, H., & Abdelhamid, R. (2015). Media portrayals of minorities: Muslims in British newspaper headlines, 2001–2012. *Journal of Ethnic and Migration Studies, 41*(6), 942–962.

Bowles, D. A., & Borden, D. L. (2000). *Creative editing*. Wadsworth.

Braun, V., & Clarke, V. (2006). Using thematic analysis in psychology. *Qualitative Research in Psychology, 3*(2), 77–101.

Bueno-Notivol, J., Gracia-García, P., Olaya, B., Lasheras, I., Lópes-Antón, R., & Santabárbara, J. (2021). Prevalence of depression during the COVID-19 outbreak: A meta-analysis of community-based studies. *International Journal of Clinical and Health Psychology, 21*(1), 100196. https://doi.org/10.1016/j.ijchp.2020.07.007

Caicedo-Moreno, A., Correa Chica, A., López-López, W., Castro-Abril, P., Barreto, I., & Rodriguez-Romero, J. D. (2022). The role of psychology in media during the COVID-19 pandemic: A cross-national study. *Psychologica Belgica, 62*(1), 136–151. https://doi.org/10.5334/pb.1054

Chikoko, R. (2020, March 21). Mutharika declares state of disaster over coronavirus. *Weekend Nation*. https://mwnation.com/mutharika-declares-state-of-disaster-over-coronavirus/

Chinoko, C. (2020, July 2). CAF gives FAM K225M Covid-19 package. *The Nation*. https://mwnation.com/caf-gives-fam-k225m-covid-19-package/

Chorwe-Sungani, G. (2021). Assessing COVID-19-related anxiety and functional impairment amongst nurses in Malawi. *African Journal for Primary Health Care and Family Medicine, 13*(1), e1–e6.

Djerf-Pierre, M., & Shehata, A. (2017). Still an agenda setter: Traditional news media and public opinion during the transition from low to high-choice media environments. *Journal of Communication, 67*(5), 733–757.

Gabielkov, M., Ramachandran, A., Chaintreau, A., & Legout, A. (2016). Social clicks: What and who gets read on Twitter? *ACM Sigmetrics Performance Evaluation Review, 44*(1), 179–192.

Garfin, D. R., Silver, R. C., & Holman, E. A. (2020). The novel coronavirus (COVID-2019) outbreak: Amplification of public health consequences by media exposure. *Health Psychology, 39*(5), 355–357. https://doi.org/10.1037/hea0000875

Greenslade, R. (2015, December 17). Where media fails on the reporting of migrants and refugees. *The Guardian*. www.theguardian.com/media/greenslade/2015/dec/17/where-media-fails-on-thereporting-of-migrants-and-refugees

Kachere, T. (2020, April 3). Former presidents speak on Covid-19. *The Daily Times*. https://times.mw/former-presidents-speak-on-covid-19/

Lha, Y. (2020, February). *Fighting the coronavirus in local languages*. Language on the Move. www.languageonthemove.com/fighting-the-coronavirus-in-local-languages/

Liu, S., Guo, L., Mays, K., Betke, M., & Wijaya, D. T. (2019). Detecting frames in news headlines and its application to analyzing news framing trends surrounding U.S. gun violence. In *Proceedings of the 23rd conference on computational natural language learning* (pp. 504–514). CONLL.

Liu, W., Yue, X., & Tchounwou, P. B. (2020). Response to the COVID-19 epidemic: The Chinese experience and implications for other countries. *International Journal of Environmental Research and Public Health, 17*(7). https://doi.org/10.3390/ijerph17072304

Motta, M., Stecula, D., & Farhart, C. (2020). How right-leaning media coverage of COVID-19 facilitated the spread of misinformation in the early stages of the pandemic in the U.S. *Canadian Journal of Political Science, 53*(2), 335–342. https://doi.org/10.1017/S0008423920000396.

Msughter, A. E., & Phillips, D. (2020). Media framing of Covid-19 pandemic: A study of daily trust and vanguard newspapers in Nigeria. *International Journal of Health, Safety and Environment, 6*(5), 588–596.

Mtumbuka, M. (2020, April 2). Applying shell planning to Covid-19. *The Nation.* https://mwnation.com/applying-shell-planning-to-covid-19/

Mzumara, G. W., Chawani, M., Sakala, M., Mwandira, L., Phiri, E., Milanzi, E., Phiri, M. D., Kazanga, I., O'Byrne, T., Zulu, E. M., Mitambo, C., Divala, T., & Squire, B. (2021). The health policy response to COVID-19 in Malawi. *BMJ Global Health, 6,* e006035. https://doi.org/10.1136/bmjgh-2021-006035

Nyasulu, J. C. Y., Munthali, R. J., Nyondo-Mipando, A. L., Pandya, H., Nyirenda, L., Nyasulu, P. S., & Manda, S. (2021). COVID-19 pandemic in Malawi: Did public sociopolitical events gatherings contribute to its first-wave local transmission? *International Journal of Infectious Diseases, 106,* 269–275. https://doi.org/10.1016/j.ijid.2021.03.055

O'Brien, S., & Cadwell, P. (2018). Translation facilitates comprehension of health-related crisis information: Kenya as an example. *Journal of Specialised Translation, 28,* 23–51.

Ogbodo, J. N., Onwe, E. C., Chukwu, J., Nwasum, C. J., Nwakpu, E. S., Nwankwo, S. U., Nwamini, S., Elem, S., & Ogbaeja, N. I. (2020). Communicating health crisis: A content analysis of global media framing of COVID-19. *Health Promotion Perspectives, 10*(3), 257–269. https://doi.org/10.34172/hpp.2020.4

Olagoke, A. A., Olagoke, O. O., & Hughes, A. M. (2020). Exposure to coronavirus news on mainstream media: The role of risk perceptions and depression. *British Journal of Health Psychology, 25*(4), e12427. https://doi.org/10.1111/bjhp.12427

Ophir, Y. (2018). Coverage of epidemics in American newspapers through the lens of the crisis and emergency risk communication framework. *Health Security, 16*(3), 147–157. https://doi.org/10.1089/hs.2017.0106

Ophir, Y., Walter, D., Arnon, D., Lokmanoglu, A., Tizzoni, M., Carota, J., D'Antiga, L., & Nicastro, E. (2021). The framing of COVID-19 in Italian media and its relationship with community mobility: A mixed-method approach. *Journal of Health Communication, 26*(3), 161–173. https://doi.org/10.1080/10810730.2021.1899344

Pasungwi, J. (2020a, April 2). COVID-19 bites. *The Nation.* https://mwnation.com/covid-19-bites/

Pasungwi, J. (2020b, July 21). Covid test kits arrive today. *The Nation,* p. 4.

Phuka, J. (2021, January 11). Chakwera denies Covid-19 laxity. *The Daily Times,* p. 1.

Reynolds, B., & Seeger, M. W. (2005). Crisis and emergency risk communication as an integrative model. *Journal of Health Communication, 10*(1), 43–55. https://doi.org/10.1080/10810730590904571

Stainback, K., Hearne, B. N., & Trieu, M. M. (2020). COVID-19 and the 24/7 news cycle: Does COVID-19 news exposure affect mental health? *Socius: Sociological Research for a Dynamic World, 6,* 1–15. https://doi.org/10.1177/2378023120969339

Su, Z., McDonnell, D., Wen, J., Kozak, M., Abbas, J., Šegalo, S., Li, X., Ahmad, J., Cheshmehzangi, A., Cai, Y., Yang, L., & Xiang, Y. (2021). Mental health consequences of COVID-19 media coverage: The need for effective crisis communication practices. *Globalization and Health*, *17*(4), 1–8. https://doi.org/10.1186/s12992-020-00654-4

Together we can win the war against Covid-19. (2020, April 18). *Weekend Nation*, pp. 4–5.

Voice of America. (2020). *Rise in Malawi suicide cases linked to COVID-19*. www.voanews.com/a/africa_rise-malawi-suicide-cases-linked-covid-19/6197220.html

Wang, Y., Pan, B., Liu, Y., Wison, A., Ou, J., & Chen, R. (2020). Health care and mental health challenges for transgender individuals during the COVID-19 pandemic. *Lancet Diabetes Endocrinol*, *8*(7), 564–665. https://doi.org/10.1016/S2213-8587(20)30182-0

World Bank. (2022, June). *Literacy rate, adult total (% of people ages 15 and above) – Malawi*. https://data.worldbank.org/indicator/SE.ADT.LITR.ZS?locations=MW

World Health Organization. (2004). *Promoting mental health: Concepts, emerging evidence, practice* (Summary Report). World Health Organization.

World Health Organization. (2020). *WHO director-general's opening remarks at the media briefing on COVID-19*. www.who.int/director-general/speeches/detail/who-director-general-s-opening-remarks-at-the-media-briefing-on-covid-19-11-march-2020

World Health Organization. (2021). *Malawi receives first shipment of COVID-19 vaccines from COVAX*. www.afro.who.int/news/malawi-receives-first-shipment-covid-19-vaccines-covax

Wu, A. W., Connors, C., & Everly, G. S. (2020). COVID-19: Peer support and crisis communication strategies to promote institutional resilience. *Annals of Internal Medicine*, *172*(12), 822–823. https://doi.org/10.7326/M20-1236

8 COVID-19 and Anxiety Constructions in African Poetry

Nick Mdika Tembo

8.1 Introduction

A tsunami of information accompanies every outbreak of an epidemic disease (Xu & Liu, 2021). This ubiquity of misinformation and conspiracy theories on social media and in the news cycle has led the director-general of the World Health Organization (WHO) to warn that we are not just fighting an epidemic but also an infodemic. According to the WHO, we live in an age where fake news spreads faster and more efficiently than this virus (WHO, 2020a). This also has made it very hard for people to find trustworthy sources and reliable guidance when they most need it (Xu & Liu, 2021). This chapter is about how the severe acute respiratory syndrome coronavirus 2 (SARS-CoV-2) – the virus that caused COVID-19 – has created much public anxiety and social panic about its spread and containment. It highlights the discourses and cultural archives on which recent and largely unknown Malawian and South African poets drew.

Finally, the chapter discusses how poets interweave psychological distress with man's irrational behaviour towards the ecosystem. Three poems from Malawi have been singled out for analysis in this chapter, namely Benedicto Malunga's "Untitled II"; William Mpina's "Down but Not Out"; and Hope Banda's "Dear Unborn Child." Four poems from South Africa were selected: Maren Bodenstein's "Green Dream"; and Phelelani Makhanya's "The Surname," "One in the Chamber," and "Vapour."

The aim is to show how the poets drew on cultural discourses and other popular archives to frame, circulate, and interrogate stories about the COVID-19 pandemic in their writing. What is unique about these poems is their dealing with the myths and conspiracy theories about COVID-19. This chapter focuses on the discourses and cultural archives surrounding the pandemic. More concretely, it focuses on how poetry mediates COVID-19 in Malawi and South Africa, as captured in the poems.

The study drew on scholarship on COVID conspiracy, understood by Achterberg (2021) as a spate of elaborate yet untested conspiracies on the origins of COVID-19. The widespread availability of these conspiracy theories

DOI: 10.4324/9781003425861-10

has led the WHO to declare that there is an infodemic about COVID-19. According to Bridgman et al. (2022), an infodemic occurs when unprecedented levels of misinformation contribute to widespread misconceptions about a novel occurrence, such as the coronavirus (Bridgman et al., 2022). The scholars further posit how "conspiracy theories, poorly sourced medical advice, and information trivialising the virus" (Bridgman et al., 2022, p. 3) have led to the quick spread of the pandemic. Other scholars invested in discourses surrounding the current infodemic are Vitriol and Marsh (2022, p. 124), who define it as "the widespread acceptance of unreliable and unverified information regarding the COVID-19 pandemic." By reading the selected poems in the light of an infodemic, therefore, my work unpicks man's proclivity to misinform in terms of what it creates in the fearful Other. I thus see the study reported here as a sustained attempt to handle sensitive facts that are "born and diffuse rapidly in times of heightened uncertainty, when high-quality information is difficult to access when trust in available sources of information is low [. . .] and when uncertainty, anxiety, threat, or fear are high" (Spitzberg, 2021, p. 15).

I proceed with three steps to fully develop how an infodemic and the resultant fear are articulated in the selected poems. (1) I begin with a discussion of the theories that informed my study; (2) I then discuss the circulation of fake news and conspiracy theories in the chosen poems as having a domino effect. I intend to show the various and nuanced ways through which an infodemic can push individuals and communities on edge and turn them into traumatised beings; (3) Finally, I focus on social and societal constructions associated with homes wrecked by the pandemic. I aim to show how the writers drew on the cultural archive to explore the intersection of the novel coronavirus with African (psycho) sociality and beliefs.

8.2 Theoretical Framework

This section adopts a theoretical perspective, drawing on critical Anthropocene studies and foundational trauma scholarship to demonstrate how ecological and psychoanalytic approaches can be applied to an understanding of the COVID-19 crisis. The term "Anthropocene" was first introduced into scholarship by Paul Crutzen and Eugene Stoermer to refer to "the major and still growing impacts of human activities on earth and atmosphere [as well as] the central role of mankind in geology and ecology" (Crutzen & Stoermer, 2000, p. 17). It was later appropriated by scholars such as Anne Fremaux, who understood the term as denoting "an ideological emblem of the new power humans have acquired over nature" (Fremaux, 2019, p. 16). The Anthropocene is, therefore, "a lens for understanding the destructive power of humanity on nature and as a warning concerning the unpredictable, long-lasting, and potentially threatening effects of human action for human and non-human life" (Fremaux, 2019, p. 42). Fremaux, however, also warns that the term does not necessarily mean so much about humankind's victory over nature but quite the opposite:

> It indicates our ecological defeat in the face of events that exceed our technical ("impotent") power. The Anthropocene – or the culmination of human dominion over nature – reveals the constitutive dependency of human life on natural ecosystems, which they are intrinsically a part of.
> (2019, p. viii; original brackets)

Understood thus, the Anthropocene is not only considered an ecological predicament but also "an era of 'non-knowledge' or rational ignorance linked to uncertainties and ontological indeterminacy than a period of human mastery and domination of earth systems" (Fremaux, 2019, pp. 46–48). The term further denotes "the helplessness (impotence) of already accumulated scientific knowledge to trigger necessary changes" (Fremaux, 2019, p. 48; original brackets). Perhaps this led Fremaux to note further that the Anthropocene is nothing but man's attempt to "live in times of pure-disasters" (2019, p. 1).

As I demonstrate later in this chapter, man's disruption of the ecosystems is cited as one of the reasons why viruses have been shaken loose from their natural habitat; humans are therefore reaping the fruits of their folly towards nature. My point, then, is that knowledge of the critical theory of the Anthropocene will help us understand man's role in the drama of his undoing, one that has brought us to the crossroads of existence as we ponder what it is that we need to do "to extricate ourselves from an era characterised by life-threatening practices" (Fremaux, 2019, p. iv) that have now come full circle to haunt and destroy us. Fremaux (2019, p. ix) is of the view that this approach – of finding a solution for our self-created problems –

> [P]rovides a reconstructive social and political project [. . .] whose purpose is to restore hope and reinvigorate the loyalty of our institutions toward the defence of the common good, encourage the reverence for life, as well as the protection of the ecospheric conditions that make the continuation of what we know and experience on Earth possible.

Regarding the emotional and psychological impact of the virus on humankind, I drew on trauma scholarship, especially the Caruthian model of trauma. Referring to Sigmund Freud, Cathy Caruth understands trauma as "an overwhelming experience of sudden or catastrophic events in which the response to the event occurs in the often delayed, uncontrolled repetitive appearance of hallucinations and other intrusive phenomena" (Caruth, 1996, p. 11). Michelle Balaev (2018, p. 360) makes an even more incisive commentary about trauma, it is "a severely disruptive experience that profoundly impacts the self's emotional organization and perception of the external world." The victim of trauma cannot fully control its effects. In this sense, the full impact of trauma is only known much later because the mind recognises the threat "one moment too late" (Caruth, 1996, p. 62), thereby missing the experience altogether. In both explications, trauma is construed to be a sudden breach in a person's life, which destroys his or her sense of protection. It makes the person either hypervigilant upon recalling or remembering what previously happened, or it causes a splitting of the ego and dissociation (Tembo, 2022b, p. 266). Trauma also immolates speech and pushes one into a wordless state because its extreme experience "fractures both language and consciousness, causing lasting damage and demanding unique narrative expressions" (Balaev, 2018, p. 363). Belatedness, latency, dissociation, the difficulties of gaining access to the traumatic story, and the unspeakability of trauma implicit in its aporetic nature are some of the essential tenets of psychological trauma. In this study, I situate COVID-19 survivors against "the trauma story" (see Mollica, 2006, pp. 48–61, 125–128; Tembo, 2014, pp. 54–62), and its effect on both the narrating I – the one who speaks in the voice of the author – and the narrated other. In that sense, the analysed poems embody what Miller and Ma (54–80) call "existential anxiety" in those left behind to tell the story. In Miller and Ma's view, the threat of death from the disastrous events encompassing the pandemic has left an indelible mark on the collective psyche of the world that has rendered many of the desperate responses wholly understandable, given how fear of death plays such a central role in human experience (2021, p. 54). This is what I cover in the penultimate section, where I discuss anxiety and psychological distress issues in COVID-19 survivors.

8.3 Poeticising COVID-spiracy in Recent Malawian and South African Poetry

The singular and most sinister exceptionality of the current COVID-19 pandemic was that it created a dizzying popular archive and generated many conspiracy theories, misinformation, and terrifying rumours, especially from social media circles into public consciousness. In Žižek's summation of the times in which we live, the ongoing spread of the coronavirus epidemic has "triggered a vast epidemic of ideological viruses which were lying dormant in our societies: fake news [and] paranoiac conspiracy theories" (Žižek, 2020, p. 39). Most of these heightened, twisted, misleading, and often harmful narratives have left more questions than answers and have provoked a lot of anxiety, especially among people who are not scientists, epidemiologists, or public health specialists (Tembo, 2022a, p. 5).

One such conspiracy theory is that the current COVID-19 crisis "was deliberately created by telecommunication companies in order to keep people at home while their engineers install 5G technology everywhere" (Erni & Striphas, 2021, p. 213). Achterberg calls this the "covid-spiracy" theory (2021, p. 17), and notes how its proponents appear to say that "behind the societal curtains, elites are trying to deal with the problem of overpopulation by means of introducing 5G and blaming COVID-19 for the negative side effects" (2021, p. 17). Indeed, Cowan and Morell (2020) advance a cluster of arguments – all with some merit and none wholly satisfactory – to explain how the coronavirus pandemic was born out of people's insatiable lust for advanced technological innovations. In their view, illness from coronavirus is highly correlated with the introduction of the fifth generation wireless (5G) in some of the world's major cities. To qualify their claim, they highlight a few cities in Asia and America that there was a spike in SARS-CoV-2 cases in some parts of Asia and the United States due to the installation of the 5G network. They even trace the birth of SAR-CoV-2 to Wuhan, China, from where they claim, the pandemic spread to other parts of the world:

> On September 26, 2019, 5G wireless was turned on in Wuhan, China (and officially launched on November 1) with a grid of about ten thousand 5G base stations [. . .] all concentrated in one city. A spike in cases occurred on February 13 – the same week that Wuhan turned on its 5G network for monitoring traffic.
> Illness has followed 5G installation in all the major cities in America, starting with New York in Fall 2019 in Manhattan, along with parts of Brooklyn, the Bronx, and Queens – all subsequent Coronavirus hot spots.

China is portrayed here as the source of a telecommunication mishap that supposedly occasioned the spread of the coronavirus – the illness that followed 5G installation – to other parts of the world. Cifre makes a similar point, charting the introduction of 5G technology in some of the popular cities in Europe. He concludes that there is "a clear and close relationship between the rate of coronavirus infections and 5G antenna location" (2020, n.p.) in these cities. The point of these controversial narratives is to trace the birth of the coronavirus to people's attempt to introduce a better and more advanced technology. The allegations have gained traction over the months and have made others wonder whether humans are not overreaching themselves.

The first poem that appears to subscribe to the notion that COVID-19 was birthed because of a mishap in technology is Malunga's "Untitled II" (2020, p. 67), a poem that scoffs at the power of man over his inventions. Indeed, the poem's poet-persona derides man's insatiable lust for technological innovation in the face of the coronavirus. The poet-persona stands at the gates of technology, taunting the "manufacturers of expensive lethal / weapons of war" for failing to see "the coming of a ruthless pandemic" (Malunga, 2020, p. 67). Malunga also highlights the corrosive and elusive nature of the pandemic, adding:

> No nuclear weapons can decimate
> No powerful leaders can evade
> No celebrities can keep at bay
> No monarchs can run away from
> No evangelists can pray against
> That's the Corona virus of our time.
> (Malunga, 2020, p. 67)

What is most striking in this passage is the growing sense of the power of the pandemic to outlast every human effort, to the extent that no ethnicity or nation is free from its excruciating grip. Understood thus, one also appreciates the virus's mutation and elusiveness. Its uncontainability becomes even more profound when one learns that not even scientists or religious leaders have managed to arrest its power. Such assertions signal how man's belief in science and religion is highly tested in the face of a raging contagion. The poet-persona further states that while we are busy trying to find ways of containing the virus, the virus in question is equally busy

> Stalking us diligently
> Claiming us one by one ruthlessly
> Making us rot as we walk
> Breaking our hearts as we
> Get separated from our beloved sick reeling under its ferocity.
> (Malunga, 2020, p. 67)

Helplessness and hopelessness dominate this passage, since they are the by-products of the cruelty and viciousness of the contagion. The lines in the passage also echo what I am calling elements of the walking dead, symbolised by the fact that the pandemic has the power of "Making us rot as we walk" and "Breaking our hearts as we/Get separated from our beloved sick." The trope of the walking dead finds a sustained resonance in the poem when one considers the deep fears that grip society as the contagion claims its victims "one by one ruthlessly" (Malunga, 2020, p. 67) and leaves them hapless and sad. Malunga's poem becomes even more poignant when one considers the millions of people that have succumbed to the pandemic worldwide, including scientists, celebrities, politicians, religious leaders, statesmen, and academics. This is what leads him to write that we are daily reeling under the ferocity of the coronavirus (Tembo, 2022a, p. 7). It does not come as a surprise when, towards the end of the poem, the poet-persona appears to say that instead of man attaining a technological breakthrough, he has ended up getting more than what he bargained for:

> That's what the world we thought
> we were remaking has become
> in the grip of Corona virus
> The king of death
> The height of panic
> The summit of plight.
> (Malunga, 2020, p. 67)

Malunga here seems to believe that the pandemic is a human creation. The words "That's what the world we thought/we were remaking" therefore, ought to be read as the poet-persona echoing scientific literature about the potential of the 5G wireless network to remake the world into a better place.

This literature argues that 5G technology "has the potential to drive numerous advancements, including digital transformation across industries, providing a platform for end-to-end IoT [Internet of Things] connectivity, enabling faster connections for consumers, and even providing a more cost-effective platform for carriers" (Deloitte, 2018, n.p.). The poet-persona thus derides those who thought they were remaking the world into a better place through the installation of the 5G technological network. He argues instead that this technological innovation has all but succeeded in plunging the world right:

[I]n the grip of Corona virus
The king of death
The height of panic
The summit of plight.
 (Malunga, 2020, p. 67)

Another conspiracy theory about the spread of the novel coronavirus is that it was passed on to human beings from mammals, such as pangolins, bats, and rats. While scientists agree that it is likely for SARS-CoV-2 to have its ancestral origins in a bat species, for example, they are quick to point out that the animal source of SARS-CoV-2 has not yet been confirmed (see, for example, Lytras et al., 2022, p. 8, 2021, p. 968; Maurin et al., 2021, p. 868; Temmam et al., 2022, p. 330). These assertions notwithstanding, writers have not stopped speculating that people's consumption of, or close contact with, animals, such as pangolins and bats, is a possible cause of the pandemic (Tembo, 2022a, pp. 8–9). We get this sense in Maren Bodenstein's "Green Dream" and Hope Banda's "Dear Unborn Child," two poems that evoke man's proclivity for eating or messing with wild (and largely endangered) mammals as the source of his own undoing. Bodenstein's poem, in particular, is poignant in the suggestion it makes that there is a probable association between the pangolin coronavirus and SARS-CoV-2. This theorisation is understandable, considering that a number of studies have also highlighted that pangolins are confirmed carriers of viruses closely related to SARS-CoV-2 (Aditya et al., 2021; Tang et al., 2020, p. 1013; Ullah et al., 2021), with some of them reporting that there is over 90% "whole genome sequence identity between pangolin coronavirus and SARS-CoV-2" (Liu et al., 2021, p. 1). Likewise, Bodenstein establishes the link between pangolins, bats, and humans in her poem, highlighting how the largely ant-eating pangolin

Sees bat and wanders
From the forest
To the marketplace
Crawls into a boiling pot
Dissolves to feed a million supplicants
Who pass the broth from lip to lip.
 (Bodenstein, 2021, p. 180)

Uneasiness runs throughout this passage in that the mammal not only "wanders/ From the forest" and "Crawls into a boiling pot" but also hands a poisoned chalice to humankind through its ability to dissolve into the pot set "to feed a million supplicants / Who pass the broth from lip to lip." The fact that the people are portrayed in the poem as "supplicants" shows that the pangolin holds some sort of ominous power over man. It does not come as a surprise, then, that the mammal is seen (in the second stanza of the poem) delivering a final death blow to all its eaters: "The streets are empty" (Bodenstein, 2021, p. 180), suggesting the kind of emptiness that comes about because the people who feasted on the mammal are probably dead. Bodenstein is also subtly concerned with the extinction of the pangolin in sanctuaries in nature. In her view, the forest can now only dream of pangolin. Bodenstein's concerns about the future of the pangolin have found validation in recent years, as we have witnessed individual countries and animal rights groups coming up with deliberate policies on pangolin conservation. This is besides according the pangolin the status of specially protected species.

Hope Banda's "Dear Unborn Child" is also concerned with the future. But unlike Bodenstein – whose poem ends with her concern for the survival of the pangolin or lack thereof – Banda's poet-persona is concerned about the future of man himself in the face of the raging novel coronavirus. Banda begins by highlighting that the spread of SARS-CoV-2 reached its peak in 2020, adding that "the year itself was untamed" and that it caught humankind "up in the slumber of jeering" (Banda, 2020, p. 42). The reason Banda gives for thinking 2020 was a difficult and traumatising year is not hard to fathom: societies all over the world were not only besieged by the pandemic but also no one seemed to know when life would return to normalcy. Next, the poet-persona states that man had been visited upon by the novel coronavirus because "Elsewhere somebody had feasted on/Bats and rats" (Banda, 2020, p. 42). The "elsewhere" in question is the Huanan Seafood Wholesale Market in Wuhan, Hubei Province, China where the coronavirus was first detected in December 2019. Banda's claim here presents itself as a layering of misinformation and also as violence against the very notion of truth. The pandemic, which has violated the fabric of our sociability, has the particularity of hitting us when "false news, conspiracy theories, magical cures and racist news are being shared at an alarming rate, with the potential to increase anxiety and stress and even lead to loss of life" (Rathore & Farooq, 2020, p. S162). It is not surprising when we see the poet-persona further allege that man is now being "screwed and schooled/Caged in protective cells" (Banda, 2020, p. 42) for feasting on bats and rats. In the poet-persona's view, human beings are architects of their own misfortunes for "touring nature sanctuaries" (Banda, p. 42), probably looking for bats and rats to consume. Banda (2020, p. 42) thus regards SARS-CoV-2 as

[T]he monster [that] had come
Laying his enamels on our melanin
Gluttonously licking his fingers
Craving for more [victims].

Man's eating proclivities are here encoded in the poet's reference to his (i.e., man's) ability to "gluttonously lick his fingers" unmindful of the danger that could be lurking in devouring bats and rats (Tembo, 2022a, p. 9).

Another COVID-spiracy theory that has found fertile ground in our society is that it is actually humanity's destruction of biodiversity that creates the conditions for new viruses and diseases, such as COVID-19, to arise. Quammen (2020) is one such person who has relentlessly advanced this line of thinking. Unlike Cowan and Morell (2020), who attribute the cause of the pandemic to so-called 5G experiments in the province of Wuhan in China (p. 7), Quammen (2020) believes there is a link between the emergence of the coronavirus and people's wanton invasion and depletion of ecosystems. For him, the bad choices human beings have been making regarding the environment over the years, have come full circle. Consequently, we are reaping the fruits of our carelessness. His observation is that humans not only "invade tropical forests and other wild landscapes, [they also] kill the animals or cage them and send them to markets." Additionally, they "disrupt ecosystems, and [. . .] shake viruses loose from their natural hosts" (Quammen, 2020, p. 7). He thus calls on humans to do everything in their power "to contain and extinguish this nCoV-2019 outbreak" (Quammen, 2020, p. 7). He concludes by saying, "when the dust settles [it will be apparent that] nCoV-2019 was not a novel event that befell us. It was – and is – part of a pattern of choices that we humans are making" (Quammen, 2020, p. 7). Similar views are echoed by Sharma (2021), who avers, "COVID-19 is a reminder of the dysfunctional relationship human beings have with Mother Nature" (p. 8). In Sharma's view, human beings have – for centuries – been invading the natural inhabitants of flora and fauna mercilessly, all the while living under the illusion that "Mother Nature cannot respond to the atrocities we inflict upon it. But it retaliated, and jolted the pseudo-victor, mankind, out of its greedy roller-coaster" (2021, p. 8). Here, man's greed and insensitivity towards the environment are being cited as the reasons for the outbreak. What stands out in both assertions is that nature is either "healing itself or taking revenge from mankind for destroying it mercilessly" (Sharma, 2021, p. 7).

The recurrent image of "destroying nature repeatedly" accompanies the opening lines of William Mpina's (2020) "Down, But Not Defeated," a poem that celebrates man's resilience and fortitude in the face of adversity. The opening seven lines are poignant in that the poet-persona insinuates that nature is protesting against man's invasion of the ecosystem:

One would think
Time is firing tears
Nature is fighting back
Catapults of darkness
Are toppling light
 (Mpina, 2020, p. 1)

References to "tears," "darkness," and "toppling light" are in fact the poet-persona's way of saying that the peace and serenity that existed before COVID-19 have been replaced by anxiety, suffering, and hopelessness. Over-all, the point that Mpina appears to make in these lines is that COVID-19 is a result of people's avaricious behaviour towards the ecosystem, which is now "fighting back." In that case, Mpina is warning human beings about the perils that await those who do not work towards restoring unto Mother Nature what they have been taking away from her. One gets the impression here, as Sharma (2021) also does, that "maybe COVID-19 is the beginning of a new chapter of a healthy relationship between mankind and nature" (p. 10), since the expectation is that the former will begin to reflect on how to interact with the latter from now on. Such sentiments – that careless and selfish human actions induce the novel coronavirus – have morphed beyond science into politics and have given rise to considerable anxiety. In the next section, I examine the implications of COVID-spiracy as reflected by the poems selected for analysis in this study. The aim is to show how COVID-19 poetry inflects psychological distress.

8.4   Haunted Selves, Fearful Lives: COVID-19 and Psychological Distress

Several studies have reported a strong correlation between psychological dis-tress and COVID-19-related stressors (Kang et al., 2020; McGinty, 2020; Qiu et al., 2020; Zhang et al., 2020). In a study conducted on United States (US) adults aged 18 years and older who responded to wave 1 of the novel coronavirus, for example, McGinty (2020) found that the longer-term dis-ruptions of the pandemic are important drivers of distress and that "more than 60% of adults with serious distress reported that pandemic-related disrup-tions to education, employment, and finances negatively affected their mental health" (p. 2555). In much the same spirit, Kang et al. (2020) observe that in battling the sudden emergence of severe acute respiratory syndrome (SARS) among medical and nursing staff in Wuhan, China, "psychological distress appeared gradually: fear and anxiety appeared immediately and decreased in the early stages of the epidemic, but depression, psychophysiological symp-toms and post-traumatic stress symptoms appeared later and lasted for a long time, leading to profound impacts" (pp. 11–12). The dichotomy undergirding the psychological distress discourse highlighted here is traceable in the open-ing remarks of the WHO director-general during a media briefing, where he formally announced the global outbreak of a new infectious disease, called COVID-19. The director-general noted that the pandemic "is not a word to use lightly or carelessly. It is a word that, if misused, can cause unreasonable fear, or unjustified acceptance that the fight is over, leading to unnecessary suffering and death" (WHO, 2020b, n.p.). This fear and distress is also trace-able in Phelelani Makhanya's three poems – "Vapour," The Surname," and "One in the Chamber" – all of which tell of cases of anxiety and loneliness among family, friends, and community members affected by the COVID-19 pandemic.

In "Vapour," Makhanya focuses on a young village boy who had lost both his grandparents to COVID-19. According to the poet-persona, since the boy's loss

> He is not with the other
> village boys on the slope
> of the weedy soccer field.
> He is not with the boys
> swimming in the murky Ququda pond.
>   (Makhanya, 2021, n.p.)

Makhanya (2021) does not reveal where the boy's biological parents are, although it is not hard to speculate that they must have been the first to die (probably from the same pandemic), leaving their son in the care of the just departed grandparents. But what is more poignant about the boy in this poem is his new plight: he keeps to himself because he realises that he is an orphan with no one to take care of him. In a country such as South Africa, where there is a deep gulf between the rich and the poor, and where over 200,000 children have lost a primary or secondary caregiver, such as a grandparent (UNICEF South Africa, 2022)[1] orphanhood is, perhaps, the worst thing that can happen to a child. According to the Centre for Disease Control and Prevention (CDC), millions of children have become orphans during the pandemic due to COVID-19-related deaths of one or both parents, and/or grandparent caregivers. These children "face risk factors that may increase the likelihood of experiencing poverty, abuse, delayed development, mental health challenges, reduced access to education, and institutionalisation" (CDC, 2022, n.p.).

What is unmistakable in the boy's behaviour is that he is grief-stricken. His keeping away from everyone, therefore, can be understood from three viewpoints. First, we sense an element of hidden pain in the boy, one that comes about because he realises that the people who should have played the role of caregiver are no longer there to give him that support. For such a child, keeping away is, therefore, his way of mourning his grief, although such an action has its own consequences. According to Treglia et al. (2021), children who keep to themselves after they have lost a parent or caregiver can suffer consequences that can persist throughout their lifetime. These consequences may include "depression, post-traumatic stress disorder (PTSD), anxiety, lower rates of academic attainment and higher dropout rates, higher rates of alcohol and other substance use, suicide, and reduced employment" (Treglia et al., 2021, p. 8). This is also what UNICEF South Africa says in their assessment of the impact of COVID-19 on orphaned children in South Africa: their lives have been devastated by the pandemic in many ways and for those who have lost parents or caregivers, the deep scars will last forever (UNICEF South Africa, 2022, n.p.). A second but related reason why the boy in Makhanya's

(2021) poem keeps to himself is that he not only feels lonesome, but he is also purposefully avoided by his village folks. We get this sense in the third and fourth stanzas of the poem, where we are told:

> When villagers see him
> approaching from a distance,
> they shout a coded signal
> to their neighbours
> They run inside their houses,
> they close the doors and windows
> like a storm is approaching.
> (Makhanya, 2021, n.p.)

In this passage, one gets the sense that myths and misinformation about people who have been in contact with COVID-19 patients are at work. One such myth is that everyone either suffering from COVID-19 or has come into contact with a COVID-19 patient dies. It is, therefore, safe to avoid such people for fear that others, too, might be infected and/or die. This is a classic case of social stigma, described by the WHO (2020a) as the negative association between a person or group of people who share certain characteristics and a specific disease. In the summation of the WHO, people tend to be labelled, stereotyped, discriminated against, treated separately, and/or experience loss of status because of a perceived link with a disease (WHO, 2020a, n.p.). Specifically focusing on the COVID-19 outbreak, the WHO observes that it "has provoked social stigma and discriminatory behaviours against people of certain ethnic backgrounds as well as anyone perceived to have been in contact with the virus" (WHO, 2020a, n.p.). We suspect similar attitudes, behaviours, and perceptions towards the boy in the poem: he is rejected, discriminated against, and kept at arm's length by his immediate community members probably because everyone thinks he might end up infecting them. The final reason why the boy keeps to himself could emanate from his "sense of insecurity and inability to cope with a traumatic past" (see Tembo, 2015, p. 71), one that forces him to remain paranoid of everyone and everything around him.

Sentiments of rejection and psychological distress equally seep through in "The Surname," a poem Makhanya wrote to celebrate his brother's recovery from COVID-19 (2021, p. 209). The poet-persona narrates how his brother "was the first to test / positive for COVID-19 on [their] side of the village" (2021, p. 209) and how his sibling and the entire community reacted after hearing the news:

> Ants already feasting on his shadow
> like a starter dish.
> I have carried many heavy stones
> in the backpack of my eyes
> but not this heavy.
> (Makhanya, 2021, p. 209)

The poet-persona feels heavy in his heart, probably fearing the worst for his brother. The words "Ants already feasting on his shadow / like a starter dish" (Makhanya, 2021, p. 209) recommend this reading. It is also possible that the persona's heart is heavy from speculating how people from his village felt when they heard that one of their own had tested positive for the novel coronavirus. This feeling is soon overtaken by "the walls and the yard of [the] home" growing "quills and spikes," a possible reference to the stigmatisation and labelling that is about to befall the poet-persona's family. By the time we get to the second stanza, the poet-persona's fears are confirmed:

> [O]ur neighbours have forged new detour pathways
> that split like a Y;
> Pathways that go deep into the woods
> They will rather crisscross with black Mamba trails
> than pass near our home.
> (Makhanya, 2021, pp. 209–210)

The poet-persona's feeling of being let down by his village folk is palpable here. The use of expressions such as "new detour pathways / that split like a Y" and "rather crisscross with black Mamba trails / than pass near our home" points to the fact that COVID-19 patients are bad news to the community. This categorisation is complete when we come to the penultimate stanza of the poem where we learn that the community writes off the poet-persona's family before it is given the benefit of doubt:

> Our neighbours no longer call our home Kwa-Makhanya
> They have given us a new surname; Kwa-Corona
> They tell their children;
> "Don't go near that yellow house, Kwa-Corona;
> We don't want to bury you."
> (Makhanya, 2021, p. 210)

The reason why the family is written off is not hard to speculate: their compound is no longer seen as a hub of life and living. Instead, it is "a black diamond ring / that eats both flesh and ring finger bones" (Makhanya, 2021, p. 210), a place of death and dying. It is interesting to note that these labels have the power to contribute to negative psychological and social outcomes, especially for individuals and communities that experience pain and suffering. This feeling of being distressed is reiterated in the last stanza of the poem, where the poet-persona states,

> We are a home with a new surname; Kwa-Corona
> A surname that has no clan name
> A surname that claims every clan name.
> (Makhanya, 2021, p. 210)

Perhaps more poignant in these lines is that the words capture the thoughts of a family at its wits end, one whose helplessness is compounded by the cold, senseless, and unfeeling attitude of its immediate community members.

Makhanya's (2021) next poem, "One in the Chamber," is a dark piece that takes the reader deep into the mind of someone who has been laid off because of COVID-19. The first stanza reads,

> Since he lost his job
> due to COVID-19,
> He spends his afternoons
> sitting under the Avocado tree
> behind the house.
>   (Makhanya, 2021,
>   pp. 210–211)

No further explanation is given why the "he" in the poem lost his job, although it is possible to speculate that the man must have lost his job either due to redundancy or because he did something that put the lives of his fellow employees at risk of contracting COVID-19. What is undeniable, however, is that the man's loss of his job had left him deflated and defeated. Central to Makhanya's (2021) "One in the Chamber," then, is the perceived connection between job loss due to COVID-19 and depression. These two factors could lead someone to feel agitated and entertain evil thoughts, including contemplating self-harm. This is the sense we get upon reading the last two stanzas of the poem:

> This is a hand miming
> the shape of a revolver.
> Every day he argues
> with the bullet in the chamber;
> lusting after the folds of his brain.
>   (Makhanya, 2021, p. 211)

The fact that the now jobless man's hand is "miming / the shape of a revolver" and that there is a "bullet in the chamber" makes us further speculate that the man is probably contemplating suicide. This speculation is not unfounded, considering that people who have lost their jobs during the COVID-19 pandemic often display tendencies of depression and struggle to cope with life. In "Job loss and mental health during the COVID-19 lockdown: Evidence from South Africa," Posel et al. (2021) observe that job loss impairs the mental well-being of an individual. The scholars further assert that people who retained paid employment during the COVID-19 lockdown in South Africa had significantly lower depression scores than those who had lost employment (Posel et al., 2021, p. 1). This entails that there is an implication of job loss for mental health because, in the scholars' view, "the source of unemployment is very likely to have been exogenous to (or beyond the control of) the individual" (Posel et al., 2021, p. 2; original brackets). To be fair, this is the defining trait for people in various other forms of pain and psychological distress: they resort to self-harm to cope with or express bottled-up emotions, feel in control, or relieve the unbearable tension that is welling within or as a response to other disturbing thoughts.

8.5 Conclusion

As argued in this chapter, an infodemic is one of the key elements that have the potential to cause profound public anxiety and social panic. It also affects public health communication, diminishes preventive measures, impedes effective crisis management, widens the gaps between races and regions, and even brings social chaos. Every poem discussed in this chapter demonstrates how an infodemic could dominate people's lives. On the one hand, we have Malunga's (2020), Bodenstein's (2021), Banda's (2020), and Mpina's (2020) poems, which highlight some of the mythologies, paranoiac conspiracy theories, and misinformation about the COVID-19 pandemic. These poets probe man's behaviour towards the ecosystem, insinuating that were it not for human irresponsibility towards Mother Nature, the world would probably have been at peace with itself, not fighting to contain the pandemic as was the case. On the other hand, Makhanya's (2021) three poems discussed in this chapter focus on the battered and troubled soul in the face of the pandemic. They also act as empathetic witnesses to the anxiety and pain the pandemic caused to individuals and communities on the African continent. This is very important, considering that pandemics have the capacity to create stress and agitation in all of us.

Note

1 These figures are based on the September 2022 data that were collated by UNICEF South Africa.

References

Achterberg, P. (2021). Covid-spiracy: Old wine in new barrels? In E. Aarts, H. Fleuren, M. Sitskoorn, & T. Wilthagen (Eds.), *The new common: How the COVID-19 pandemic is transforming society* (pp. 17–22). Springer. https://doi.org/10.1007/978-3-030-65355-2

Aditya, V., Goswami, R., Mendis, A., & Roopa, R. (2021). Scale of the issue: Mapping the impact of the COVID-19 lockdown on pangolin trade across India. *Biological Conservation, 257*, 1–5. https://doi.org/10.1016/j.biocon.2021.109136

Balaev, M. (2018). Trauma studies. In D. Richter (Ed.), *A companion to literary theory* (pp. 360–371). Wiley.

Banda, H. C. (2020). Dear unborn child. In M. C. Juwa, W. K. Mpina, & B. Galafa (Eds.), *Walking the battlefield: An anthology of Malawian poetry on the COVID-19 pandemic* (pp. 42–24). JC Creations.

Bodenstein, M. (2021). Green dream. *English Studies in Africa, 64*(1–2), 180. https://doi.org/10.1080/00138398.2021.1969119

Bridgman, A., Merkley, E., Zhilin, O., Loewen, P. J., Owen, T., & Ruths, D. (2022). Infodemic pathways: Evaluating the role that traditional and social media play in cross-national information transfer. In A. de Angelis, C. E. Farhart, E. Merkley, & D. A. Stecula (Eds.), *Political misinformation in the digital age during a pandemic: Partisanship, propaganda, and democratic decision-making* (pp. 33–43). Frontiers Media SA. https://doi.org/10.3389/978-2-88976-454-9

Caruth, C. (1996). *Unclaimed experience: Trauma, narrative, and history.* The John Hopkins University Press.

Centres for Disease Control and Prevention. (2022). *Global orphanhood associated with COVID-19.* www.cdc.gov/globalhealth/topics/orphanhood/index.html

Cifre, B. P. I. (2020, March–April). *Estudio de la correlación entre casos de Coronavirus y la presencia de redes 5G [Study of the correlation between cases of coronavirus and the presence of 5G network]* (C. Edwards, Trans.). www.stop5gticino.ch/wp-content/uploads/2020/04/Study-of-correlation-Coronavirus-5G-Bartomeu-Payeras-i-Cifre.pdf

Cowan, T. S., & Morell, S. F. (2020). *The contagion myth: Why viruses (including "coronavirus") are not the cause of disease.* Skyhorse.

Crutzen, P. J., & Stoermer, E. F. (2000). The "anthropocene". *IGBP Newsletter, 41,* 17–18. https://inters.org/files/crutzenstoermer2000.pdf

De Coninck, D., Frissen, T., Matthijs, K., d'Haenens, I., Lits, G., Champagne-Poiriers, O., Carignan, M.-E., David, M. D., Pignard-Cheynel, N., Salerno, S., & Généreux, M. (2022). Beliefs in conspiracy theories and misinformation about COVID-19: Comparative perspectives on the role of anxiety, depression and exposure to and trust in information sources. In A. de Angelis, C. E. Farhart, E. Merkley, & D. A. Stecula (Eds.), *Political misinformation in the digital age during a pandemic: Partisanship, propaganda, and democratic decision-making* (pp. 47–59). Frontiers Media SA. https://doi.org/10.3389/978-2-88976-454-9

Deloitte. (2018). *Will 5G remake the world or just make it a little faster?"* Deloitte Center for Technology, Media and Telecommunications. https://www2.deloitte.com/content/dam/Deloitte/global/Documents/Technology-Media-Telecommunications/gx-tmt-will-5g-remake-the-world.pdf

Erni, J. N., & Striphas, T. (2021). Introduction: COVID-19, the multiplier. *Cultural Studies, 35*(2–3), 211–237. https://doi.org/10.1080/09502386.2021.1903957

Fernando, J. L. (2020). The virocene epoch: The vulnerability nexus of viruses, capitalism and racism. *Journal of Political Ecology, 27*(1), 635–684.

Fremaux, A. (2019). *After the anthropocene: Green republicanism in a post-capitalist world.* Palgrave.

Kang, L., Ma, S., Chen, M., Yang, J., Wang, Y., Li, R., Yao, L., Bai, H., Cai, Z., Yang, B. X., Hu, S., Zhang, K., Wang, G., Ma, C., & Liu, Z. (2020). Impact on mental health and perceptions of psychological care among medical and nursing staff in Wuhan during the 2019 novel Coronavirus disease outbreak: A cross-sectional study. *Brain, Behavior, and Immunity, 87,* 11–17. https://doi.org/10.1016/j.bbi.2020.03.028

Liu, P., Jiang, J.-Z., Wan, X.-F., Hua, Y., Li, L., Zhou, J., Wang, X., Hou, F., Chen, J., Zou, J., & Chen, J. (2021). Correction: Are pangolins the intermediate host of the 2019 novel coronavirus (SARS-CoV-2)? *PLOS Pathogens, 17*(6), e1009664. https://doi.org/10.1371/journal.ppat.1009664

Lupton, D. (2022). *Covid societies: Theorising the coronavirus.* Routledge.

Lytras, P., Hughes, J., Martin, D., Swanepoel, P., de Klerk, A., Lourens, R., Pond, S. L. K., Xia, W., Jiang, X., & Robertson, D. L. (2022). Exploring the natural origins of SARS-CoV-2 in the light of recombination. *Genome Biology and Evolution, 14*(2), 1–14. https://doi.org/10.1093/gbe/evac018

Lytras, S., Xia, W., Hughes, J., Jiang, X., & Robertson, D. L. (2021). The animal origin of SARS-CoV-2: Trading of animals susceptible to bat coronaviruses is the likely cause of the COVID-19 pandemic. *Science, 373*(6558), 968–970.

Makhanya, P. (2021). Two poems by Phelelani Makhanya. *English Studies in Africa, 64*(1–2), 209–211. https://doi.org/10.1080/00138398.2021.1969123

Malunga, B. (2020). Untitled II. In M. C. Juwa, W. K. Mpina, & B. Galafa (Eds.), *Walking the battlefield: An anthology of Malawian poetry on the COVID-19 pandemic* (p. 67). JC Creations.

Maurin, M., Fenollar, F., Mediannikov, O., Davoust, B., Devaux, C., & Raoult, D. (2021). Current status of putative animal sources of SARS-CoV-2 infection in humans: Wildlife, domestic animals and pets. *Microorganisms, 9*(4), 868. https://doi.org/10.3390/microorganisms9040868

McGinty, E. (2020). Psychological distress and COVID-19–related stressors reported in a longitudinal cohort of US adults in April and July 2020. *JAMA, 324*(24), 2555–2557. https://doi.org/10.1001/jama.2020.21231

Miller, C. H., & Ma, H. (2021). How existential anxiety shapes communication in coping with the coronavirus pandemic: A terror management theory perspective. In D. O'Hair & M. J. O'Hair (Eds.), *Communicating science in times of crisis: The COVID-19 pandemic* (Vol. 1, pp. 54–80). Wiley Blackwell.

Mollica, R. F. (2006). *Healing invisible wounds: Paths to hope and recovery in a violent world.* Harcourt.

Morell, S. F. (2020). Preface. In T. Cowan & S. Morell (Eds.), *The contagion myth: Why viruses (including "coronavirus") are not the cause of disease* (pp. i–v). Skyhorse.

Mpina, W. K. (2020). Down, but not defeated. In M. C. Juwa, W. K. Mpina, & B. Galafa (Eds.), *Walking the battlefield: An anthology of Malawian poetry on the COVID-19 pandemic* (pp. 1–2). JC Creations.

Posel, D., Oyenubi, A., & Kollamparambil, U. (2021). Job loss and mental health during the COVID-19 lockdown: Evidence from South Africa. *PLOS One, 16*(3), 1–15. https://doi.org/10.1371/journal.pone.0249352

Qiu, J., Shen, B., Zhao, M., Wang, Z., Xie, B., & Xu, Y. (2020). A nationwide survey of psychological distress among Chinese people in the COVID-19 epidemic: Implications and policy recommendations. *General Psychiatry, 33*, e100213. https://doi.org/10.1136/gpsych-2020-100213

Quammen, D. (2020, April 4). How we made the Coronavirus pandemic. *The Times of India.* https://timesofindia.indiatimes.com/times-evoke/photo/74977081.cms

Rathore, F. A., & Farooq, F. (2020). Information overload and infodemic in the COVID-19 pandemic. *Journal of the Pakistan Medical Association, 70*(3), S162–S165. https://doi.org/10.5455/JPMA.38

Sharma, D. (2021). Reading and rewriting poetry on life to survive the COVID-19 pandemic. *Journal of Poetry Therapy, 34*(2), 95–108. https://doi.org/10.1080/08893675.2021.1899631

Spitzberg, B. H. (2021). Comprehending covidiocy communication: Dismisinformation, conspiracy theory and fake news. In D. O'Hair & M. J. O'Hair (Eds.),

Communicating science in times of crisis: The COVID-19 pandemic (pp. 15–53). Wiley Blackwell.

Tang, X., Wu, C., Li, X., Song, Y., Yao, Y., Wu, X., Duan, Y., Zhang, H., Wang, Y., Qian, Z., Cui, J., & Lu, J. (2020). On the origin and continuing evolution of SARS-CoV-2. *National Science Review, 7*(6), 1012–1023. https://doi.org/10.1093/nsr/nwaa036

Tembo, N. M. (2014). Traumatic memory and "scriptotherapy" in Malawian poetry: The case of Bright Molande's *Seasons. English Academy Review, 31*(1), 51–65. https://doi.org/10.1080/10131752.2014.909003

Tembo, N. M. (2015). Paranoia, "chosen trauma" and forgiveness in Leah Chishugi's *A Long Way from Paradise. English Academy Review, 32*(2), 70–87.

Tembo, N. M. (2022a). Anxious competition: Exploring the poetic imaginarium of the SARS-CoV-2 pandemic in Malawi. *Journal of Literary Studies, 38*(1), 1–18. https://doi.org/10.25159/1753-5387/10418

Tembo, N. M. (2022b). Confronting apartheid's revenants: Trevor Noah's *Born a Crime* and/as traumedy. *a/b: Auto/Biography Studies, 37*(2), 263–283. https://doi.org/10.1080/08989575.2022.2135241

Temmam, S., Vongphayloth, K., Baquero, E., Munier, S., Bonomi, M., Regnault, B., Douangboubpha, B., Karami, Y., Chrétien, D., Sanamxay, D., Xayaphet, V., Paphaphanh, P., Lacoste, V., Somlor, S., Lakeomany, K., Phommavanh, N., Pérot, P., Dehan, O., Amara, F., . . . Eloit, M. (2022). Bat coronavirus related to SARS-CoV-2 and infectious human cells. *Nature, 604*, 330–336. https://doi.org/10.1038/s41586-022-04532-4

Treglia, D., Cutuli, J. J., & Arasteh, K. (2021). *Hidden pain: Children who lost a parent or caregiver to COVID-19 and what the nation can do to help them.* COVID Collaborative. www.covidcollaborative.us/assets/uploads/img/HIDDEN-PAIN-FINAL.pdf

Ullah, A., Ahmad, S., Ur Rahman, G., Alqarni, M. M., & Mahmoud, E. E. (2021). Impact of pangolin bootleg market on the dynamics of COVID-19 model. *Results in Physics, 23*. https://doi.org/10.1016/j.rinp.2021.103913

UNICEF South Africa. (2022). *Number of COVID-19 orphans nears 150,000 in South Africa.* www.unicef.org/southafrica/press-releases/number-covid-19-orphans-nears-150000-south-africa

Vitriol, J. A., & Marsh, J. K. (2022). A pandemic of misbelief: How beliefs promote or undermine COVID-19 mitigation. In A. De Angelis, C. E. Farhart, E. Merkley, & D. A. Stecula (Eds.), *Political misinformation in the digital age during a pandemic: Partisanship, propaganda, and democratic decision-making* (pp. 123–136). Frontiers Media SA. https://doi.org/10.3389/978-2-88976-454-9

World Health Organization. (2020a). *A guide to preventing and addressing social stigma associate with COVID-19.* https://cdn.who.int/media/docs/default-source/epi-win/stigma/covid19-stigma-guide.pdf?sfvrsn=48f6ac1_2&download=true

World Health Organization. (2020b, March 11). *WHO director-general's opening remarks at the media briefing on COVID-19.* www.who.int/director-general/speeches/detail/who-director-general-s-opening-remarks-at-the-media-briefing-on-covid-19-11-march-2020

Xu, J., & Liu, C. (2021). Infodemic vs. pandemic factors associated to public anxiety in the early stage of the COVID-19 outbreak: A cross-sectional study in China. *Frontiers in Public Health, 9*, 1–10.

Zhang, J., Lu, H., Zeng, H., Zhang, S., Du, Q., Jiang, T., & Du, B. (2020). The differential psychological distress of populations affected by the COVID-19 pandemic. *Brain, Behaviour, and Immunity, 87*, 49–50. https://doi.org/10.1016/j.bbi.2020.04.031

Žižek, S. (2020). *Pandemic! COVID-19 shakes the world.* OR Books.

9 Psychological Toll of COVID-19 Communication Patterns in Malawi

Peter Mhagama

9.1 Introduction

During the first phase of the COVID-19 outbreak, the media in Malawi abounded with infodemics, misinformation, and disinformation about the disease to the extent that many people were left wondering which information to believe. Whenever there is a pandemic, people respond differently due to the information they receive concerning the disease and its effects. How people respond to the information they receive about the disease could have psychological consequences for their mental health, such as anxiety and emotional distress (Su et al., 2021). This could further affect how they adhere to the preventive measures of the disease and how they might react after contracting it. Mental health is defined as "a state of well-being in which the individual realises their abilities, can cope with normal stresses of life, can work productively and fruitfully, and can make a contribution to his or her community" (World Health Organization [WHO], 2004, p. 14). Studies have shown that psychological factors could also affect how a pandemic is managed and how people cope with infection and the fear of death (Cullen et al., 2020; Mach et al., 2021; Zhou et al., 2020). For instance, Cullen et al. (2020, p. 311) argue, "During an outbreak of an infectious disease, the population's psychological reactions play a critical role in shaping both the spread of the disease and the occurrence of emotional distress and social disorder during and after the outbreak." In light of the nature and effect of COVID-19, it was expected that information dissemination about the pandemic would be regular as the government and other stakeholders took measures to mitigate its effect. This is where the role of the media in curbing the spread of a pandemic manifested.

The media serve as a primary source of health information, which could help curb disease transmission and could bring health professionals, policymakers, and the general public together to have a common understanding in the fight against the pandemic (Laing, 2011). The media disseminate risks to their audiences and shape public perceptions of them through the volume of information, the content, and the tone of reporting (Mach et al., 2021). However, during the initial stages of the pandemic, there was a considerable amount of information, misinformation, and disinformation about COVID-19

DOI: 10.4324/9781003425861-11

in Malawi. This created panic, fear, mental distress and disorder, and anxiety among the people to the extent that their mental health was affected negatively. News biased, negative, and misleading could adversely affect mental health (Su et al., 2021).

Several studies have been done, which have found a positive correlation between the consumption of negative COVID-19 news and the mental health of the people. For instance, a study conducted among university students in France by Wathelet et al. (2020) found that individuals who reported spending much time seeking COVID-19 news daily during the lockdown developed high levels of anxiety, distress, stress, and depression. This evidence confirms the view that the media negatively affect the mental health of their audiences. Similarly, a study by Buchanan et al. (2021) found that as little as two minutes of exposure to negative news about COVID-19 can have negative effects and that research on social media exposure to COVID-related news has been correlational, leaving open the possibility that unhappy people are more likely to seek out negative news. The COVID-19 news mainly focused on negatives and rumours, making people unhappy because of the fear it created. To find the truth about the disease, they resorted to seeking information from any available source that could either confirm or dispel the rumours. A study conducted to examine the relationship between happiness and the rise of media consumption during COVID-19 confinement by Muñiz-Velázquez et al. (2021) found that far from cultivating greater happiness, those who engaged in heavy consumption of media during confinement were less happy than those who did so more moderately and spent more time performing other activities (p. 146). Being unhappy can be one of the signs or causes of stress or mental depression. For instance, Li et al. (2022) investigated the effect of media use among the elderly during the COVID-19 era and found that more frequent media use increased the rate of depression.

It is clear from the foregoing that seeking news or information on COVID-19 from different news sources was a common habit among many people during the pandemic, and this had the potential to affect people's psychological well-being. To help understand how the media affected people's mental well-being during the COVID-19 pandemic, the current study was informed by media effects theory, which explains how the mass media influence the attitudes and perceptions of their audience. According to Valkenburg et al. (2016), the media effects theory has two features concerning how people consume news. First, people only attend to a limited number of messages out of a myriad that could attract their attention. The second is that only those messages people select have the potential to influence them (see also Knobloch-Westerwick, 2015). Under the media effects theory, we can further identify two theories to help us understand how news about COVID-19 affects people.

The agenda-setting theory of media states that the mass media determine the issues that concern the public rather than the public's views. This theory posits that the issues that receive the most attention from the media become those that people discuss and debate (Hanson, 2009). In the process, readers become affected by such issues. A study by McCombs and Shaw (1972) on how the day-to-day selection of news influences the public agenda found a high correlation between the importance of issues on the media agenda and how those issues become the public agenda. Concerning COVID-19 news, it was noted that the media focused much attention on negative news and that this overcrowded people's thinking and affected their behaviour. It is further argued that by shaping their own selective media use (deliberately or not), individuals also somehow shape their own media effects (Valkenburg et al., 2016). In times of a pandemic, such as COVID-19, it is normal for people to seek information. However, the type of information they sought or to which they were exposed during COVID-19 brought a whole range of effects.

During the COVID-19 pandemic, people did not deliberately seek negative news. Still, because there were few facts available about the disease, it was inevitable for anyone to land on negative stories about COVID-19 because the media were full of them, and unfortunately, this is what hurt people's well-being – directly or indirectly. According to Buchanan et al. (2021, p. 2), "Indeed, information seeking during a pandemic may prove problematic because negative information is ubiquitous and unending, and no amount of information can eliminate the pervasive sense of uncertainty." In agenda-setting theory, the relative salience of a news item determines how the audience will be affected or influenced by it (Dearing & Rogers, 1996). By frequently broadcasting some news items, the media give salience to such news, which makes people attracted to it and, in the process, influenced or affected by it either positively or negatively.

Another media effects theory is the uses and gratifications theory, which states that consumers use the media to satisfy specific needs or desires (Lule, 2016). Many people use the media for several purposes, such as entertainment or relaxation, social interaction, education, or information. Whatever the purpose might be, Papacharissi (2009) observes that each of the uses satisfies a particular need (i.e., gives gratification), and the needs determine the way in which people use the media. The severity of COVID-19 forced people to seek more information about prevention and control in the news media, including social media. Informed by media reports, people were able to change their behaviours. They took corrective measures, such as frequent hand washing with soap, wearing masks, observing social distancing, and observing social isolation at home to avoid passing on or contracting the infection from others (Zhou et al., 2020). This is one of the positive effects that the media had on various audiences during the COVID-19 pandemic. However, understanding the effects of media on audiences has become increasingly complicated over the years as more and more people are now relying on social media for their news. According to Buchanan et al. (2021, p. 8), "People seek out social media for many reasons other than news consumption and may not realise that minimal exposure to negative news on these platforms can have such negative consequences." This was particularly the case during the COVID period because social media provided conflicting information, infodemics, and disinformation, confusing many people and creating fatalistic beliefs regarding their mental well-being (Spiteri, 2021).

Some research found that the benefits of using social media were satisfying the basic human need for belonging, increasing life satisfaction, and reducing loneliness (McLaughlin & Sillence, 2018; Zhan et al., 2016). However, other studies found that excessive use of social media has been linked to serious mental health issues, such as depression and anxiety (Primack et al., 2017; Reer et al., 2019; Van der Velden et al., 2019). The emphasis is placed on excessive use of social media as a contributing factor to negative mental health, implying that if people reduced their consumption of social media content or did not believe everything to which they had been exposed, there would have been fewer cases of depression and anxiety among the populations. Nonetheless, it must be appreciated that the need to be updated with new information – possibly of hope – about the disease raised the people's desire to seek more information using any available means, obliviously becoming mentally affected.

However, according to Cushion (2019), some studies have dismissed the simplistic correlations between media consumption and audience responses, arguing that media effects cannot only be measured in many direct and indirect ways, but that sociocultural, political, and economic factors also contribute to shaping human behaviour (see also Preiss et al., 2007). Considering that the media effects theory is not enough to explain how the media influence people, the social cognitive theory was also used to inform this study. According to Fiske and Taylor (1991), the effects of the media can be understood from the perspective of social cognition, which generally emphasises how people gain, understand, interpret, store, and apply social information. These processes often involve relying on limited and sometimes biased information, especially from the media, by drawing people's attention to specific knowledge, ideas, values, and behaviours, oftentimes at the exclusion of others (Dhanani & Franz, 2020). Such exclusion could be intentional or not. According to Bandura (2001), human behaviour can be explained as one-way causation, in which behaviour is shaped and affected by environmental influences or inherent qualities or factors.

The social cognitive theory postulates that most external influences, such as consumption of media content, affect behaviour through cognitive processes rather than directly. Cognitive processes determine, to an extent, which external factors will be observed, what meaning will be derived from them, what behavioural effects they will have, what emotional impact they will have, and how the information they convey will be used (Bandura, 2001, p. 267). In summary, Bandura (2001) believes "unless people believe that they can produce desired effects and forestall undesired ones by their actions, they have little incentive to act" (p. 267). This implies that self-efficacy is the driving force that can determine whether one is affected negatively or positively by the media content one consumes as opposed to the direct effect propagated by the media effects theory. This argument presents two groups of people, namely passive and active media audiences. Passive audiences can easily be affected by the news they consume because they believe it without question. At the same time, the active group has the ability to question the news and then decide what to do with it.

The arguments presented earlier point to one thing, and that is that the way the media reported about the COVID-19 pandemic had the potential to cause psychological distress among various population groups. Therefore, the current study aimed to examine the psychological effects of COVID-19 information dissemination on people's emotional well-being in Malawi and how they reacted to the information.

Key informant interviews were conducted with editors and reporters from media houses across Malawi. Four people – two editors and two reporters – in each media outlet were interviewed. These were media personnel involved in conceiving, designing, producing, and disseminating COVID-19 news reports and programmes. These media personnel were drawn from the following media houses: *The Nation Newspaper* (national), *Daily Times* (national), MBC Radio 1 (national) and MBC Television (national), Times Television (national), Zodiak Radio Station (national), Lilanguka Community Radio, Mudzi Wathu Community Radio, Tuntufye Community Radio, Nkhotakota Community Radio, Mzimba Community Radio, and Gaka Community Radio. The study also conducted eight focus group discussions (FGDs) with community members across the country's three regions. The FGDs were conducted in Mangochi and Chiradzulu in the southern region, Salima and Mchinji in the central region, and Mzimba and Karonga in the northern region.

9.2 Initial Reaction to the News about COVID-19

In the initial stages of the pandemic, many people in Malawi thought that COVID-19 would not last for long and would not reach countries such as Malawi, but to everyone's surprise, the disease spread fast, and the death toll rose in the same fashion. Many people are still wondering about the disease because there has been no disease like this before in recent years. Very little information was available about the disease through the media, and a few people knew and understood it. One respondent in a focus group discussion said, "[a]t first, we took COVID-19 for granted, just like a hearsay, but later we started believing after officials raised our awareness and encouraged us to be wearing masks." The disease took everyone by surprise and destabilised people's daily living, which in itself, was a cause for concern. In their article, Moreno et al. (2020, p. 814) observe that the general public displayed "increased symptoms of depression, anxiety and stress related to COVID-19, as a result of psychological stressors such as life disruption, fear of illness, or fear of negative economic effects." A participant in one focus group discussion lamented:

> At first it reduced our affection for one another, people stopped greeting each other through the normal affectionate way of shaking hands and hugging; people could leave dead bodies alone in the vigil room/house,

and people stopped using public transport which led to loss of business for the vehicle owners.

The lack of contact with family members during the time of quarantine, failure to observe funeral rites and to properly mourn loved ones and accord them a dignified burial could have a long-lasting psychological effect on people's mental health and could be traumatising as well. News that the government was going to impose a lockdown was even worse. "It was like telling us to go and die in our homes," someone reported in a focus group discussion. This corresponds with what is available in the literature, namely that restrictive measures in the form of lockdowns, isolation, and quarantine have psychological effects on people's well-being and the way they respond to the pandemic itself (Taylor, 2019; Talevi et al., 2020; Brooks et al., 2020; Rubin, 2020). The restrictive measures were blamed for exacerbating the risk factors and causing adverse health behaviours among people (Tsao et al., 2021; Su et al., 2021). Similarly, research studies conducted in West Africa on psychological response to quarantine during the Ebola outbreak confirm that there was fear, anger, and anxiety-induced insomnia among the people (Talevi et al., 2020).

During the COVID-19 pandemic, many people lost their jobs or businesses, which had been their sole source of income, and this caused emotional stress not only among those directly affected but also for those who depended on them. Loss of one's job or business meant an increase in the unemployment rate, financial insecurity, and an inability to meet basic needs. According to Moreno et al. (2020, p. 813), "these economic factors can induce mental health problems in previously healthy people and negatively affect those with pre-existing mental disorders." The number of infected people and the death toll as a result of the disease was another major cause of emotional distress, as everyone thought that once they had been diagnosed with COVID-19, it would eventually lead to death, since there was no cure for it. Studies have shown that "seemingly endless newsfeeds related to Covid-19 infection and death rates could considerably increase the risk of mental health problems" (Su et al., 2021, p. 1). The rate at which people were dying and the speed with which the disease took away people's lives were so alarming that most people thought that the disease would not spare anyone. Fears of death of oneself or one's close relatives and friends were enough to trigger emotional distress and depression among the population. Many people came to know about all that was happening through the media, and it can be concluded that it was the information coming through the media about COVID-19 that was responsible for causing the mental distress.

Furthermore, during the initial stages of the pandemic, many people did not know how to differentiate COVID-19 or its main signs and symptoms from other diseases, especially respiratory diseases. Mere knowledge that one had signs and symptoms similar to those of COVID-19 was cause for anxiety and depression. Testing positive for COVID-19 was like getting a death sentence because in people's view, that meant that one was going to die, considering the fact that the disease had no cure and also looking at the high fatality rate attributed to it. For this reason, some people stopped going to the hospital to be treated for other illnesses or to access other health services for fear that they might end up being told that they were COVID-19 positive. For instance, one participant in a focus group discussion reported

> People stopped going to the hospital for fear that doctors would end up killing them because we have seen people who were strong but after going to the hospital, they were told that they had corona virus and then they died immediately.

It was also due to the same fears that some people refused to go for COVID-19 testing and also refused to receive the vaccine because they were afraid that they might end up being killed. According to Su et al. (2021, p. 2), there were "rumours circulating that hospitals were told to inflate covid cases so that the government can receive more funding from international bodies to assist with the fight against Covid-19." These rumours were also heard in Malawi. For instance, one participant reported

> There were stories going round [in social media] that health workers were getting allowances for every dead person who succumbed to COVID-19. So, it was like doctors were deliberately killing people so that they can get more allowances. For this reason, people stopped going to the hospital.

Such was one piece of misinformation that raised fears and caused stress in people. This is where the media needed to come in to quell such fake news and misinformation. However, as reported later, journalists, too, were as ignorant about the disease as everyone else was, and dispelling such news without valid facts was a challenge.

There was also hesitancy among some health experts in commenting on the disease. At the very beginning of the pandemic, some health experts had little information about the disease. They, too, relied on the international media before commenting on the pandemic. The same was the case with the vaccine. Journalists, too, did not have the right information with regard to the pandemic and the vaccine, and so they could not provide the correct information to the people. In other words, journalists' confidence levels in reporting about COVID-19 were low, and sources of information with regard to COVID-19 were limited. Journalists, therefore, had a difficult time getting the right information. Most media houses relied on information given by sponsors and donors through already produced programmes. Because of this, it was difficult to get feedback.

As if that was not enough of a problem, one journalist reported, "[t]here are too many jargons associated with COVID-19, which makes it difficult to dilute the message in such a way that the common man or woman may grasp the issues." The lack of adequate scientific knowledge about a pandemic, such as COVID-19, by journalists is risky and results in poor coverage of the disease and failure to inform the masses about preventive measures. Mach et al. (2021) observe that pandemic-related coverage with low scientific quality and which also fails to raise public awareness exacerbate public health effects of the disease. This could have psychological effects on people's decision-making processes, particularly when immediate solutions are needed but not enough information is given. Such reporting can also worsen the disease outcomes and cause unnecessary fear in relation to other factors that shape people's perceptions (Hoffman & Justicz, 2016; Laing, 2011). In times like these, people resort to any available channel that can fill the gap. Unfortunately, this is where social media came in. However, some social media sites have quality control limitations on what is published and, sometimes, the source.

That being the case, it was difficult to give feedback to the audience because the public was asking questions for which the reporters did not have the answers. The mere lack of information amidst a pandemic that threatened to wipe out a population had a lot of potential to cause panic, fear, mental distress, and impatience, as reported by the participants in this study. In one of the focus group discussions, a participant said, "[w]e were afraid because we were receiving news that once infected by COVID-19 virus, we would die very quickly." The fear factor created around the dissemination of COVID-19 messages was further exacerbated by the media's focus on negative news. Research studies on media effects have documented that negative news could result in mild to severe mental health problems among public members (Su et al., 2021). Audiences complained that the media were focusing too much on negative issues around COVID-19, much to the detriment of news focusing on prevention, raising hope, and the fight against the pandemic. The focus on negative news obscured the progress and other successes registered in the war against COVID-19. In relation to media effects, it has been argued, "the novelty of the virus has required the public to formulate new ideas and attitudes about the virus, which have taken shape in the context of the media messages one has been exposed to" (Dhanani & Franz, 2020, p. 64). Many people were exposed to negative news about COVID-19 in the media. By doing so, the media were constructing a social reality about the nature of the disease, which consequently created fears in the people.

The major theme emerging from the study was that during the initial period of COVID-19, communities experienced what they saw as contradictions and inconsistencies in COVID-19 information. For communities living in areas bordering Tanzania, this was particularly the case because of the stand taken by the former Tanzanian president, John Magufuli, who went against common knowledge on COVID-19. He believed and told Tanzanians that there was no such thing as COVID-19. A participant in a focus group discussion said,

We live near the border with Tanzania whose president [he late John Magufuli] believed and said it openly that there was no coronavirus. So,

it was difficult for us to believe that COVID-19 was real since our neigh-
bours never closed schools. So, we didn't believe the truth. In Tanzania,
the people were not observing the COVID-19 restrictions.

Malawians in these areas had access to Tanzanian media and, therefore, received
such contradictory messages. However, over time and because of increasing levels
of awareness, the information became more consistent. People's initial reactions
to news about COVID-19 generally centred on fear, panic, and apprehension.

It must also be pointed out that at the time of conducting this study
(March 2021), vaccines for COVID-19 had been developed, and countries,
including Malawi, were vaccinating their people. This was when Malawi was in
the third wave of the pandemic. The introduction of the COVID-19 vaccine
was met with mixed reactions from different groups of people. Some people
voluntarily received the jab while others hesitated until they had enough information, while yet others refused outright to receive the jab. The hesitancy
and refusal to receive the jab were due to the conspiracy theories circulating,
especially on social media, concerning COVID-19 and its vaccines.

9.3 Infodemics of COVID-19

At the time, various media houses were giving out conflicting and excessive
amounts of information (causing an infodemic) concerning the pandemic,
such that mitigating its effect was being made much more difficult. Infodemics have to do with the "purposeful spread of misinformation and disinformation via the media, particularly social media platforms" (Su et al., 2021,
p. 3). In this chapter, an infodemic refers to an overload of dangerous misinformation circulating around the COVID-19 pandemic. It further relates to
an overabundance of information (infodemics), some accurate and some not,
making it hard for people to find trustworthy sources and guidance. Usually, there is a wide range of topics on which misinformation and disinformation are based and disseminated via social media platforms, such as Twitter,
Facebook and WhatsApp – under the sponsorship of influential individuals
and groups – to achieve political and economic gains (Brennen et al., 2020).
In a situation like that, people may feel anxious, depressed, overwhelmed,
emotionally drained, and unable to meet important demands. According to
Buchanan et al. (2021), there is evidence suggesting that, in the initial stages
of the pandemic, many people were increasingly spending time searching for
COVID-19-related information as a result of being caught in a barrage of
unending negative news, arguing that such behaviour is a sign of poor mental health. When asked whether they felt that the information they received
about COVID-19 was too much, one participant had this to say, "[y]es, we
were overloaded with information. The information was too much and it was
scary." Receiving information that is too much, conflicting, and scary – all at
the same time and about a pandemic – could cause mental distress because of
failure to digest it and know what to believe.

Infodemics could derail government's efforts to curb the transmission of the disease and might ignite public fear and mistrust, which could result in serious personal and economic repercussions (Brennen et al., 2020; Orso et al., 2020). Another participant said, "[y]es, there were fears. Sometimes we just ignored the messages." Ignoring excessive and scary messages about COVID-19 should be seen as a coping or defence mechanism. When one cannot process all the messages being received and does not know who or what to believe, it is safe to ignore the messages or pretend that they are not true. This also points to the fact that in times of a pandemic, people select news that satisfies their need as postulated in the media effects theory. However, according to the social cognitive theory, "people typically avoid discomforting cognitive dissonance caused by information that is incompatible with their existing dispositions (e.g., beliefs, attitudes)" (Valkenburg et al., 2016, p. 321; see also Festinger, 1957). Talevi et al. (2020) provide different types of psychological reactions to pandemics, namely maladaptive behaviours, emotional distress, and defensive responses, such as anxiety, fear, frustration, loneliness, anger, boredom, depression, stress, and avoidance behaviours. Although it was difficult to tell what might have happened if one decided to ignore COVID-19 news (Su et al., 2021), ignoring COVID-19 infodemics should be looked at as a defensive mechanism or avoidance to reduce levels of stress and depression in difficult times, such as the pandemic. To avoid discomforting news or state of cognitive dissonance, people "actively seek information that reinforces their dispositions, and they avoid potentially contradictory information that would exacerbate dissonance" (Valkenburg et al., 2016, p. 321).

When probed on the kind of messages that were scary and raised fear, one participant responded, "we were scared because we heard that COVID-19 mostly affects old people and so, I was afraid that if my parents were to be found COVID-19 positive, they would die and leave us alone." Some of the information disseminated through the media was that older people – aged 50 and above – were at most risk of contracting COVID-19. These kinds of messages formed the basis of the fears that people had. Fear of losing loved ones, parents, relatives, or friends caused panic, uncertainty, and stress among the people, especially if the one affected was a breadwinner. The death of a breadwinner might mean a bleak future for those left behind, hence the fears.

9.4 Specific COVID-19 Information Received

From the FGDs, the COVID-19 information that participants had received centred on the following areas:

- nature, origins, causes, and transmission of COVID-19;
- preventive measures (e.g., washing of hands with soap, wearing masks, social distancing, isolation, quarantine);
- going to the hospital when one became sick;

- eating citrus fruits and other foods for prevention and treatment, such as oranges, lemons, ginger, and garlic;
- immunity boosters – as there was no specific cure or medicines for the disease, treatment was through addressing the known symptoms, such as cough and sore throat;
- old people were more likely to be attacked by COVID-19 than children; and
- people with known ailments, such as diabetes and HIV/AIDS could die quickly of COVID-19.

These responses from the participants show that many people were aware of the pandemic and ways of preventing its spread, which is another positive effect the media had on the people by raising their awareness to preventive measures. What made matters worse were the fake news and misinformation spread through social media, which many people tended to believe.

9.5 Myths and Misconceptions around COVID-19 Pandemic and COVID-19 Vaccine

The lack of correct information about COVID-19 and its vaccine resulted in a number of myths, misinformation, and disinformation, some of which were conflicting. Misinformation and fake news emerged as one of the major themes shaping the discourse on COVID-19. The discussion around COVID-19 misinformation focused mostly on the role of social media in spreading such information. With regard to media audiences, across all FGDs, participants said the major sources of misinformation were social media platforms and not the mainstream media. One participant had this to say:

> The media are playing their rightful role but it is social media which is misleading people. All the misinformation has been spread through WhatsApp, for example, news that one would die after one year of getting the vaccine. All this comes through social media and not the radio stations.

"When news is biased and misleading, the adverse effects of Covid-19 media coverage on personal and population health and wellbeing could be more pronounced" (Su et al., 2021, p. 3). Another participant said, "[s]ocial media, especially WhatsApp, was the main culprit in spreading misinformation; nevertheless, people believed what was circulating on it." This corroborates the postulates of media effects theory that people seek information to satisfy a particular need. However, in relation to excessive use of social media, it has been reported that its use could cause elevated psychological and social meltdown (Bollen & Gonçalves, 2018).

Some of the myths surrounding COVID-19 were, for instance, that COVID-19 was meant to reduce the world population; that men would become impotent and so women would not get pregnant; and that the population would be reduced by the year 2024. Buchanan et al. (2021, p. 2) remark, "individuals who reported spending more time consulting Covid-19 related news each day also reported higher levels of anxiety, distress, and depression." The myths about the COVID-19 vaccine that also created fear and psychological distress among the people were, among others,

- those who received the vaccine would die or be wiped out by 2024;
- COVID-19 could be spread through sexual intercourse;
- if you got vaccinated you were going to die within two years because vaccines were aimed at wiping out the population;
- vaccines were a satanic practice;
- one became impotent after being vaccinated;
- vaccines caused clotting of the blood; and
- only people aged 18 and above were eligible to receive the vaccines.

A respondent at an FDG in Mzuzu said this in relation to inconsistencies, "I didn't get vaccinated because there were rumours that once you get vaccinated you will not bear any children, and that the aim is to reduce the population."

Such myths and misinformation created anxiety among members of the general public, as they did not have anywhere to turn to for credible facts about the disease. This problem was exacerbated when sources of information were not available on time to give news, or were not open enough to provide accurate information. In such situations, people turned to social media to fill the gap but not without negative consequences. Social media were the major culprit spreading misinformation and fake news. Media attention was disproportionately skewed towards COVID-19 infodemics with little regard for its effects on people's mental health (Su et al., 2021). According to one reporter, fake news led to the citizenry's scepticism on anything to do with COVID-19, especially because people thought that COVID-19 was a social construction created by Western conspirators to decimate the African population. Any voice of reason from the media was quickly drowned out in waves of suspicion, and this negatively affected the role of the media in dissemination of COVID-19-related messages. Many people we interviewed reported that social media were responsible for increasingly spreading fake news, which was confusing them. The fake news was creating misconceptions that made people afraid of getting vaccinated. Social media were considered to have affected the fight against the spread of the disease negatively. In instances of receiving fake news and misinformation, people developed anxiety and fear because most of them believed the myth that COVID-19 vaccine was meant to wipe out the population, so they refused to be vaccinated.

Another respondent reported:

> There was also fear, especially when we thought of our children. We didn't want to leave them behind as orphans. They [the media] say that

children cannot die with the disease but that they can transmit it to adults who can die from it. This caused panic in us because we were afraid of dying and leaving our children behind as orphans.

Fears of becoming impotent upon receiving the COVID-19 vaccine were also commonplace because that is what was circulating in social media. Use of social media or accessing social media sites is not bad in itself, but media effects theory can explain its influence on people's mental attitude in terms of its excessive use, which resulted in spreading panic, fear, and misinformation during the COVID-19 pandemic. This also made people to fear COVID-19. A respondent in the focus group discussion said, "I didn't get vaccinated because there were rumours that once you get vaccinated you will not bear any children and that the aim is to reduce the population." Such rumours prevented some people from getting vaccinated because they were afraid that they would leave no offspring behind, and this fear was a major cause of hesitancy among the people to get vaccinated.

Furthermore, there was more information about COVID-19 circulating in the urban areas than in the rural areas. People in the rural areas were the ones who believed the fake news, myths, and misinformation about COVID-19 because of a lack of access to information. The pandemic was considered the disease of the urban area. However, people in the rural areas were dying from the disease without knowing.

One specific way to understand how the media have the ability to affect and influence the audience is by looking at how the media focus on the most salient aspect of the news. The results discussed previously can best be understood from that perspective. In view of the social cognitive theory and media effects theory, it has been argued that people tend to rely on the information they are most likely to recall through repeated messaging by the media, which reinforces chosen aspects of a topic (Happer & Philo, 2013). In so doing, the media exert sociocultural pressure on audiences to conform to the values, norms, or behaviours (Dhanani & Franz, 2020) disseminated, which causes mental disorders, especially when the news content is negative.

9.6 Conclusion

Based on the findings, it is clear that a wide range of information on COVID-19 was disseminated. The media disseminated both negative and positive stories about COVID-19. However, some of the information audiences received was from unreliable sources, such as social media, perpetuating fake news on COVID-19. Given the nature of the disease and its dramatic effect, people's reaction by displaying psychological disorders to information about COVID-19 was normal. Potentially, feelings of dying and leaving orphans behind could cause anxiety and mental distress in people, and this is what the current study has established. This was particularly the case when during the initial stages of COVID-19, information, knowledge, and awareness had not spread sufficiently enough. Most of the information that communities viewed as contradictions concerned the COVID-19 vaccines. As the results show, social media was the main source of inconsistencies in COVID-19 information. People's daily consumption of infodemics, misinformation, and disinformation and being distressed by it were caused by how the media paid particular attention to the negative aspects of the pandemic. This is understandable, given the nature of the disease and its dramatic effect. It was recommended that efforts to curb the disease should also be directed at dealing with mental health issues, and the media should also focus on raising hope and progress made in the fight against the pandemic instead of dwelling on negative news.

Although the mainstream media had been able to provide a broad range of information on COVID-19, more information could have helped to reinforce the messages and to address persistent knowledge gaps around some areas of the disease, thereby reducing the anxiety and mental distress from which people were suffering. Furthermore, most journalists in Malawi were not trained in reporting about pandemics. There was also a lack of specialisation. Those who were called health or science journalists were general reporters with minimal skills on issues of pandemics. The journalists needed more profound knowledge and understanding of the pandemic to enable them to report issues of importance to the layperson confidently. COVID-19, therefore, exposed the ill-preparedness of the media to report on pandemics.

References

Bandura, A. (2001). Social cognitive theory of mass communication. *Media Psychology*, *3*, 265–299.
Bollen, J., & Gonçalves, B. (2018). Network happiness: How online social interactions relate to our well-being. In S. Lehmann & Y.-Y. Ahn (Eds.), *Complex spreading phenomena in social systems* (pp. 257–268). Springer.
Brennen, J. S., Simon, F. M., Howard, P. N., & Nielsen, R. K. (2020). *Types, sources, and claims of Covid-19 misinformation* (Vol. 7, p. 3). Reuters Institute.
Brooks, S. K., Webster, R. K., Smith, L. E., Woodland, L., Wessely, S., Greenberg, N., & Rubin, G. J. (2020). The psychological impact of quarantine and how to reduce it: Rapid review of the evidence. *Lancet*, *395*, 912–920.
Buchanan, K., Aknin, L. B., Lotun, S., & Sandstrom, G. M. (2021). Brief exposure to social media during the COVID-19 pandemic: Doomscrolling has negative emotional consequences, but kindness-scrolling does not. *PLOS One*, *16*(10), e0257728. https://doi.org/10.1371/journal.pone.0257728
Cullen, W., Gulati, G., & Kelly, B. D. (2020). Mental health in the COVID-19 pandemic (commentary). *QJM: An International Journal of Medicine*, *113*(5), 311–312. https://doi.org/10.1093/qjmed/hcaa110
Cushion, S. (2019). The political impact of media. In J. Curran & D. Hesmondhalgh (Eds.), *Media and society* (6th ed., pp. 303–322). Bloomsbury. https://doi.org/10.5040/9781501340765.ch-016
Dearing, J., & Rogers, E. (1996). *Agenda-setting*. Sage.
Dhanani, L. Y., & Franz, B. (2020). The role of news consumption and trust in public health leadership in shaping Covid-19 knowledge and prejudice. *Frontiers in Psychology*, *11*, 63–75. https://doi.org/10.3389/fpsyg.2020.560828

Festinger, L. (1957). *A theory of cognitive dissonance.* Stanford University Press.

Fiske, S. T., & Taylor, S. E. (Eds.). (1991). *Social cognition* (2nd ed.). McGraw-Hill.

Hanson, R. (2009). *Mass communication: Living in a media world.* CQ Press.

Happer, C., & Philo, G. (2013). The role of the media in the construction of public belief and social change. *Journal of Social and Political Psychology, 1,* 321–336. https://doi.org/10.5964/jspp.v1i1.96

Hoffman, S. J., & Justicz, V. (2016). Automatically quantifying the scientific quality and sensationalism of news records mentioning pandemics: Validating a maximum entropy machine-learning model. *Journal of Clinical Epidemiology, 75,* 47–55. https://doi.org/10.1016/j.jclinepi.2015.12.010

Knobloch-Westerwick, S. (2015). *Choice and preference in media use.* Routledge.

Laing, A. (2011). The H1N1 crisis: Roles played by government communicators, the public and the media. *Journal of Professional Communication, 1,* 123–149. https://doi.org/10.15173/jpc.v1i1.88

Li, Y., Lin, Z., & Wu, Y. (2022). Exploring depression among the elderly during the Covid-19 pandemic: The effects of the big five, media use, and perceived social support. *International Journal of Environmental Research and Public Health, 19*(20), 1–12. https:// doi.org/10.3390/ijerph192013534

Lule, J. (2016). *Understanding media and culture: An introduction to mass communication.* University of Minnesota.

Mach, K. J., Reyes, R. S., Pentz, B., Taylor, J., Costa, C. A., Cruz, S. G., Thomas, K. E., Arnott, J. C., Donald, R., Jagannathan, K., Kirchhoff, C. J., Rosella, L. C & Klenk, N. (2021). News media coverage of COVID-19 public health and policy information. *Humanities and Social Sciences Communications, 8*(1), 1–11. https:// doi.org/10.1057/s41599-021-00900-z

McCombs, M. E., & Shaw, D. L. (1972). The agenda-setting function of mass media. *Public Opinion Quarterly, 36*(2), 176–187.

McLaughlin, C. J., & Sillence, E. (2018). Buffering against academic loneliness: The benefits of social media-based peer support during postgraduate study. *Active Learning in Higher Education, 19,* 1–14. https://doi.org/10.1177/146978741879 9185

Moreno, C., Wykes, T., Galderisi, S., Nordentoft, M., Crossley, N., Jones, N., Cannon, M., Correll, C. U., Byrne, L., Carr, S., Chen, E. Y. H., Gorwood, P., Johnson, S., Kärkkäinen, H., Krystal, J. H., Lee, J., Lieberman, J., López-Jaramillo, C., Männikkö, M., . . . Arango, C. (2020). How mental health care should change as a consequence of the COVID-19 pandemic. *Lancet Psychiatry, 7,* 813–824.

Muñiz-Velázquez, J. A., Gómez-Baya, D., & Lozano Delmar, J. (2021). Exploratory study of the relationship between happiness and the rise of media consumption during Covid-19 confinement. *Frontiers in Psychology, 12,* 146–155. https://doi.org/10.3389/fpsyg.2021.566517

Orso, D., Federici, N., Copetti, R., Vetrugno, L., & Bove, T. (2020). Infodemic and the spread of fake news in the COVID-19-era. *European Journal of Emergency Medicine, xxx.* https://doi.org/10.1097/MEJ.0000000000000713

Papacharissi, Z. (2009). Uses and gratifications. In D. Stacks & M. Salwen (Eds.), *An integrated approach to communication theory and research* (pp. 280–298). Routledge.

Preiss, R. W., Gayle, B. M., Burrell, N., Allen, M., & Bryant, J. (Eds.). (2007). *Mass media effects research: Advances through meta-analysis.* Erlbaum.

Primack, B. A., Shensa, A., Escobar-Viera, C. G., Barrett, E. L., Sidani, J. E., Colditz, J. B., & James, A. E. (2017). Use of multiple social media platforms and symptoms of depression and anxiety: A nationally-representative study among U.S. young adults. *Computers in Human. Behaviour*, *69*, 1–9. https://doi.org/10.1016/j. chb.2016.11.013

Reer, F., Tang, W. Y., & Quandt, T. (2019). Psychosocial well-being and social media engagement: The mediating roles of social comparison orientation and fear of missing out. *New Media and Society*, *21*, 1486–1505. https://doi.org/10.1177/1461444818823719

Rubin, J. G. (2020). The psychological effects of quarantining a city. *BMJ Journal*, *368*, m313.

Spiteri, J. (2021). Media bias exposure and the incidence of COVID-19 in the USA. *BMJ Global Health*, *6*, e006798. https://doi.org/10.1136/ bmjgh-2021–006798

Su, Z., McDonnell, D., Wen, J., Kozak, M., Abbas, J., Šegalo, S., Li, X., Ahmad, J., Cheshmehzangi, A., Cai, Y., Yang, L., & Xiang, Y. (2021). Mental health consequences of COVID-19 media coverage: The need for effective crisis communication practices. *Globalization and Health*, *17*(4) https://doi.org/10.1186/s12992-020-00654-4

Talevi, D., Socci, V., Carai, M., Carnaghi, G., Serena Faleri, S., Trebbi, E., Bernardo, A. D., & Capelli, F. (2020). Mental health outcomes of the COVID-19 pandemic. *Rivista di Psichiatria*, *55*(3), 137–144.

Taylor, S. (2019). *The psychology of pandemics: Preparing for the next global outbreak of infectious disease*. Cambridge Scholars Publishing.

Tsao, S., Chen, H., Tisseverasinghe, T., Yang, Y., Li, L., & Butt, Z. A. (2021). Public health measures: What social media told us in the time of COVID-19 – a scoping review. *Lancet Digital Health*, *3*, e175–e194. https://doi.org/10.1016/S2589-7500(20)30315-0

Valkenburg, P. M., Peter, J., & Walther, J. B. (2016). Media effects: Theory and research. *Annual Review of Psychology*, *67*, 315–338. https://doi.org/10.1146/annurev-psych-122414-033608

Van der Velden, P. G., Setti, I., Van der Meulen, E., & Das, M. (2019). Do social networking sites use predict mental health and sleep problems when prior problems and loneliness are taken into account? A population-based prospective study. *Computers in Human. Behaviour*, *93*, 200–209. https://doi.org/10.1016/j.chb.2018.11.047

Wathelet, M., Duhem, S., Vaiva, G., Baubet, T., Habran, E., Veerapa, E., Debien, C., Molenda, S., Horn, M., Grandgenèvre, P., Notredame, C. E., & D'Hondt, F. (2020). Factors associated with mental health disorders among university students in France confined during the COVID-19 pandemic. *JAMA Network Open*, *3*(10), e2025591. https://doi.org/10.1001/jamanetworkopen.2020.25591

World Health Organization. (2004). *Promoting mental health: Concepts, emerging evidence, practice* (Summary Report). World Health Organization.

Zhan, L., Sun, Y., Wang, N., & Zhang, X. (2016). Understanding the influence of social media on people's life satisfaction through two competing explanatory mechanisms. *Aslib Journal of Information Management*, *68*, 347–361. https://doiorg/10.1108/ajim-12-2015-0195

Zhou, W., Wang, A, Xia, F., Xiao, Y., & Tang, S. (2020). Effects of media reporting on mitigating spread of COVID-19 in the early phase of the outbreak. *Mathematical Biosciences and Engineering*, *17*(3), 2693–2707. https://doi.org/10.3934/mbe.2020147

Part 3

From Confusion to Anxiety

10 Proliferation and Impacts of Health Misinformation on Social Media During COVID-19 in Kenya

Hellen Jepkemoi Magut and Richard Guto

10.1 Introduction

COVID-19 has been viewed in different contexts by different people – often due to misinformation. Many people received much information about COVID-19 from various media, some false information that misled them. Misinformation is bound to be introduced by many agencies, such as individuals, media news, gossip, and works of fiction. Misinformation spreads faster and more profoundly than factual information, and it causes significant crises in many setups, the health sector not excluded. Nyhan and Reifler (2010) remark that misinformation is incorrect information without scientific proof or evidence and can be passed on through different modes of communication. However, sometimes misinformation may continue without contradicting the factual information (Kata, 2010). Some accurate or untruthful phenomena can be changed within the logical environment with proof and accord from experts or researchers (Vraga & Bode, 2020). Scholars have also attempted to distinguish between misinformation, misperception, and disinformation. According to Southwell et al. (2018), misperception is holding a belief that is incorrect or false, whereas disinformation is driven by the intention to deceive (see Wardle, 2017), while misinformation is passing on false information through various media, which can be deliberate or unintentional (Southwell et al., 2018).

The COVID-19 epidemic has posed an unmatched threat to humanity's overall welfare. Countless people rely on the Internet to gain some health information to learn more about safeguarding themselves and their households from the impending health hazard. COVID-19 was a novel case of disease, and due to its uniqueness, it was necessary to know its originality (Bento et al., 2020; Garfin, 2020). There are numerous sources of false data about the prevention of COVID-19 and therapy circulating on the Internet, but these sources must be supported by scientific proof. This concept is crucial since depending on unreliable information could cause harmful health and encourage the public to participate in futile and harmful activities.

DOI: 10.4324/9781003425861-13

Amidst the outbreak of infectious diseases, there is a high likelihood of misinformation, for instance,

[A] Zika virus study established that half of the top 10 news items were grounded on false information or gossip and that those stories were three times more likely to be shared on social mass media than ones grounded on truths.

(Sommariva et al., 2018, p. 3)

False materials were tweeted and accessed more frequently than information backed by science or created by public health professionals, according to other studies on COVID-19 (Bridgman et al., 2020).

The emergence of COVID-19 has seen the spread of information revolving around its causes and treatment, leading to misinformation. Since the outbreak of COVID-19, much information has been generated and disseminated to the extent that one can no longer differentiate true from false information. COVID-19 misinformation has affected healthcare systems and services globally. In Kenya, COVID-19 health misinformation created challenges for health systems and the provision of health services. Because of the vast amount of information obtained online, many Kenyans were reluctant to take up the COVID-19 vaccination and, more so, avoided visiting healthcare systems for medical assistance. In attempts to treat COVID-19, people have been found taking self-made medication that had not been tested medically. Different people put forward several myths, primarily through social media platforms, on who was behind COVID-19, how it spread, and how to cure it. The increase in misinformation about COVID-19 necessitated the technical communication and social media teams of the World Health Organization (WHO) to work together to track and respond to these myths and rumours. According to Swire-Thompson and Lazer (2019), misinformation is information that goes against the principles of a scientific community relating to an occurrence.

Swire-Thompson and Lazer (2019) further indicate that the Internet is a powerful instrument for learning about health, and much information is passed through various podiums, such as Facebook, WhatsApp, and Twitter. Unfortunately, some of this information is inaccurate; hence, people get misinformed. The Director-General of the WHO, Tedros Adhanom Ghebreyesus, indicated that the COVID-19 pandemic went through an infodemic of misinformation (The Lancet Infectious Diseases, 2020). Infodemic implies an information epidemic (Barua et al., 2020). In addition, health workers have also noted that much information about COVID-19 was being produced and consumed at an alarming rate on social media, and instances of false information were heavily documented.

The COVID-19 pandemic was associated with an infodemic. In addition to Barua et al.'s (2020) definition, an infodemic is seen as a situation where false information spreads rapidly through various online sites, such as Facebook, Twitter, WhatsApp, and others. The continuous spreading of unverified information over these platforms caused health crises. This agrees with a publication by Park Chan-Kyong (2020), which indicated that a church in Gyeonggi Province in Indonesia sprayed saltwater into the mouths of Christians, believing it would kill COVID-19. Still, many people contracted the disease in the process because the same bottle was used.

Misinformation further resulted in stigmatisation, fear, and even death. The spread of false information about COVID-19 instilled fear of contracting the disease, misconceptions, and myths about the virus. In Kenya, responses to COVID-19, such as restriction of movements and the fear of contracting the disease in healthcare facilities, led to people avoiding preventive visits to healthcare systems, affecting healthcare services (Kiarie et al., 2022).

Misinformation contributed to detrimental effects on healthcare systems and services use during the COVID-19 pandemic. Therefore, healthcare practitioners faced competition from the Internet to provide accurate information about COVID-19. The mission of the Ministry of Health in Kenya is to build a sustainable healthcare system that will ensure the attainment of the highest standards of healthcare services for all Kenyans. However, due to misinformation during COVID-19, this objective was not attained, as many people feared visiting healthcare systems. Healthcare systems were assumed to be the hot spots for contracting the virus (Ng'ang'a, 2021). In addition, health workers too feared handling patients because of a lack of personal protective equipment. This led to the referral of patients from lower-level facilities to higher-level facilities; hence, congesting these and ultimately affecting service delivery. Besides, information on social media about COVID-19 and vaccine uptake was not filtered and contributed to vaccine hesitancy among people (Shah et al., 2022). This issue of misinformation was a concern for the Ministry of Health in Kenya. The then cabinet secretary in charge of health in Kenya, Mutahi Kagwe, indicated that lies and half-truths made people fear attending hospitals. He made those remarks during the UNESCO webinar conference on 26 May 2021. He pointed out that such misinformation made it difficult for healthcare providers to monitor and manage diseases, including cancer, diabetes, hypertension, and other non-communicable diseases (NCDs). The health cabinet secretary lamented that misinformation is a monstrous enemy that threatens to undermine progress made in the health sector in Africa and, more critically, on providing healthcare services in Kenya during the pandemic. This study, therefore, explored the effects of online misinformation on the healthcare systems and services in Kenya.

The study used a systematic literature review of publications on the effects of online misinformation during the COVID-19 pandemic. The articles reviewed were from Google Scholar, Emerald Insight, Taylor and Francis, the Wiley Online Library, and the EBSCOhost research database. The targeted articles were published in September 2021 and September 2022. Similar keywords were used across all the databases. The keywords used were "online misinformation," "COVID-19 and health services," "COVID-19 and healthcare systems," and "COVID-19 and Kenya." The five databases were chosen because they allowed the researchers to find articles that would inform the current study, find conference proceedings, reports, and even grey literature. Using the keywords mentioned earlier, 78 articles were identified. After removing duplicates and reviewing abstracts for relevance, the researchers assessed the selected articles for inclusion in the systematic review process. A total of 23 articles were found relevant to address the objectives of the current study.

10.2 Sources of COVID-19 Information Disorders

From the data collected, several results were found on COVID-19 and online misinformation and how this has affected healthcare services and systems. The results from the 23 articles indicated that various social media tools were used by citizens to spread false information during the COVID-19 pandemic. False information on social media was spread faster, deeper, and wider than true information, and was often one of the most popular social media posts. Chuai and Zhao (2022) note that surprise and anger spreads faster among people than regular content. This kind of viral information is realised during times of pandemic, such as diseases and economic crises. A study on the use of Twitter for communication showed that when a message contained immoral and emotional words, the penetration rate increased by 20% for each additional word (Guarino et al., 2020).

The reviewed literature revealed that the digital era not only radically sped up the distribution and dissemination of information but also exposed human beings to all sorts of information disorders both solicited and unsolicited from varied sources. The information explosion has made it difficult for the general public to find original sources and reliable guidance when required, especially during the COVID-19 pandemic period (World Health Organization & Pan American Health Organization, 2020).

The findings of the study indicated that social media was used during the COVID-19 pandemic to spread misinformation. This agrees with the analysed literature where social media emerged as the main source of the information disorder. According to Dizikes (2018), incorrect information is prevalent on social media because it is simple to produce and propagate. Sharing false information is now commonplace and has increased the spread of inaccurate medical information (Perakslis & Califf, 2019). Further, according to Sharma et al. (2017), false posts are always more popular than those that share pertinent and correct public health information regarding a particular disease. Conspiracy theories about COVID-19, therefore, abounded despite being debunked over and over by legitimate information providers.

The analysis of the data provided evidence of social media tools as sources of misinformation. The findings of all the selected and reviewed articles agreed on social media being the source of misinformation. The current study, therefore, agrees with previous findings that social media tools play a role as sources of information disorder. During the pandemic, social media sites, such as Facebook, Twitter, and WhatsApp were crucial sources for gathering and dissemination of information. Because of this, the use of social media platforms has expanded globally by 20%–87% (Bruno Kessler Foundation, 2020).

The top social media sites for monitoring false information and debunking rumours have been identified as Facebook, Twitter, and online newspapers. In a survey conducted in March by the Illinois Centre for Health Information (Illinois, 2022), the terms "coronavirus," "COVID-19," and "pandemic" were found to have been used in around 550 million tweets. The study found that the volume of tweets increased exponentially around the start of the Italian lockdown and peaked around the time the United States declared the pandemic a national emergency. Of the tweets, 35% originated in the United States, followed by the United Kingdom (7%), Brazil (6%), Spain (5%). and India (4%). This indicates that online unproven information is on the rise. This poses a danger to the dissemination of correct information on health-related matters to the public. From the reviewed articles, the authors conclude that there is a need for further studies on social media and the role they play in spreading misinformation, and to identify best practices that would control the kind of information shared through social media. If social media are used correctly to provide the right COVID-19 information, then healthcare systems would not face stiff competition from the Internet; on the contrary, people would not be hesitant to seek healthcare services from various healthcare systems (Roozenbeek et al., 2020).

10.3 Effects of Health-Related Misinformation

Five of the reviewed articles presented evidence of negative effects of health-related misinformation. Some of these negative effects were linked to resistance to COVID-19 vaccination, stress and mental health problems, isolation, misinterpretation of information, misplaced health resources, fear and panic, and a lack of trust in health providers and systems.

Amidst the COVID-19 pandemic, people all over the world were exposed to various types of information, such as news, research, opinions, myths, rumours, and infographics about COVID-19. While information was supposed to help people know about the disease and how to prevent it, the vast amounts of information led to confusion, stigmatisation, isolation, and even harassment. Since COVID-19 is a new disease, much research is still going on, and major changes are expected in the health sector in terms of public health recommendations and patient assessment. The findings of the five reviewed articles indicated that there is a lack of clarity on who is responsible for health-related misinformation, and the specific strategies to be put in place to curb such misinformation. Without clarity of information, it becomes difficult for people to understand COVID-19 as a disease, ways to minimise its spreading, which source of information to trust, and where to get help in case of attacks. With all this information emanating from diverse sources, people have been misinformed. They have received false health information, resulting in major effects in the health sector comprising healthcare providers, the facilities themselves, and other frontline workers in the medical field. More so, health emergencies have posed challenges in the provision of healthcare services, hence increasing death rates during the COVID-19 pandemic.

In agreement with the reviewed literature is the study of De Figueiredo et al. (2020) which found that there is well-documented evidence of COVID-19 vaccine resistance all over the world. Because of the resistance, reaching the necessary immunisation levels were not to be taken for granted. Resistance is driven by online and offline misinformation questioning the necessity, safety, and effectiveness of vaccinations (Bellaby, 2003). Much false information about the pandemic has been shared on social media, including that the virus is connected to 5G mobile networks.

An analysis of the effects of health-related misinformation revealed an urgent need to build resilient healthcare systems that will holistically meet the healthcare needs of all citizens by not only providing healthcare services but also by acting as frontlines in providing the right information to all people. During the COVID-19 pandemic, death rates increased due to a lack of the right information. The inadequacy of the right information resulted in hesitancy to receiving COVID-19 vaccines, and a lack of trust in healthcare providers and systems. As a result, some people were mentally affected.

In addition, the study found that online health misinformation has an impact on psychological and mental disorder in people. This was the result of the financial and economic crisis, fear of the unknown, and anxiety. The introduction of lockdown brought about psychological disorder, since many people could not continue with their usual chores. In addition, isolated and quarantined people relied on social media for information on COVID-19, such as its treatment and remedies. Some of the information consumed in the process induced fear, anxiety, and stress, leading to psychological and mental disorders.

10.4 Measures to Minimise Health-Related Misinformation During a Pandemic

One of the main reasons for increased health-related misinformation surrounding COVID-19 is that the disease was unknown, and many facts about it were not known. As such, everyone was trying to come up with possible ways of treatment based on unproved facts. All the reviewed articles presented some measures, such as

- policymakers and social media administrators should consider targeted interventions to curb the spread of COVID-19 misinformation (Office of the Assistant Secretary for Planning and Evaluation, 2022);
- health practitioners should utilise digital health approaches and not underestimate the role of social media in circulating unproven information;
- stakeholders within the health sector need to be trained on health-related fake news; and
- health misinformation needs to be taken into consideration to minimise its effects on people (Banerjee & Meena, 2021).

In addition to the measures presented in the reviewed articles, the World Health Assembly held in May 2020 passed resolutions on COVID-19 health misinformation (WHO, 2020a). The resolutions emphasised the need to control misinformation during the COVID-19 pandemic. Member states were called upon to provide reliable information about COVID-19 and to control digital technologies used to pass information. The WHO also emphasised the need to prevent harmful digital activities that would undermine factual health responses. Further, states, countries, multinational organisations, and individuals were asked to join forces to create strong actions to manage misinformation (WHO, 2020a)

Several agencies, such as government, public health practitioners, mass media, and health systems should come together to ensure provision of reliable information to the public. The government of Kenya should launch platforms where people can report, verify, and get information. Moreover, the public need to be informed about reliable information and from which sources to get this information. Such credible sources can be published on the websites of the Kenyan Ministry of Health and the WHO. In addition, the public need to be made aware of the effects of consuming fake information regarding their health, especially during pandemics such as COVID-19. That way people will be keen to use the correct information they obtain and can rely on the sources of such information. However, of importance is to give healthcare systems an opportunity to provide health information without interference from social media and mass media. Such opportunities will enable healthcare systems to thrive, as many people seek healthcare services.

10.5 Conclusion

Social media are not only posing serious problems for healthcare systems around the world, but they are also giving rise to a profusion of myths, hoaxes, and incorrect information about the aetiology, symptoms, causes, prevention, and treatment of COVID-19. By disseminating false information, the use of healthcare systems and utilisation of healthcare services are being affected. The reluctance to seek medical advice made the virus spread faster and ultimately harmed people's physical and mental health. In addition, the emergence of COVID-19 was a shock to everyone, and this contributed to a decline in the number of people seeking medical attention. This move had a significant negative effect on healthcare systems and services. For many people, the fear of contracting the disease caused them to avoid visiting healthcare systems, and for some people, restrictions put forward by the government prevented them from visiting healthcare facilities.

The study concluded that social media were sources of information disorder during the COVID-19 pandemic. Social media brought more harm than good, and proper control measures on information dissemination through social media should be put in place. The major organs to ensure control are healthcare systems, the Ministry of Health, private organisations, individuals, and government. If stringent measures are put in place and those found sending fake information punished, credible information is likely to exist. Further, it is possible to minimise misinformation through enactment of policies to streamline misinformation. Finally, if misinformation around COVID-19 is tamed, healthcare systems will fully provide their services to the public, hence reducing death rates during pandemics.

References

Ahmed, W., Vidal-Alaball, J., Downing, J., & Seguí, F. L. (2020). COVID-19 and the 5G conspiracy theory: Social network analysis of Twitter data. *Journal of Medical Internet Research*, *22*(5), e19458. https://doi.org/10.2196/19458.

Altmann, D. M., Douek, D. C., & Boyton, R. J. (2020). What policymakers need to know about COVID-19 protective immunity. *Lancet*, *395*, 1527–1529.

Avram, M., Micallef, N., Patil, S., & Menczer, F. (2020, July 28). Exposure to social engagement metrics increases vulnerability to misinformation. *Harvard Kennedy School Misinformation Review*, *1*. https://doi.org/10.37016/mr-2020-033.

Banerjee, D., & Meena, K. S. (2021). COVID-19 as an "infodemic" in public health: Critical role of the social media. *Frontiers in Public Health*, *9*, 1–8. https://doi.org/10.3389/fpubh.2021.610623

Barua, Z., Barua, S., Aktar, S., Kabir, N., & Li, M. (2020). Effects of misinformation on COVID-19 individual responses and recommendations for the resilience of disastrous consequences of misinformation. *Progress in Disaster Science*, *8*. https://doi.org/10.1016/j.pdisas.2020.100119

BBC News. (2021, August 12 day). "Hundreds dead" because of Covid-19 misinformation. *BBC News*. www.bbc.com/news/world-53755067.

Bellaby, P. (2003). Communication and miscommunication of risk: Understanding UK parents' attitudes to combined MMR vaccination. *BMJ Journal*, *327*, 725–728.

Bento, A. I., Nguyen, T., Wing, C., Lozano-Rojas, F., Ahn, Y. Y., & Simon, K. (2020). Evidence from internet search data shows information-seeking responses to news of local COVID-19 cases. *Proceedings of the National Academy of Sciences of the United States of America*, *117*(21), 2–4. https://doi.org/10.1073/pnas.2005335117

Bin Naeem, S., Bhatti, R., & Khan, A. (2021). An exploration of how fake news is taking over social media and putting public health at risk. *Health Information and Libraries Journal*, *38*(2), 143–149. https://doi.org/10.1111/hir.12320.

Bin Naeem, S., & Kamel Boulos, M. N. (2021). COVID-19 misinformation online and health literacy: A brief overview. *International Journal of Environmental Research and Public Health*, *18*, 15. https://doi.org/10.3390/ijerph18158091.

Bridgman, A., Merkley, E., Loewen, P. J., Owen, T., Ruths, D., Teichmann, L., & Zhilin, O. (2020, June 18). The causes and consequences of COVID-19 misperceptions: Understanding the role of news and social media. *Harvard Kennedy School Misinformation Review*, *1*(3). https://doi.org/10.37016/mr-2020-028

Bruno Kessler Foundation. (2020). *COVID-19 and fake news in the social media*. www.fbk.eu/en/press-releases/covid-19-and-fake-news-in-the-social-media/

Center for Preparedness and Response. (2020). Responding to rumours and misinformation. *The American Journal of Tropical Medicine and Hygiene*. https://doi.org/10.4269/ajtmh.20-0812

Chan-kyong, P. (2020, March 16). Coronavirus: Saltwater spray infects 46 churchgoers in South Korea. *Health & Environment News*. www.scmp.com/week-asia/health-environment

Chuai, Y., & Zhao, J. (2022). Anger can make fake news viral online. *Frontiers in Physics*, *10*, 1–12. https://doi.org/10.3389/fphy.2022.970174

The COVID-19 infodemic. (2020). *The Lancet Infectious Diseases*, *20*(8), 875. https://doi.org/10.1016/S1473-3099(20)30565-X

Cuan-Baltazar, J. Y., Muñoz-Perez, M. J., Robledo-Vega, C., Pérez-Zepeda, M. F., & SotoVega, E. (2020). Misinformation of COVID-19 on the Internet: Infodemiology study. *JMIR Public Health and Surveillance*, *6*(2), 1–9. https://doi.org/10.2196/18444.

De Figueiredo, A., Simas, C., Karafllakis, E., Paterson, P., & Larson, H. J. (2020). Mapping global trends in vaccine confidence and investigating barriers to vaccine uptake: A large-scale retrospective temporal modeling study. *Lancet*, *396*, 898–908.

Dizikes, P. (2018, March 8). On Twitter, false news travels faster than true stories. *MIT News*. https://news.mit.edu/2018/study-twitter-false-news-travels-faster-true-stories-0308

Fleming, N. (2020). Coronavirus misinformation, and how scientists can help to fight it. *Nature*, *583*(7814), 155–156. https://doi.org/10.1038/d41586-020-01834-3.

Garfin, D. R. (2020). Technology as a coping tool during the coronavirus disease 2019 (COVID-19) pandemic: Implications and recommendations. *Stress and Health*, *36*(4), 555–559. https://doi.org/10.1002/smi.2975

Guarino, S., Trino, N., Celestini, A., Chessa, A., & Riotta, G. (2020). Characterising networks of propaganda on twitter: A case study. *Applied Network Science*, *5*(1), 1–22. https://doi.org/10.1007/s41109-020-00286-y

Han, Q., Zheng, B., Cristea, M., Agostini, M., Belanger, J. J., Gutzkow, B., & Kreienkamp, J. (2021). Trust in government regarding COVID-19 and its associations with preventive health behavior and prosocial behavior during the pandemic: A cross-sectional and longitudinal study. *Psychological Medicine*, *53*(1), 149–159. https://doi.org/10.1017/S0033291721001306.

Illinois Center for Health Information. (2022). *Covid-19 briefing* (Covid-19 Briefing Series). University of Illinois.

International Telecommunication Union. (2020). *Measuring digital development: Facts and figures 2020*. www.itu.int/en/ITU-D/Statistics.

Islam, M. S., Sarkar, T., Khan, S. H., Kamal, A. H. M., Murshid Hasan, S. M., Kabir, A., Yeasmin, D., Islam, M. A., Chowdhury, K. I. A., Anwar, K. S., Chughtai, A. A., & Seale, H. (2020). COVID-19-related infodemic and its impact on public health: A global social media analysis. *American Journal of Tropical Medicine and Hygiene*, *103*(4), 1621–1629. https://doi.org/10.4269/ajtmh.20-0812.

Joshi, A., Sparks, R., Karimi, S., Yan, S.-L. J., Chughtai, A. A., Paris, C., & Macintyre, R. (2020). Automated monitoring of tweets for early detection of the 2014 Ebola epidemic. *PLOS One*, *15*(3), e0230322. https://doi.org/10.1371/journal.pone.0230322.

Kata, A. (2010). A postmodern Pandora's box: Anti-vaccination misinformation on the Internet. *Vaccine*, *28*(7), 1709–1716. https://doi.org/10.1016/j.vaccine.2009.12.022

Kiarie, H., Temmerman, M., Nyamai, M., Liku, N., Thuo, W., Oramisi, V., Nyaga, L., Karimi, J., Wamalwa, P., Gatheca, G., Mwenda, V., Ombajo, L. A., Thumbi, S. M., Cosmas, L., Kiarie, J., Soe, K., Munyao, O., Gathiti, Z., Maina, L., . . . Gitau, S. (2022). The COVID-19 pandemic and disruptions to essential health services in Kenya: A retrospective time-series analysis. *The Lancet Global Health*, *10*(9), e1257–e1267. https://doi.org/10.1016/S2214-109X(22)00285-6

Kickbusch, I., Pelikan, J. M., Apfel, F., & Tsouros, A. D. (2013). *Health literacy: The solid facts*. WHO Regional Office for Europe. https://apps.who.int/iris/bitstream/handle/10665/128703/e96854.pdf.

Lewandowsky, S., & Cook, J. (2020). *The conspiracy theory handbook*. George Mason University Center for Climate Change Communication. www.climatechangecommunication.org/conspiracy-theory-handbook/.

Megha, S. (2017). Zika virus pandemic: Analysis of Facebook as a social media health information platform. *American Journal of Infection Control, 45*(3), 301–302. https://doi.org/10.1016/j.ajic.2016.08.022.

Ng'ang'a, T. K. (2021). *Impact of COVID-19 measures on Kenya's health system* (African Economic Research Consortium Working Paper COVID-19 012). http://publication.aercafricalibrary.org/handle/123456789/2873

Nsoesie, E. O., & Oladeji, O. (2020, April 27). Identifying patterns to prevent the spread of misinformation during epidemics. *Harvard Kennedy School Misinformation Review*. https://doi.org/10.37016/mr-2020-014.

Nyhan, B., & Reifler, J. (2010). When corrections fail: The persistence of political misperceptions. *Political Behavior, 32*(2), 303–330. https://doi.org/10.1007/s11109-010-9112-2

Office of the Assistant Secretary for Planning and Evaluation. (2022). *Impact of the COVID-19 pandemic on the hospital and outpatient clinician workforce: Challenges and policy responses* (Issue Brief No. HP-2022-13, pp. 1–27). ASPE. https://aspe.hhs.gov/sites/default/files/migrated_legacy_files//196851/COVIDNH.

Office of the Surgeon General. (2021). *Confronting health misinformation: The U.S. surgeon general's advisory on building a healthy information environment*. US Department of Health and Human Services.

Osakwe, Z. T., & Cortés, Y. I. (2021). Impact of COVID-19: A text mining analysis of Twitter data in the Spanish language. *Hispanic Health Care International, 19*(4), 239–245. https://doi.org/10.1177/15404153211020453.

Pennycook, G., McPhetres, J., Zhang, Y., Lu, J. G., & Rand, D. G. (2020). Fighting COVID-19 misinformation on social media: Experimental evidence for a scalable accuracy-nudge intervention. *Psychological Science, 31*(7), 770–780. https://doi.org/10.1177/0956797620939054.

Perakslis, E., & Califf, R. M. (2019). Employ cybersecurity techniques against the threat of medical misinformation. *JAMA, 322*(3), 207–208. https://doi.org/10.1001/jama.2019.6857

Rootman, I., & Gordon-El-Bihbety, D. (2008). *A vision for a health literate Canada*. www.cpha.ca/sites/default/files.

Roozenbeek, J., Schneider, C. R., Dryhurst, S., Kerr, J., Freeman, A. L. J., Recchia, G., Van der Bles, A. M., & Van der Linden, S. (2020). Susceptibility to misinformation about COVID-19 around the world: Susceptibility to COVID misinformation. *Royal Society Open Science, 7*(10), 2–15. https://doi.org/10.1098/rsos.201199

Sanche, S., Lin, Y. T., Xu, C., Romero-Severson, E., Hengartner, N., & Ke, R. (2020). High contagiousness and rapid spread of severe acute respiratory syndrome coronavirus2. *Emerging Infectious Diseases, 26*(7), 1470–1477. https://doi.org/10.3201/eid2607.200282.

Sandada, M., & Kambarami, P. (2016). The determinants of the compliance to public procurement policy requirements among public enterprises in Zimbabwe. *Acta Universitatis Danubius, Administratio, 8*(1), 2–15.

Selden, C. R., Zorn, M., Ratzan, S., & Parker, R. M. (2000). *Health literacy*. National Institutes of Health, US Department of Health and Human Services. www.ruhruni-bochum.de/healthliteracy/NIHhliteracy.pdf.

Shah, J., Abeid, A., Sharma, K., Manji, S., Nambafu, J., Korom, R., Patel, K., Said, M., Mohamed, M. A., Sood, M., Karani, V., Kamandi, P., Kiptinness, S., Rego, R. T., Patel, R., Shah, R., Talib, Z., & Ali, S. K. (2022). Perceptions and knowledge towards COVID-19 vaccine hesitancy among a subpopulation of adults in Kenya: An English survey at six healthcare facilities. *Vaccines, 10*(5), 1–15. https://doi. org/10.3390/vaccines10050705

Sharma, M., Yadav, K., Yadav, N., & Ferdinand, K. C. (2017). Zika virus pandemic: Analysis of Facebook as a social media health information platform. *American Journal of Infection Control, 45*(3), 301–302. https://doi.org/10.1016/j.ajic.2016.08.022

Silverman, C. (2016, November 17). This analysis shows how viral fake election news stories outperformed real news on Facebook. *BuzzFeed News*. www.buzzfeednews. com/article.

Sommariva, S., Vamos, C., Mantzarlis, A., Đào, L. U.-L., & Martinez Tyson, D. (2018). Spreading the (fake) news: Exploring health messages on social media and the implications for health professionals using a case study. *American Journal of Health Education, 49*(4), 246–255. https://doi.org/10.1080/1932503 7.2018.1473178

Southwell, B. G., Thorson, E. A., & Sheble, L. (2018). Misinformation among mass audiences is a focus for inquiry. In B. G. Southwell, E. A. Thorson, & L. Sheble (Eds.), *Misinformation and mass audiences* (pp. 1–14). University of Texas Press.

Srijan, K., & Neil, S. (2018, April). *False information on web and social media: A survey* (p. 35). https://arxiv.org/pdf/1804.08559.pdf.

Suarez-Lledo, V., & Alvarez-Galvez, J. (2021). Prevalence of health misinformation on social media: Systematic review. *Journal of Medical Internet Research, 23*(1), 2–17. https://doi.org/10.2196/17187.

Swire-Thompson, B., & Lazer, D. (2019). Public health and online misinformation: Challenges and recommendations. *Annual Review of Public Health, 41*, 433–451. https://doi.org/10.1146/annurev-publhealth-040119-094127

Tan, S. S., & Goonawardene, N. (2017). Internet health information seeking and the patient-physician relationship: A systematic review. *Journal of Medical Internet Research, 19*(1), e9. https://doi.org/10.2196/jmir.5729.

Vraga, E. K., & Bode, L. (2020). Defining misinformation and understanding its bounded nature: Using expertise and evidence for describing misinformation. *Political Communication, 37*(1), 136–144. https://doi.org/10.1080/10584609.20 20.1716500

Wardle, C. (2017, February 17). Fake news: It's complicated. *Medium*. https:// medium.com/1st-draft/fakenews-its-complicated-d0f77376

Wardle, C., & Derakhshan, H. (2017). *Information disorder: Toward an interdisciplinary framework for research and policymaking*. Council of Europe.

World Health Organization. (1980). WHO guideline. *Food and Nutrition Bulletin, 2*(1). https://doi.org/10.1177/156482658000200103.

World Health Organization. (2019). *Ebola virus disease – Democratic Republic of the Congo*. www.who.int/csr/don/28-november-2019-ebola-drc/en/.

World Health Organization. (2020a). *Coronavirus disease 2019 (COVID-19) situation report 13*. www.who.int/emergencies/diseases/novel-coronavirus-2019

World Health Organization. (2020b). *Managing the COVID-19 infodemic: Promoting healthy behaviours and mitigating the harm from misinformation and disinformation*. www.who.int/news/item/23-09-2020

World Health Organization, & Pan American Health Organization. (2020). *Understanding the infodemic and misinformation in the fight against COVID-19.*

Digital Transformation Toolkit. https://iris.paho.org/bitstream/handle/10665.2/52052/Factsheet-infodemic_eng.pdf

Yusuf, I., Adam, R., Ahmad, S., & Yee, P. (2014). Ebola and compliance with infection prevention measures in Nigeria. *The Lancet Infectious Diseases, 14*(11), 1045–1046. https://doi.org/10.1016/s1473-3099(14)70954-5.

Zarocostas, J. (2020). How to fight an infodemic. *Lancet, World Report, 395*(10225), 676. https://doi.org/10.1016/S0140-636(20)30461-X.

11 African Hybridity, Information, and Psychological Distress During COVID-19

Joshua Isaac Kumwenda

11.1 Introduction

In its long history, Africa has reportedly experienced a series of pandemics – ranging from leprosy to smallpox, measles, polio, Ebola, AIDS, and COVID-19. In their encounter with each pandemic, the reactions of black Africans and their fight against the pandemics have always been affected by their unique sense of being, which in this chapter is referred to as "Africanness" or "black African hybridity." In their encounter with COVID-19 around 2020 to 2022, when this pandemic was at its peak, for example, Africanness emerged as one of the aspects that either impeded the fight against COVID-19 or made it more accessible. According to Chigangaidze et al. (2022), Africanness is a broad term which refers to various aspects of the African culture, which may encompass a communal way of perceiving humanity and an integrated world view, supported by certain beliefs, customs, and practices that constitute the Ubuntu philosophy coupled with a unique historical sense of forced victimisation.

Historically, Africanness has been the main source of conflict between Africans and non-Africans, especially in the West, and it has also been the main source of differences in approaches between African and Western societies to many things, including pandemics. Negritude of Leopold Sedar Senghor, the Ubuntu of Desmond Tutu, the blackness of Femi Abodunrin, and the Pan-Africanism of Kwame Nkrumah are some of the ideologies through which the uniqueness of the African personality manifests. As regards negritude as championed by Senghor (1964), Africans have a unique reality of existence closely associated with the African cosmology where there is no demarcation between the physical and the supernatural world to such an extent that what is regarded as mere objects in the West, embody supernatural powers in Africa. For Tutu (2011), the African personality trait known by the term "Ubuntu" entails that care for others and a sense of communality make the individual a human being because, as far as Tutu is concerned, a person is a human due to the presence of others without whom his or her humanity evaporates. And as for blackness as conceptualised by Abodunrin (2006), being African is a concept describing an identity created by the historicity of the black condition since pre-colonial

DOI: 10.4324/9781003425861-14

times, which is characterised by subjugation, exploitation, and enslavement leading to endemic mistrust of the other. What black Africans do, what they believe in, their reaction to information about a pandemic in their midst, its veracity in causing death or what to do about it, all reflect their unique way of understanding the world. Africanness or black African hybridity influences African people's judgements, perceptions, and emotions during crucial times of life or death. As a marker of their Africanness, black people south of the Sahara believe they live in a very complex, evil, dangerous, and hostile world responsible for their endless suffering and death, requiring collective energy to survive.

This chapter presents a discussion on the role that Africanness played in the interpretation of information about COVID-19, which proliferated between 2020 and 2022, whether valid or not, and how this was instrumental in determining the psychological well-being of COVID patients and caregivers or the lack of such well-being. Data were collected through narratives where 50 respondents – comprising 25 former COVID-19 patients and 25 caregivers – recounted their stories, detailing their encounters with COVID-19 and the (mis)information circulating at that time. These respondents were purposefully sampled and referred to the researcher by the hospitals or fellow respondents in a snowball sampling. Face-to-face interviews followed up narrations of their experiences with the same respondents. The interviews directed them to discuss the relationship between their interpretation of (mis)information about COVID-19, their Africanness, and the psychological distress they suffered either as patients or as caregivers to COVID-19 patients. The study generated two types of data: anecdotes and information gathered through interviews.

The study employed the content analysis method of data interpretation for data generated through interviews and dialogic narrative analysis for data in the form of anecdotes. Content analysis is interested in the contexts, meanings, intentions, and sub-texts contained in the data (Luo, 2022) and was considered the most appropriate method of extracting meanings patients and caregivers attached to the information related to COVID-19 with which they came into contact. The dialogic narrative analysis focused on what the anecdotes reveal about the narrator's perceptions, fears, and even their thinking (see Frank, 2015). This method was instrumental in determining the respondents' psychological distress, considering that a narrative offers a window into a person's experiences and mental state (Frank, 2015). As Rocha et al. (2021) observe, psychological distress as a mark of psychological malaise is an umbrella term standing for all conditions that show a troubled state of the human psyche and encompasses fear, anxiety, a sense of rejection, psychological trauma, depression, panic, uncertainty, and insomnia.

The study used grounded theory since the researcher focused on understanding the experiences of the COVID-19 patients and caregivers from which he discerned the role played by Africanness in the interpretation of (mis)information from their point of view as Africans, and how that process promoted psychological distress or minimised it. Grounded theory is a bottom-up approach, where data are approached without preconceptions (Holton, 2008). In the current study, the researcher tried to root COVID-19 in the local culture and understand the people under study. According to Tie et al. (2019), the results of a study where the researcher is using grounded theory are descriptive, but what is needed are the insights and conclusions the researcher draws from what is happening on the ground. In using grounded theory, people's experiences and consciousness are understood from the point of view of those experiencing the phenomenon because, traditionally speaking, black Africans have their way of understanding and approaching diseases, which is determined by their unique sense of being.

11.2 Black African Culture and the Fight Against COVID-19

Africa has had pandemics before experiencing waves of COVID-19 in 2020 to 2022. While all the previous pandemics were equally deadly, COVID-19 was not only the world's most serious airborne disease of the last two centuries, but it also had the most conspiracy theories that served to cause panic and anxiety among the world's populations, more especially the black African population on the mother continent (De Coninck et al., 2021). A further major contextual difference is that COVID-19 emerged in an era of uncontrolled flow of information due to the active presence of social and mainstream media. Globalisation entails that what is happening in one corner of the globe is immediately known by the rest of the world due to sophisticated technology in instant communication transfer (Gabriel & MacDonald, 2018). In the same vein, diseases and conspiracy theories can spread quickly from one part of the world to the rest due to high mobility of goods, people, and services. The same applies to valuable knowledge, innovations, threats of extinction, and utter falsehoods. Resistance to globalisation as noted by Spivak (2003), however, implies that most societies are slowly but surely becoming inward-looking instead of outward-looking as they try to strengthen their own essential values, cultures, and identities in order to survive as nations or ethnic communities. For black Africa, the colonial experience, the legacy of enslavement, and resistance of their traditional culture have left the people with a hybrid cultural identity that allows them to draw knowledge from more than one source in the face of a social threat to existence (Amamio, 2021).

Another difference is that COVID-19 emerged at a time when suspicions between Africa and the West were at an all-time high according to Young (2021). These suspicions run deep as they emanate from historical experiences of colonisation of African people by European countries and bloody independence struggles. Unfortunately, the bloody independence struggles were followed by sabotaging of African economies by the West, which until now is responsible for high levels of unemployment and poverty among the populations of most formerly colonised lands through imposition of neoliberal capitalist economic policies (see Rodney, 1972). Further to that, with reports that the world's population is growing at an unsustainable rate, there have been YouTube videos propagated by Young (2021) and other conspiracy theorists that the white race is trying to come up with mechanisms with which to eliminate the other races, especially the black race and the elderly. Besides, the rise of prophetic Christian ministries fuelled speculations that COVID-19 was perhaps the beginning of the end of times as prophesied in the Holy Scriptures. This is so because, although most countries did not call for compulsory COVID-19 vaccination, they nevertheless placed unprecedented restrictions on the unvaccinated individuals to prevent them from entering public buildings, travelling outside their immediate environments, or accessing vital social services worldwide unless they got vaccinated. This echoed the biblical projections of the end of times, where it is indicated that those who will resist the Devil's machinations will experience untold restrictions and suffering in the world.

11.3 The Hybrid Nature of Black African Culture and its Role in the Interpretation of Social Experiences

Some scholars have questioned whether there exists an authentic African culture, considering that Africa is very hybrid, broad, and differentiated (see Mphahlele, 1980; Mbembe, 2007; Durán-Almarza et al., 2017). Amongst other things, they point out that the Muslim society in the northern countries of the African continent is very different culturally speaking from that of the predominantly black Christian south, or even West Africa comprising Nigeria, French-speaking African countries of Côte d'Ivoire or Cameroon. With these cultural disparities, one would easily conclude that it is, therefore, improper to talk about African culture in general but that African culture should be demarcated into black African culture and other African cultures, such as the African Muslim culture north of the Sahara.

Coming to black Africa, it must be recognised that this is not necessarily a cultural-geographical territory per se but rather a concept denoting a particular spirit, for although black African identity is characterised by linguistic and cultural diversity at regional and national level, there are elements which bind all black Africans together (Dabiri, 2015). Common historical experiences of slavery, racism, colonisation, and the fight against European colonisation plus common beliefs, black socialism, world image as economically and technologically backward, and world view are some of the vital elements that indisputably bind all black Africans together regardless of their internal religious, geographical, and economic differences (Ede, 2016).

Collectively, black Africans see themselves as victims of Western imperialism and endemic subjugation and exploitation, and they also believe in the power of their ancestral spirits regardless of the religious faith to which they subscribe. As Legum (1964) contends, the black African mentality as a mark of their Africanness runs very deep, and it is a mentality of suspicion towards world powers, such as the West and the communists. Africans also hold that the work of invisible forces (miracles, witchcraft, extraordinary phenomena, the power of ancestral spirits, and superstitions) would attack them if provoked or conversely bail them out of difficult situations if evoked (Tengatenga et al., 2021). Since COVID-19 originated outside of Africa and considering the fact that the West has been at the forefront producing vaccines, there was bound to be some complications on how black Africans would interpret information about COVID-19 or its vaccines. Issues of trust and the fact that the media in whatever form were more active and widely dispersed than ever before, could have enhanced the hype, could have stoked fears, and could have shaken the core of African existence more than ever before. For once, African socialism and the Ubuntu ideology – both of which hinge on communality and care for one another – were challenged due to the high transmissibility of the coronavirus, resulting in very un-African ways of caring for one another in times of sicknesses and bereavement as noted by Kainja et al. (2022) and Masina (2021).

In the sub-Saharan Africa, when one member of the community is sick, it is commonly understood that the entire community is sick (Wright & Jayawickram, 2021). What is also unique, according to one respondent, is that cheering the sick up at home or in hospital and having physical contact with them and the bereaved are regarded as gestures of paramount significance than sending them money, flowers, or other expressions of goodwill. In fact, societal expectations are that members of the community should cheer up the sick and the bereaved if they are to feel better. Physical presence is extended even to the time an individual passes on when the remains of the dead are bathed and the face is viewed for the last time as it lies in state in the coffin just before taking it away for burial as a way of bidding farewell to him or her. In some of these countries in the sub-Saharan Africa, such as Malawi, the dead person is referred to as "the king" or "the queen," for upon dying, the person is believed to take on more significant roles of looking after the living or warning them through dreams as all ancestors do. The other thing to note is that since the black African reality consists of both real facts and fantasy, unfounded information is easily believed. Rumours travel very fast, since the line separating facts from fiction is usually blurred as magical realism or extraordinary phenomena are treated in the same manner that facts are treated, that is, usually without questioning or scrutinising their possibility or rationality.

11.4 The Role of Africanness in Limiting Psychological Distress

During the COVID-19 pandemic, Africanness played a constructive role in the interpretation of news from social media as it provided assurances to caregivers that they would survive the ordeal. At the peak of the pandemic, the social as well as mainstream media were awash with instructions on which traditional remedies people should apply on a regular basis such as the mixture of ginger, lemon, and garlic, but also steaming using blue gum leaves and other traditional herbs. These assured them, as caregivers or COVID-free people, that they would not contract the coronavirus while looking after their patients, since black Africans view these as concoctions that had served them and their ancestors well for centuries. The information shared through social media was that those traditional remedies were quite effective in neutralising coronaviruses in the trachea before it could start damaging the lungs. This is a case where scientific explanations reinforced traditionally held knowledge for the creation of a positive feeling. What is noteworthy is the fact that most COVID-19 patients were being cared for by their immediate family members at home since quarantine centres at the hospitals were either full or the patients were scared of being treated at the hospital. However, due to the confidence they drew from their Africanness, it is not surprisingly that most caregivers who were interviewed indicated that they were not worried that they could end up contracting the coronavirus themselves since they trusted the protection from traditional herbs.

The news about the efficacy of these concoctions was very assuring and soothing at a time when caregivers were in daily contact with their relations or loved ones who were suffering from COVID-19, considering that total quarantine of the patients they were looking after was not feasible at home where most of the COVID-19 patients were recuperating. What was actually circulating in the communities was that there was no designated Western medicine to cure COVID-19 but that the disease could easily be prevented and even cured using traditional concoctions and prayers. Such information regarding the efficacy of traditional remedies and medicine created the impression that COVID-19 could be defeated using African means. Such news was very assuring considering that traditional medicine was easy to find.

In a study by Lichey et al. (2021), use of traditional African herbal medicine to cure COVID-19 reflected a Pan-African spirit in Tanzania and several other African countries, namely that Africans could look after themselves and survive. Perhaps that was one of the reasons why most Africans shunned Western vaccines and opted for regular steaming and use of traditional remedies instead as a way of protecting themselves from contracting COVID-19.

When COVID-19 just emerged, a narrative was born which claimed that COVID-19 was not meant for black Africans. This narrative emerged after noticing that African resistance defied all odds having beaten the West's prediction of doom for Africa in the wake of the emerging COVID-19. In Africa in general, the number of patients who were hospitalised or died of COVID-19 was much lower compared to that of Europe, Asia, and North America according to reports by the World Health Organization. This information by itself was quite assuring to the African personality that he or she was the strongest breed of people God had created. One former COVID-19 patient who was interviewed had this to say:

> I think the media over-exaggerated the transmissibility and deadliness of COVID-19. How come I lived in a compound of over twenty immediate family members during my COVID-19 sickness that lasted for more

than two weeks and no one else in the family contracted it? I think the West forgets that we are black people with the blood very close to that of monkeys in resisting most diseases.

The caregiver of one former patient also indicated that she was not very worried about the prospects of contracting COVID-19 because it was not the disease for Africans. What is intriguing is the conviction that the coronavirus would have little effect on them simply because they were Africans. Such narratives circulating in the community assured most Malawians of their survival in the wake of the emerging pandemic called COVID-19. The information created hope that the COVID-19 wave would go away without causing much devastation in their communities compared to communities in Europe, Asia, and America. Although belief needs to be matched with reality, the truth of the matter is that the lower COVID-19 deaths in African communities in comparison to communities outside Africa as reported by the media gave most Africans hope that COVID-19 was not meant for them; hence, it could not kill them.

Patients belonging to certain religious institutions, such as Seventh Day Reformists, claimed that although they contracted COVID-19, they had hope that they would survive because their leader prophesied in 2017 that there would come a corona disease but that the righteous would not die of it. In preparation for the yet-to-come COVID-19 then, one respondent reported that the leader of the Seventh Day Reformist Church to which he belonged assembled members in designated places throughout Malawi to pray for them so as "to remove the corona of death and give them the corona of life." That started in 2017, two years before COVID-19 emerged. Such prophesies gave members hope that all they needed to do was to confess their sins and engage in continuous prayer and fasting in order to survive God's wrath that had come allegedly due to growing wickedness in the world.

Although the pandemic had come for everyone, members of Seventh Day Reformist Church learned at their church that the righteous would not die from it because God would heal them. As one member of that church and a former COVID-19 patient asserted, prophesy gave her hope that even if she were to contract coronavirus, she was not going to die even though a lot of people were dying of COVID-19 at the time. But to some members of the same denomination who ended up contracting the coronavirus, this information that came in form of a prophesy caused considerable anxieties due to self-blame, as this chapter later explains, since to them, contracting coronavirus meant that they were not spiritually doing well in the eyes of God. Pentecostalism has become part and parcel of black African identity today, and it is influencing the manner its practitioners interpret things – whether with good or bad outcomes.

Apart from prophesy, dreams also provided information that became a source of hope for survival to the patients by creating previews of how COVID-19 would end in people's lives. This particular 40-year-old respondent who became sick and recovered from COVID-19, narrated that throughout his life, each time he became very sick, he usually dreamed singing a particular hymn throughout the sleep. The next day he would start feeling better and was on the road to full recovery. In total, this happened twice before COVID-19 emerged in 2020. When he contracted the coronavirus and in the midst of his COVID-19 pandemic, he experienced a similar dream. To him, this was a sign that he had turned the corner. Interestingly, the following day he started experiencing signs of active healing. In that dream, the song was about the biblical Sodom and Gomora where God destroyed the city and only three people survived. The message of the song gave this patient hope that he would be healed at a time when many people were succumbing to COVID-19. Traditionally, dreams are regarded highly among black Africans when they are sick as well as when they are healthy. This even applies when they are waiting for the outcome of examinations, job interviews, or contractual bids. Through dreams, most Africans get premonitions of the things to come as they await the results.

11.5 The Role of Africanness in Exacerbating Psychological Distress

Despite their Africanness, the information that was circulating about COVID-19, whether valid or invalid, had severe and negative effects at the time of sickness on COVID patients and their caregivers. Hospitalisation due to COVID-19 exerted undue fear and anxieties on patients and caregivers because the rumour circulating in some of the countries in the Southern Africa Development Community (SADC) region was that hospitals were given huge sums of money for each COVID-19 death they reported to their international donors. As a result, it was rumoured that some doctors were deliberately causing deaths, since the donor monies were trickling down to them. This particular caregiver interviewed had lost her husband to COVID-19 under mysterious circumstances. She did not mince words in suspecting that the hospital to which her husband had been admitted and where he died had engaged in foul play. Their Africanness made them entertain ideas that enemies had taken advantage of the man's hospitalisation to bewitch him. News circulating in most black African communities was that witches and wizards were hiding behind COVID-19 to eliminate their targets. When the man therefore died, his relatives did not accept that he had died of COVID-19 but pointed fingers at foul play by the hospital or the witches. When black Africans are perplexed by a situation or piece of information, they trust their culturally rooted explanation, which in this case only led to growing fear and anxiety that the patient would never get healed.

In Africa, people find a mythical explanation for every death that occurs. The previous case where the patient had a range of health problems, it fell prey to black African myth-making culture where reality and fantasy work together. The fact that there was no definite cause of the patient's death gave rise to superstition-based speculations, including witchcraft, in a typical African fashion. As proof that the caregiver was psychologically traumatised by her husband's death, she is reported to have seen the ghost of her late husband twice asking her for food following his burial. In sub-Saharan Africa, people believe that there must be one distinct illness that can later be cited as the cause of the patient's death in order for that death to be regarded as a natural one. When the patient says he or she is suffering from several sicknesses at once, it is indicative of the work of witches and wizards, according to black African people's beliefs. Since this patient had diabetes and accidentally fell into a pit and broke his leg, he was hospitalised. He was later briefly discharged before he started purging blood, and was re-admitted to hospital. He was finally diagnosed with COVID-19 and died. This sequence of events raised everybody's suspicion that the man had been bewitched. This created a situation of loss of hope for survival in the patient himself as well as the caregiver. Scepticism and rumours play out on African people's psyches more than anything else since, at community level, the dominant reports about COVID-19 were negative news of people dying and witches taking advantage of COVID-19 to achieve their sinister aims, thereby causing much psychological torture on COVID-19 patients, their relatives, and caregivers. Had the black Africans taken a more scientific approach, they would have been more objective in accepting many COVID-19 deaths as natural, and would have suffered less anxiety.

News that COVID-19 spread very quickly and was extremely lethal prevented many relatives and friends from visiting the sick, which created feelings of rejection and the conclusion within the patient's mind that perhaps he or she was indeed dying. In African culture, one sign that the patient is on the verge of death is a sharp reduction in the number of people coming to see him or her on the deathbed. This can be very threatening to the patient. One of the patients interviewed reiterated that he felt abandoned and rejected because, although none of the twenty members of his family members that were living with him in the same compound contracted the coronavirus from him, media hype over-exaggerated the threats of transmission, a scenario that created fear of imminent death in him. Other former patients reported that, as they lay in quarantine centres in hospital, they were bothered constantly that perhaps the information circulating out there that doctors were deliberately killing people in the name of COVID-19 in order to receive huge sums of money from international organisations, was true. She lamented, "I asked myself, what if what people out there are saying is true?" This shows that she viewed getting treated in hospitals as a risky exercise, which created much anxiety and fear among COVID-19 patients because of the rumours that were going around. Suspicions between black Africans and people from the West run very deep with the former always entertaining thoughts that the latter want to wipe them off the face of the earth to depopulate it through pandemics, sterilising vaccines, and tricking them into accepting some birth control measures (Olatunji et al., 2022).

As already indicated, the narrative about COVID-19 was that it was lethal. However, daily national updates consistently showed that in all black African countries, more people were recovering compared to those who were dying of COVID-19. The over-exaggerations equated the contraction of the coronavirus to death. School-going children from a family struck with COVID-19 were barred from going to school, and one of the sick members complained that friends and members of the community were avoiding him even on WhatsApp. This increased his depression. By being communal, Africanness prevents depression of the sick and the bereaved (Jamieson & Van Blerk, 2021). However, the isolation that COVID-19 preventive measures encouraged coupled with a general feeling of abandonment, to which most patients were forcibly subjected, became the main causes of depression among Africans who rely on African harmony and solidarity for their psychological well-being during difficult times, including life-threatening sicknesses (Patterson & Balogan, 2021). This state of feeling abandoned implied that, in the patient's mind, people out there had already concluded his or her death to COVID-19 even before his or her time. For Ndhlovu (2022), there is a need to add the desire to go out and mingle as another cause of depression among Africans during COVID-19 lockdowns or sickness because black Africans are essentially communal. All these added to the patients' psychological distress. Africanness weighed on all these regulations to conclude that society deemed concerned black Africans as undesirable or on the verge of death while someone in the West who was used to a life of isolation would never have been adversely affected by these restrictive regulations.

According to Joffe (2021) and Baird et al. (2022), the exaggerated manner in which COVID-19 was presented caused great psychological distress in black African communities for both the patients and their caregivers. The pandemic crippled their very economic livelihoods, especially in countries that offered no relief support to their populations during the most crucial period when jobs were lost or businesses were closed. However, for another respondent who was interviewed, conspiracy theories played a greater role in causing psychological trauma than anything else due to his hybrid African identity. The man had received one out of the two vaccinations before contracting the coronavirus. His major fears arose due to the numerous conspiracy theories circulating in the community regarding COVID-19 vaccines. Some rumours had it that getting the COVID-19 vaccine was akin to attracting the coronavirus itself into one's body, and that all those who had received the vaccine were surely going to die immediately or within the next five years. What compounded his fears was the rumour that the COVID-19 vaccines sent to their part of Africa were different from those administered in the West because the overall agenda of the West was to reduce the population of black Africa or even worse. This had prompted some African governments, such as Tanzania, to dissuade their citizens from taking Western vaccines (Lichey et al., 2021). As already stated, Africanness often makes black Africans to have great mistrust of anything coming from the West.

Generally, Africans do not trust easily stemming from their culture and historical experiences as a people. That is part of their culture, which is highly embedded in their ideology, which purports to depict the world as full of evil intentions. Historical experiences of being enslaved, colonised, externally motivated and funded armed conflicts and economic exploitation have consolidated that ideology of mistrust among black Africans. Some of the respondents who had contracted the coronavirus could not turn a deaf ear to the numerous rumours surrounding COVID-19 vaccines. Vaccines threatened them while death threatened them even more. For the sick, anxiety developed because they felt like they were trapped with nowhere to escape. One of the rumours was that vaccines led to sexual dysfunctionality in men. For black African men, sexual performance is of paramount significance in maintaining their social dignity and respect as men. It is equated to life itself. As a result, this patient who contracted the coronavirus after getting one of the two vaccinations had even more reason to worry. Firstly, he worried that he was going to die, and secondly, that even if he was to survive, the COVID-19 vaccine had perhaps tampered with his sexual prowess permanently, which would not auger well with his status as a polygamous man (husband to three wives). As Schmidt et al. (2022) concur, in most African countries and beyond, there proliferated a lot of false information, myths, and misconceptions associated with COVID-19. In a big blow to the South African government, efforts to carry out door-to-door COVID-19 screening, false and threatening information kept circulating on social media, creating fear among those who had already received the COVID-19 vaccine. What is intriguing about Africa, according to Okereke et al. (2021), was the fact that culturally, black Africa always seems to be detached from official information on important matters, a scenario that breeds misinformation, rumours, and conspiracy theories. During COVID-19, false narratives – which, unfortunately, were accepted in the black African communities, which thrive on such unverified, mythical stories – were dominant.

One of the new developments, which Malawians encountered during COVID-19 era, were daily updates on COVID-19 cases that were broadcast on the national television and several radio stations. Every morning, the television and radio stations reported figures coming from the Ministry of Health showing new infections, deaths, and recoveries. In their study on the role of information on psychological distress, Ruiz-Frutos et al. (2020) observed that both information and a lack of it have the potential of affecting people's levels of psychological distress. In particular, it was noted that the quality of information could cause even more distress. According to one former COVID-19 patient, disclosing the number of those who had died in the course of the night was very threatening to her as a patient and it was "un-African." "Those figures were very threatening," she lamented on reflection reportedly because it gave her the impression that she was next in line. However, for professionals of which the patients and caregivers were not, such psychological distress is minimised by exposure to a variety of crucial information types, such as updates on new cases, expert opinions, frontline reports, global scopes, and journal articles, which have the capacity to minimise misinformation and, in the process, psychological distress.

In Africa, death and its approach are supposed to be kept mysterious, secretive, and dignified, all of which the prevailing approach during COVID-19 pandemic could not guarantee. Regular media updates were strange to traditional African approaches, and in fact, they were a threat to the patient as they created heightened anxiety that he or she was next in line to die. News updates also created a sense of helplessness upon learning the demise of someone the patient knew. Most former COVID-19 patients interviewed in this study testified that news about the death of two cabinet ministers due to COVID-19 on that fateful day in June 2021 shook their hope of survival to the bone. It made them conclude in their minds that they too were dying, since the two cabinet ministers were considered to be both physically strong and wealthy; hence, they could have withstood COVID-19 better than most people in the community. One thing that characterises African mentality is the ability to segment things or bring things in comparison. The communal mentality entails that one always considers oneself as a member of a particular group rather than as an individual. Therefore, even when it comes to the question of survival during a pandemic, for example, most black Africans would say those in the top class of society would die last while the poorest of the poor would die first. This exposes the thinking that money can buy anything because with it comes connections in society (social capital), which can be beneficial to the rich person.

As one respondent insisted, COVID-19 came as punishment from God due to prevalence of too many sins here on earth. Many religious institutions propagated this narrative. For a person who had contracted the coronavirus, the impression created was that he or she was a sinner in a typical game of self-blame. Church leaders in the Seventh Day Reformist Church, for example, had prophesied that there would come a corona virus but that God would protect his children from it. The sick, therefore, asked themselves many questions amidst their praying and fasting. One former COVID-19 patient lamented that she asked herself questions such as

> Have I been conducting myself in ways that have not pleased you God to allow this to happen to me? Are you Lord going to allow that I die; Is the promise you gave us that you would protect us a lie?

This barrage of questions gives credence to the fact that such patients were in great distress during the COVID-19 pandemic. In interpreting the religious prophesy, black African religiosity played the role of making black people doubt their faith in the Christian God's promises. And as death was drawing closer, it also made them question their conviction that their race was the strong breed. Even for some Christians, the assurance that those who had a good relationship with God would not die, was a tricky one. In Africa, for the majority of the people, living conditions are dire, leading to many sins, such as corruption, telling lies, theft, jealousy, and infidelity. Due to their black African religiosity and as a mark of their hybrid black identity, contracting the coronavirus therefore automatically forced patients to start worrying about their standing in the eyes of God and that if they were found wanting, that they would go to Hell. That was the root cause of their fear. There were doubts that the Western culture would influence white people in the same manner when they are faced with life-threatening situations.

According to respondents, news about variants also caused great anxiety amongst black African patients and caregivers, as it enhanced the intergenerational suspicions that exist between black Africans and the West. Due to their Africanness, news about variants created an impression that Satanists were adjusting the efficacy of the coronavirus in the laboratory aimed at eliminating black Africans. What worried them most was the thinking that they were victims of an international conspiracy that had set its eyes on them as a target of elimination. One former COVID-19 patient explained:

> When a more lethal variant called Delta Variant came to the scene, it caused so much anxiety but real fear grabbed me when the hospital told me that I had COVID-19 a few weeks after the nation was told of the emergence of this new and deadlier variant called Delta.

This patient lamented that to him it was very clear that someone was adjusting the efficacy of the coronavirus in the laboratory to kill more people. He wondered how it had been possible that people had predicted the month when the new variant would emerge, including its efficacy. This element of predicting COVID-19 made it bear the image of an artificial disease championed by forces of darkness. Such pieces of information led black Africans to conclude that they had been targeted by evil forces and that their chances of survival in this world were non-existent. Africanness enables black Africans to accept endless suffering until death, but it also regards black Africans as victims of hatred, exploitation, and manipulation by the West. Looking at how most respondents interpreted news about variants, one is left with no doubt that when really puzzling information emerges, most black Africans draw on their rich repertoire of the African past, suspicions, and traditional reasoning, which – in most cases – is not scientific. This is used to justify what is happening to them as black people. With this kind of thinking, black African COVID-19 patients regarded themselves as the unfortunate group of people caught in the crossfire of a big spiritual war between forces of goodness and those of darkness – and they asked themselves, why them. This question bothered many patients and caregivers throughout the period they were battling with COVID-19, and it enhanced their psychological distress.

Those Malawians who were not strict followers of modern religions believed in maintaining a good relationship with their ancestors whom they believed could facilitate their protection, success, recovery during sickness, and even protect them from death. This kind of thinking, rather than looking at diseases as natural, creates great anxiety among Africans when they have been diagnosed with a life-threatening illness, such as COVID-19. As Isoko (2020) notes, from the African perspective, Africans have continuously attached a spiritual explanation to almost everything that happens in society, including diseases. As a result, there are numerous Afrocentric explanations of what lies behind many pandemics in Africa, including COVID-19. News propagated mostly by traditionalists was that COVID-19 had come in their midst because Malawians had abandoned their ancestral worship or due to witchcraft.

As Tengatenga et al. (2021) argue, no sickness in Africa can be explained without pointing fingers at another human or the spiritual realm as the cause because Africans inhabit the natural, supernatural, and spiritual worlds at the same time (p. 4). As news about emerging COVID-19 variants forced most Malawians to compare COVID-19 with malaria, the number one killer disease in the country, more suspicions were raised as malaria has had no known variants that have caused havoc in the public health sphere. As a result, many patients and caregivers conjured a question such as "[w]hat was so special with COVID-19?" Such questions raised suspicions that perhaps it was true that the coronavirus was an artificially created virus by evil people in the West aimed at eliminating humanity in general and Africans in particular. This led to even more psychological distress. It is hard to dismiss their conclusions, suspicions, and interpretations of the information or what they thought was happening to them, for that constituted their reality in line with grounded theory.

Dreams too, as sources of information, were root causes of fear and anxiety among Malawian COVID-19 patients and their caregivers due to their Africanness. One particular caregiver who lost her husband, claimed that dreams played very important roles in her husband's two struggles against COVID-19 until his eventual demise. She narrated that in the first COVID-19 attack, her husband told her that when the sickness was at its peak, he dreamed seeing his late grandfather leading a long queue of people into a tall white building. In that dream, the patient was standing in that queue but upon seeing him, his grandfather took him out the queue while shouting angrily at him to go back because his time had not yet come; he was in the next batch. The patient turned back recovered from COVID-19 following this rejection of admission into that building by his late grandfather. However, when he was hospitalised again months later as the Delta variant was at its peak, the patient told his wife that he was not going to make it since he was having the same dream of being in a long queue. This second time, his grandfather, though having seen him, was just busy letting people into that white building without uttering a word to him like someone totally unknown to him. Unfortunately, the patient indeed passed on. To this day, most black Africans believe that their ancestors still play a role in their lives. It is, therefore, common belief among black Africans that the persistent dream about this patient's late grandfather had a deep meaning about the course of events. One can only imagine the amount of fear and psychological trauma these dreams inflicted especially on the patient but also on the caregiver in their encounter with COVID-19.

11.7 Conclusion

In interpreting information about COVID-19 to which patients and caregivers of black Africans were exposed, Africanness played both positive and negative roles of minimising and enhancing the psychological distress of patients and caregivers. Some of that information strengthened their hope for survival and soothed them, but most of it unsettled them psychologically, as it confounded long-held mistrusts that, as black Africans, the patients and caregivers already had that made them interpret information about the source, the efficacy and status of the COVID-19 as a disease. Regular updates, although desirable in this modern era of social media, for instance, created an impression that Satanists were perhaps adjusting the efficacy of the coronavirus in the laboratory in order to eliminate black Africans. This led to great psychological anguish amongst patients and caregivers. The information in certain instances confirmed the patients and caregivers' widely held belief that as Africans they are members of a strong race while in others it challenged that belief.

Since most of the information confused black Africans people's imagination, they tapped on the rich repertoire of their black hybrid identity to make sense of it. Unfortunately, most of those interpretations were not based on objective science, and therefore only worsened the situation by making both COVID-19 patients and caregivers experience heightened fear, anxiety, and a sense of rejection, psychological trauma, depression, panic, uncertainty, and insomnia. Africanness featured prominently while processing the barrage of information about COVID-19 amongst black African patients and caregivers, as everything was interpreted in relation to the black African cosmology, values, and historical experiences that had shaped them as black Africans. This shows that Africans experience pandemics in their own unique way contrary to how their counterparts in the West experience them; thus, leading to speculations that diseases are not just biological or pathological but cultural too and must be approached as such.

References

Abodunrin, F. (2006). *Blackness: Culture, ideology and discourse*. African Book Collective.

Amamio, R. (2021). Hybridity and the shape of the new African woman. *Journal of Language and Literature, 21*(2), 349–361.

Assefa, N., Soura, A., Hemler, E., Korte, M., Wang, D., Abdullahi, Y., Lankoande, B., Millogo, O., Chukwu, A., Workneh, F., Sie, A., Berhane, Y., Baernighausen, T., Oduola, A., & Fawzi, W. (2021). Covid-19 knowledge, perception, preventive measures, stigma and mental health among healthcare workers in three sub-Saharan African countries: A phone survey. *The American Society of Tropical Medicine and Hygiene, 10921*, 342–350.

Baird, M., Cantor, J., Troxel, W. M., & Dubowitz, T. (2022). Job loss and psychological distress during Covid-19 pandemic: Longitudinal analysis from residents in the nine predominantly African American low-income neighbourhoods. *Health Economics, 31,* 1844–1861.

Belayachi, D. (2021, January 15). Doctor claiming Bill Gates wants to kill 3 billion people. *France 24 News.* https://observers.france24.com/en/africa/20210119-bill-gates-kill-three-billion-people-video-conspiracy.

Chigangaidze, R. K., Mafa, I., Simango, T. G., & Mudehwe, E. (2022). Establishing the relevance of the Ubuntu philosophy in social work practice: Inspired by the Ubuntu world social work day, 2021 celebrations and the IFSW and IASSW's (2014) global definition of social work. *International Social Work, 66*(2). https://doi.org/10.1177/00208728221078374.

Dabiri, E. (2015). Why I am (still) not an Afropolitan. *Journal of African Cultural Studies, 28*(1), 104–108.

De Coninck, D., Frissen, T., Matthijs, K., Lits, G., Carignan, M., David, M. D., Salerno, S., & Généreux, M. (2021). Beliefs in conspiracy theories and misinformation about COVID-19: Comparative perspectives on the role of anxiety, depression and exposure to and trust in information sources. *Frontiers in Psychology, 12,* 646394. https://doi.org/10.3389/fpsyg.2021.646394.

Durán-Almarza, E. M., Kabir, A. J., & Rodríguez González, C. (2017). Introduction: Debating the Afropolitan. *European Journal of English Studies, 21*(2), 107–114. https://doi.org/10.1080/13825577.2017.1344471.

Ede, A. (2016). The politics of Afropolitanism. *Journal of African Cultural Studies, 28*(1), 88–100.

Frank, A. (2015). *Dialogical narrative analysis.* Sage Publication.

Gabriel, C., & MacDonald, L. (2018). After the international organization for migration: Recruitment of guatemalan temporary agricultural workers to Canada. *Journal of Ethnic and Migration Studies, 44*(10), 1700–1724. https://doi.org/10.1080/1369183x.2017.1354062.

Holton, J. (2008). Grounded theory as a general research methodology. *The Grounded Theory Review, 7*(2), 67–94.

Isoko, P. A. (2020). Religious construction of disease: An exploratory appraisal of religious response to the Covid-19 pandemic in Uganda. *Journal of African Studies and Development, 12*(3), 77–96.

Jamieson, L., & Van Blerk, L. (2021). Responding to Covid-19 in South African social solidarity and social assistance. *Children's Geographies, 20*(4), 1–10.

Joffe, A. (2021). Covid-19 and the African cultural economy: Opportunity to re-imagine and re-invigorate? *Cultural Trends, 30*(1), 28–39.

Kainja, J., Ndasauka, Y., Mchenga, M., Kondowe, F., M'manga, C., Maliwichi, L., & Nyamali, S. (2022, October 31). *Umunthu,* Covid-19 and mental health in Malawi. *Heliyon, 8*(11), e11316. https://doi.org/10.1016/j.heliyon.2022.e11316. PMID: 36353175; PMCID: PMC9638767.

Legum, C. (1964). *Pan-Africanism: A short political guide* (Revised ed.). Frederick A. Praeger Publishers.

Lichey, A. L., Gissel, L. E., Kweka, O. L., Bærendtsen, P., Kragelund, P., Hambati, H. Q., & Mwamfupe, A. (2021). South-South humanitarianism: The case of Covid-organics in Tanzania. *World Development, 141*(105375), 1–11.

Luo, A. (2022). Content Analysis | A Step-by-Step Guide with Examples. Scribbr. Retrieved 8 November 2023, from https://www.scribbr.co.uk/research-methods/content-analysis-explained.

Masina, L. (2021, February 12). Malawi health workers face harassment over Covid-19 deaths. *Voice of America News.* www.voanews.com/a/covid-19-pandemic_malawi-health-workers-face-harassment-over-covid-19-deaths/6201961.html

Mbembe, A. (2007). Afropolitanism. In S. Njami & L. Durán (Eds.), *Africa remix: Contemporary art of a continent* (pp. 26–29). Jacana Media.

Mphahlele, E. (1980, June 7). On negritude in literature. In A. L. McLeod & M. B. McLeod (Eds.), *Power above power: Representative South African speeches, the rhetoric of race and religion*. University of Mysore Press.

Ndhlovu, T. (2022). Writing a South African pandemic moment: Inequality and violence in the lockdown collection. *Journal of Literary Studies*, *38*(1), 1–16.

Okereke, M., Ashinedu, N. U., Muthoni, L. N., Mwansa, C., Mohammed, S. A., Ogunkola, I. O., Jaber, H. M., Mashkur, A. I., Ekpenyong, A., & Lucero-Prisno, D. E. (2021). Covid-19 misinformation and infodemic in rural Africa. *The American Journal of Tropical Medicine and Hygiene*, *104*(2), 453–456.

Olasemi, A., Akinsola, O. S., Samson, F., Agberotimi, S. F., & Oguntayo, R. (2020). Psychological distress experiences of Nigerians during Covid-19 pandemic: The gender difference. *Social Sciences and Humanities Open*, *2*, 1–7.

Olatunji, O., Ayandele, O., Ashirudeen, D., & Olaniru, O. S. (2022). "Infodemic" in a pandemic: Covid-19 conspiracy theories in an African country. *Social Health and Behaviour*, *3*(4), 152–157.

Patterson, A., & Balogan, E. (2021). African response to Covid-19: The reckoning of agency. *The African Studies Review*, *64*(1), 144–167.

Rocha, Y. M., de Moura, G. A., Desidério, G. A., de Oliveira, C. H., Lourenço, F. D., & Nicolete, L. D. (2021, October). The impact of fake news on social media and its influence on health during Covid-19 pandemic: A systematic review. *Journal of Public Health from Theory to Practice*, *9*, 1–10.

Rodney, W. (1972). *How Europe underdeveloped Africa*. Bogle-L'ouverture Publications.

Ruiz-Frutos, C., Ortega-Moreno, M., Dias, A., Bernardes, J. M., García-Iglesias, J. J., & Gómez-Salgado, J. (2020). Information on Covid-19 and psychological distress in a sample of non-health workers during Covid-19 pandemic period. *International Journal of Environment Research and Public Health*, *17*, 2–18.

Schmidt, T., Cloete, A., Davids, A., Makola, L., Zondi, N., & Jantjies, M. (2022). Myths, misconceptions, othering and stigmatising responses to Covid-19 in South Africa. *PLOS One*, *15*(12), e0244420. https://doi.org/10.1371/journal.pone.0244420

Selaise, T. (2005, March 3). Bye-bye Babar. *The Lip Magazine*. http://thelip.robert-sharp.co.uk/?p=76.

Senghor, L. S. (1964). *Liberté I, Négritude et humanisme*. Seuil.

Spivak, G. C. (2003). *Death of a discipline*. Columbia University Press.

Tengatenga, J., Duley, S. T., & Tengatenga, C. J. (2021). Zimitsani moto: Understanding the Malawian Covid-19 response. *Laws*, *10*(20), 1–14.

Tie Chung, Y., Birk, M., & Francis, K. (2019). *Grounded theory research: A design framework for novice researchers*. Sage.

Tutu, D. M. (2011). *God is not a Christian and other provocations*. HarperOne.

Wright, J., & Jayawickram, J. (2021). We need other human beings in order to be human: Examining the indigenous philosophy of umuthu and strengthening mental health interventions. *Culture, Medicine and Psychiatry*, *45*(4), 613–628.

Young, R. O. (2021). *Sterilization and population control*. www.YouTube.be/gKjnEz5s37o?t=5584.

12 Utilitarian Perspectives on Curbing Online Abuse of Women During the COVID-19 Crisis

Wasilat Opeoluwa Lasisi

12.1 Introduction

Although the number of confirmed cases of people infected with COVID-19 in Africa is nothing compared to the rest of the world, it has still left an indelible effect on the lives of many Africans (Bissoonauth, 2020). Social vices, such as bullying of women, have soared to an all-time high due to the pandemic. The factors leading to this bullying are (but not limited to) verbal abuse and dumping one partner for another. However, during the pandemic, many women still face violence arising from bullying, which extends to body shaming, cyberbullying, sex exploitation and blackmailing.

Social media was a powerful medium for communicating and disseminating vital information during the pandemic. However, it also left lasting implications on the mental health of many women. Although some women who became redundant during that period could utilise the opportunity availed to them by the Internet to learn soft skills, many others created online stores for their businesses. However, the overreliance on this type of business harmed their mental health and well-being as many of them now live online and find it difficult to move away from the new normal.

Reports on gender-based violence across the globe show a correlation between the forced lockdown during COVID-19 and physical violence against women (see Bradleye et al., 2020; World Health Organisation [WHO], 2020). Consequently, many social vices were targeted at women (especially married women). Many had no choice but to be locked down with their husbands, who were often abusive (United Nations [UN], 2020). Many women had to resort to social media to get themselves busy during the COVID-19 lockdown.

Social media are interactive technologies that facilitate creating and sharing information, ideas, interests, and other forms of expression through virtual communities and networks. There are many forms of social media, such as blogs, micro blogs, wikis, social networking sites, photo-sharing sites, instant messaging apps, video sharing sites and apps, podcasts, widget, virtual words, and more.

The mental health issue is as huge as that related to social media use. Mental health reflects our well-being and encompasses our psychological, social, and emotional well-being. It affects how we think, feel, and act, helps us determine

DOI: 10.4324/9781003425861-15

how we handle stress in every situation and interpersonal relationship, and how to make healthy choices. Our mental health is determined by individual, social, and structural determinants, which may combine to protect or undermine our mental health (WHO, 2022). One social factor, for instance, verbal and physical assaults on women trending on news media, often cause women who had lost their livelihood or had been caught in infidelity by their male partners to fall into a devastating mental state. Some then post their confidential issues on social media.

In Robert Nozick's (1974) view, libertarianism seeks to justify individual liberty and all forms of coercion are unacceptable, wherever they might come from. John Hospers (1971) argues that every individual is entitled to his or her life, and everyone has the right to live as he or she chooses insofar as that freedom does not infringe on the freedom of others. Libertarians argue for the permissibility of individual freedom of choice to live as one pleases without external interference.

Digital libertarians believe in a technology world where censorship is restrained, and individual liberty should be guaranteed (see Dahlberg, 2017). Neither the creators of the content nor the viewers are restricted in any way because they are supposed to inhabit a free world.

The current study assessed the libertarianism principle that upholds the condemnation of any infringement of individual freedoms, especially that of women. The survey reported here was conducted in 2022. The variables used were West African women and their digital experiences. The participants completed a survey that reflected age range, social media apps used, and questions on the effect of the COVID-19 pandemic on the participants. Another survey was conducted of 50 women aged 36–45 (76% were married and working-class women).

12.2 Utilitarianism

Utilitarianism is the ethical theory that holds that morally right actions are those that maximise good for the greatest number and minimise the bad things such as pain (West & Duignan, 2023). If the number of people who would benefit from such actions is smaller than the number that would be harmed by it, then such actions are morally acceptable (Uduigwomen, 2006). The principle of the greatest happiness for the greatest number holds that right actions promote happiness, while wrong actions tend otherwise. Utilitarianism upholds that, whatever the action, the happiness or unhappiness that would be accrued from it, has to be taken into consideration (West & Duignan, 2023). Everyone's well-being is thus accounted for.

According to Bentham (1907, p. 1), mankind has been placed under the governance of two controllers: pain and pleasure. Mankind then has to determine which one they ought to seek and which one they should do (Bentham, 1907, p. 1). In the current context, utilitarianism upholds the social value of actions, for it considers the greater number of people. This social benefit of utilitarianism would support the use of social media by African women. Even though many women were distressed due the COVID-19 pandemic, the positive outcome gained from the use of social media as shown by this research, surpassed the negative effect. Invariably, use of social media, therefore, served its utilitarian purpose.

John Stuart Mill (2007) urges individuals to refrain from acts that infringe on the liberties of others. This autonomous act gives weight to an individual's freedom to choose and to determine how to live his or her life by avoiding pain and at the same time refraining from harming others. The responsibility for ensuring happiness and avoiding pain, therefore, lies on the shoulders of the agents of acts. For Mills (2007), pleasure is the outcome of happiness and the absence of pain. Hare (1981) considered a utilitarian concept where two levels of moral thinking are applied. He states that the two levels of intuition (characterised by emotions) and critical reflection (which subscribes to the doctrine of the mean), carried out by archangels, are required in determining the consequences of actions (Hare, 1981). In this case, the value of actions is taken into consideration, and agents are able to make alternatives in ethical decision-making. Intuitively, there are some moral thoughts that come to mind, such as refraining from killing, stealing, or lying, which guide our daily lives. Critically, utilitarianism advocates that when all facts are checked, choosing actions that will maximise the good cannot be but be embraced. Hare's utilitarian decision-maker "archangel" is aware of the possible outcomes of all available options (Price, 2019). This decision-maker adopts the reflective critical method and queries which actions are acceptable (Price, 2019).

12.3 Women's Use of Social Media During the Pandemic

A hundred West African women from Ghana, Nigeria, and Benin aged 19–35 (around 51% of whom were single working-class women, 43% were single non-working-class women who believed that they felt freer using social media for friendship than in physical form, and 6% who did not specify) participated in the study. These women were users who spent some of their time on social media. Of these, 48% used Instagram and TikTok only (because TikTok has numerous filters that help them edit their photos or video content, while Instagram helps them attract large numbers of followers and customers), 40% used Facebook, and 6% used Twitter. Generally, 60% reported increased loneliness because their expectations of finding the right suitor seemed utopian. These participants also showed symptoms of smartphone addiction. Some claimed that they posted video content online to shed their suicidal thoughts as they still hoped to be wooed by potential future partners. Others lauded the platforms as they had served and were still serving at the time as avenues for them to make a daily living. Social media plays a vital role in the advancement of female representation and visibility in the global world and has offered many women opportunities to advertise their businesses during COVID-10 pandemic (see Rah et al., 2021).

Social media use by women in Africa is one of the most criticised phenomena that have influenced lives positively and negatively, and one can never forget its deficiency on the cultural aspect of life (Okorie, 2021). On the vastness of mental health and the pervasiveness of social media in Africa, especially during and after COVID-19, I confine my exposition to examples in which women's health and cybersecurity met at an angle where they interacted and at another angle where there is a divergence.

COVID-19 dealt a heavy blow to African women who were moving from gender inequality towards liberation, especially in the workforce (Barua, 2022). Many independent young women who became redundant due the pandemic were also faced with economic shock. In this case, many had to resort to other means of survival. Economic uncertainty, increased substance abuse, and changes to daily family lives as a result of the pandemic also increased tensions within households, compounding violent situations (Parsitau, 2021). African women have faced and are still facing the obvious effects of societal acceptability due to their skin colour, especially women of the sub-Saharan African region who are dark-skinned. The inferiority complex they feel when they make comparisons with women of white or red skin colours compounded their mental health issues. As if that was not enough, the problem of a pandemic ravaging the world led to increased aggressive behaviour in some homes, especially aggression erupting from fear of infection, frustration due to a lack of the necessary supplies, depression arising from the inability to find a husband, unemployment, and financial loss. In addition to this, there has been an overall decrease in women's mental health (Loades et al., 2020; Condry et al., 2020). Due to immobility caused by the lockdown imposed on residents by the government, for instance in Nigeria, many promising young women became disappointed and depressed as the pandemic shattered their hopes of success due to heightened pressure from their parents and society either to abandon schooling, find a life partner, or source for survival means (Bissoonauth, 2020).

The importance of the Internet – especially social media – during the pandemic cannot be overemphasised. That the cyberspace had helped women in terms of self-identity and confidence due to its swiftness and connectivity, is unavoidably true (Madhavi & Hima, 2019). Many African women saw the pandemic period as a stage in their lives during which they strived to establish a sense of breaking free from societal mandates on the female gender and establishing self-identity, as well as struggling to fit in, and receiving attention from their peers and society at large. It was a critical time when health-risk behaviours by the opposite sex and even by some of their peers – in the form of verbal abuse and cyberbullying – were initiated. The reason is not far-fetched. Indigenous African societies are perceived to be androcentric, and women hardly have a say in most African societies. During the pandemic, when many of them had ample time to study on the Internet how other women in the world were faring, they took the chance to show to the world that they are also intelligent, hardworking, and creative.

> I've always used social media. I have a Facebook page that I employ in selling my hair products, but I must say that I got more traffic in late 2022 because many of those that visited my page now patronise me.
> (Participant, Lagos, Nigeria, October 2022)

> Before the pandemic outbreak, I used to waste data posting pictures on Instagram and Facebook. My parents used to give me pocket money so it was easy. But when coronavirus came and government mandated a lockdown policy, my dad lost his job and mama, who was a teacher couldn't go to work but had to do online teaching which didn't fetch her much. A friend of mine introduced me to Jobberman and Allison free soft skills training so I grabbed the opportunity to learn digital marketing.
> (Participant, Lagos State University, Nigeria)

> I learnt baking from an online outlet via Facebook video and now, I can bake and even make pastries.
> (Participant, Accra, Ghana, 2022)

> The lockdown provided us with learning opportunities. When I could not go to work, I started making short videos and posting them on YouTube. The channel is yet to be monetised but I am happy that I didn't waste the whole time.
> (Participant, Accra, Ghana, 2022)

> I learnt how to edit videos with different filters, thanks to online teaching that my school adopted. That period of lockdown, I made lovely videos for my pupils and learning became fun.
> (Participant, Lagos, Nigeria, 2022)

Some of them, however, lamented bitterly due their inability to use the Internet or unavailability of funds.

> I am a trader. I sell dried fish. Coronavirus did not allow me go out to sell because I fear that I may be arrested. I had only primary education and I do not know how to use the Internet. That was when I know that it is important to know how to use Facebook, maybe I could have sold my fish there like you suggested [referring to the interviewer].
> (Participant, Cotonou, Benin Republic, 2022)

> I didn't learn anything online, in fact, I couldn't. The reason is because I barely afforded call credits talk more of data. There was no money for such.
> (Participant, Egbeda, Ibadan, Nigeria, 2022)

I do not have a browsing phone, so how can I use it for social media?
(Participant, Lagos, Nigeria, 2022)

Not only is social media a point of economic development in recent times, it also sometimes determines the extent to which women can live their lives and the quality of life expectancy. To some, it is a form of recreational activity (learning driving, dance skills, recipes for food, weight reduction – which is one of the major problems facing African women, especially in Nigeria) (Eke et al., 2014); others use it to get the latest information and news (Fasae & Adegbilero-Iwari, 2016; Statistica, 2018); do shopping; go job searching; or enjoy it as a leisure activity (Lenhart et al., 2010). However, due to its obvious relevance to women, it also carries with it considerable responsibility. Over-reliance on it has caused some level of misfortune for women. Women should, therefore, consider the social value of integrity and dignity in censoring contents before posting anything on social media, and also consider staying off cyberspace should it show any sign of a negative effect on their well-being.

Arguably, in Africa, women now believe that they have the choice to explore cyberspace, but it is also noteworthy that resilient social media use, emotional investment in social media – for instance, the inability to find a suitor on Instagram or Facebook – may cause distress. Excessive use of social media at nighttime may result in insomnia and probably hallucination, which in turn might lead to weight gain or loss (thereby causing body shaming). Some studies have found correlations between increased use of social media and mental health issues, such as depression, addiction, cravings, lower self-esteem, and even suicide (Turel et al., 2018). Many women nowadays compare their lifestyles to the flamboyant lifestyles of social media influencers, and they become depressed when they are unable to live such life. Recently, the media space has been fed with a series of clips of women's intimate tapes shared by blackmailers (Kingsley, 2021). As if this is not enough, many women have to deal with comments passed by social media users on their physical appearances. They no longer eat well nor live the way they wish to live because they are always conscious of what society has to say about their physique (Elsesser, 2021).

In Nigeria, women who felt that they needed to be in vogue on social media posted content that exposed them to the risk of sharing intimate photos or highly personal stories, which resulted in them being bullied and blackmailed (Kingsley, 2021). Such content has particularly concerning implications, as it increases sexual expectations when women use social media to evaluate potential partners and also to compare themselves with other women in the world who might have the freedom of sharing intimate content online without mass condemnation. Conversely, many women have been blackmailed and assaulted due to the content they shared or that was leaked by some sociopaths on Facebook, YouTube and Instagram (consider the series of intimate clips of Nigerian female celebrities during the COVID-19 pandemic (Kingsley, 2021). What baffles one is that instead of condemning both parties when a social vice is committed, African society is apt to crucify the women involved because they consider females as being inferior and weak (Nealon & Giroux, 2011;

Leon-Guerrero, 2009)). This act of severe condemnation and rejection has had negative consequences for the health of African women. Why should they be condemned for sharing content about their personal lives on chat apps, and why should anyone infringe on their freedom as human beings to act according to their will?

Furthermore, the exposure of African women to online marketing and advertising on Instagram, Facebook, and Twitter has been seen by many as one of the most significant positive outcomes of the COVID-19 pandemic period because it saved the lives of many breadwinning young women in danger of becoming redundant (many of them now operate online stores selling handbags, shoes, clothes, or food items). Although this may sound simple, it surely paved the way for boosting sales and visibility. Moreover, many working-class women utilised the social media to seek better employment. This made it easier for them to pursue their growth and development. These women could use the existing social media apps for personal benefits to solve the new problem ushered in by the pandemic, such as layoffs and lockdowns. However, such unavoidable dependence on social media also resulted in recent abuse of women and its intending effect on their mental health, spilling over to other aspects of their lives.

12.4 Digital Libertarianism and African Women

Libertarianism holds that, without much interference from the government or state, individuals are free to choose the kind of lives they desire (Wolff, 2006). However, the government might make regulations so that some individuals do not infringe on the freedom of others.

"This is my world, so do let me be" seems to be the motto of libertarians. Individual freedom is essential and paramount. Libertarians place substantial value on individual freedom and frown upon any form of coercion by individuals or the government (Van der Vossen, 2019). Although laws might be put in place to limit infringement on the freedom of others, people cannot be forced to consider the overall good of society. Individual liberty relates to private ownership of property, equal opportunities for people of different lifestyles (including LGBTQ lifestyles), and so on (Van der Vossen, 2019).

Whether individuals are free to post content on cyberspace or whether their posts should be regulated by society or government is controversial (see Samples, 2019). Should moral judgement pertaining to cyberspace autonomy be based on moral uprightness or on interest? (see Lasisi, 2022, p. 84) Who should lay claim to the ownership of cyberspace? Cyberspace appears to be just as it were, for its origins are concealed and whether those origins are state-sponsored schemes or market-structured order remains obscured (Boyle, 1997, p. 177). Cyberspace seems to have been created on a libertarian principle if one considers how Internet corporations, such as Google and Facebook, operate (Dahlberg, 2010). This is evident in the unsuccessful attempts by some governments to ban some activities online. For instance, when the federal government of Nigeria banned Twitter operations from June 2021 through January 2022 (Princewill & Busari, 2021), many users employed virtual private networks (VPNs), which enabled them to operate freely (Nwosu, 2021).

It is evident that the adverse effects of the pandemic escalated into society and resulted in mental health issues, especially among women – inconsistencies in policymaking, censorship and banning of some social media apps by the government (such as the ban on Twitter in 2021–2022 by the Nigerian government), economic meltdown, and violence, which hitherto contradicted individual liberty. In my opinion, every individual freedom matters, and any other principle that goes against that ought to be unacceptable.

Digital libertarianism emphasises the commitment to liberty; therefore, it will encourage women to be free to use cyberspace at will insofar as their usage does not interfere with the freedom of other users (here, I consider others as men who may be sexually aroused by sultry contents and children who may be exposed to disturbing contents). I believe that women have the liberty to own private property – their products of whatever nature – and to post content online. Over time, women have been abused whenever they showcase their free choice to use cyberspace because of the patriarch nature of many African societies (Venditto et al., 2022; Loum, 2022). Women now believe that the digital space should be explored without hindrance from anywhere whatsoever, and they believe they have the individual right to utilise it in any form they deem fit. This, however, gives rise to their objectification and harassment (Zainal, 2022).

Many Nigerian women have embraced the digital space positively. The cyberspace has helped many married women who are yet to conceive to subsume their fears because they could share their challenges with women worldwide (on chat apps like *FemaleIN* on Facebook). Also, violence against females, especially girls, received wide attention on social media. Consider, for instance, *#BringBackOurGirls* in Nigeria (see Tomchak, 2014). This is also true of many abused women who have now summoned the courage to speak up whenever they face any form of emotional and physical violence. Pages, such as Female IN and RantHQ on Facebook, hashtags such as *#Blackgirl-magic* on Twitter, and the Harassmap online tool launched in Egypt encourage women to report any case of sexual harassment via their mobile phones (Young, 2014), and through non-governmental organisation, Women at Risk International Foundation [WARIF] (in Nigeria). Many disheartening reports on women's bullying are, however, still being seen and read daily.

Although women have the free choice to post any content on cyberspace or emulate social media influencers, some of the existing literature on social media usage suggests that there are many social comparisons, like appearance comparison (Jason, 2022). When one looks at other people's lives, mostly on Instagram and Twitter, it might be pretty easy to conclude that everyone else's life is better than one's own. Comparing oneself not only to people one thinks are more elegant or smarter but also to people who are less wealthy or pretty can be linked to poorer well-being. Inauthentic life has become the order of the day, and the integrity of many has been watered down because they wish to live the kind of life many influencers showcase online. This problem, in turn, makes it essential for users to rely on their ability to navigate online risks and opportunities by making wise and responsible decisions that would maximise their pleasure without undermining others.

12.5 Towards A Utilitarian Route Map for Cyberspace Usage

Utilitarianism implies upholding happiness and despising pain (Dimmock & Fisher, 2017). The maximisation of the good is impartially considered (Driver, 2014). The pleasure I seek from using the Internet is no different from that other members of society seek. Everyone should possess the right to promote the greatest good for the same reason (Driver, 2014). The use of social media should not be handled light-heartedly because it is a complex system – cultural, political, social, and intellectual – manifested in virtually every aspect of our lives (Teich, 1972, p. 1). It should be noted that women in Africa using cyberspace should do this with the necessary ethical attitude and relevant physical, mental, and social attitude necessary to apply it safely, effectively, and appropriately (Rodger & Dietz, 2014). Although women can choose their actions, they should also desist from content that may affect their personality. They should adopt social media to produce a well-informed and well-balanced individual through adequate sensitisation. They should also use social media in order to perform tasks and function effectively in a world filled with a collection of chat apps.

Hare argues that, depending on circumstances, we can switch between intuitive and critical forms of utilitarianism (Hare, 1981). Concerning social media use by women in Africa and its mental health implications, Hare would want us to think critically, and by that, we would understand that the use of special media has helped a lot of women in terms of empowerment and liberation especially during the COVID-19 pandemic (Dempere & Grassa, 2023). African women have been overwhelmed by the COVID-19 pandemic, coupled with the backlash from using social media. To maximise utility, there is, however, a need to give priority to the many women who have been able to find their voices or who have been empowered by considering critically and intuitively the social value of social media (Nwaolikpe, 2021, p. 1).

In principle, utilitarianism (especially Mill's 2007 version) calls us to be morally responsible for our actions to the extent that we can foretell and control the possible effects of our actions. Although the consequences of such actions may be unintended, the fact that they may be foretold and avoided makes us inadvertently responsible for them. Invariably, engaging in actions that may prevent the outcome of more promising is the same as causing such things to happen intentionally.

It follows logically that the adverse mental health of African women does not arise mainly from their use of social media to satisfy recreational purposes or due its economic importance during the COVID-19 pandemic, but also because women rely so much on it now that they no longer know the limits of its usage and the societal factors to be considered. African women ought to employ social media for social, recreational, and business purposes to tackle problems, and to have adequate information on happenings in their communities that will enhance the improvement of their qualitative lives the way they did during the height of the COVID-19 pandemic; otherwise, they should be held liable for their overreliance on social media.

Notably, African women's overreliance on social media has affected them negatively because it has led to the proliferation of a submerged, manipulated, and dehumanised culture, which is alien to the African people (see Okorie, 2021). In Africa, virtually all aspects of life are related to society, and people embrace communal lifestyles that seek the greatest happiness for all (Menkiti, 1984, p. 171), akin to Bentham's (1907) version of utilitarianism. However, in a bid to shed off any suffocating societal norms, African women thought that they were free to search, argue, and dare to share their thoughts and private lives publicly (see Twongyeirwel, 2012). However, since utilitarianism considers how well the majority lives, the quality of lives lived by women is more important than any negative comments or backlash they may get from the society.

In traditional African society, women were considered subjects to their men, as they were seen as vessels who could not do things on their own, and they had to rely on the men. This factor has contributed greatly to the marginalisation and subjugation of women (Olusola, 2023, p. 81). However, the principle of the greatest pleasure for the greatest number will indeed work for African women using social media because the number of women who benefit from it surpasses those who experience negativity. Many women have become entrepreneurs, while some have gained employment and scholarship opportunities using the digital space. I believe the happiness these women get from cyberspace ought to nullify any sociocultural barriers.

12.6 Conclusion

Mental health is a complicated social phenomenon that should be treated as urgent, especially during this period following the pandemic. African women should be given the respect and liberty of utilising media, but, in turn, they should maximise using it for the benefit of all. They should consider their mental health and refrain from content that may attract bad energy and backlash from society. They should also be moderate in their actions by avoiding over-dependence on cyberspace. Suppose any woman experiences depression due to cyberbullying, the inability to find a suitor, or disappointment due to not having the kind of lifestyle she envisages. In that case, it will affect her family members and society. Despite its usefulness, issues disturbing social values, communal responsibilities, and the dignity of women in Africa remain. On the other hand, the evident positive side of women's use of social media outweighs the criticism that might be levelled against these in society as some of the examples cited in this work on social media use and women eloquently uphold a healthy relationship between social media use and societal values.

Acknowledgement

I would like to thank my students, Adamson, Caroline, and others, for assisting in collating my research data.

References

Barua, A. (2022). *Gender equality, dealt a blow by COVID-19, still has much ground to cover: At the brink of squandering past gains.* Deloitte. https://www2.deloitte.com/us/en/insights/economy/impact-of-covid-on-women.html

Bentham, J. (1907). *An introduction to the principles of morals and legislation.* Clarendon Press.

Bissoonauth, R. (2020). *Addressing the impact of Covid-19 on girls and women's education in Africa.* African Union International Center for Girls and Women's Education in Africa. www.globalpartnership.org/blog/addressing-impact-covid-19-girls-and-womens-education-africa

Boyle, J. (1997). Foucault in cyberspace: Surveillance, sovereignty, and hardwired censors. *University of Cincinnati Law Review, 66,* 177–205.

Bradley, N., DiPasquale, A., Dillabough, K., & Schneider, P. (2020). Health care practitioners' responsibility to address intimate partner violence related to the COVID-19 pandemic. *Canadian Medical Association Journal, 192*(22), e609–e610.

Condry, R., Caroline, M., Brunton-Douglas, T., & Oladapo, A. (2020). *Experiences of child and adolescent to parent violence in the Covid-19 pandemic.* www.law.ox.ac.uk/sites/files/oxlaw/final_report_capv_in_covid_aug20.pdf

Dahlberg, L. (2010). Cyber-libertarianism 2.0: A discourse theory/critical political economy examination. *Cultural Politics: An International Journal, 6*(3), 331–356.

Dahlberg, L. (2017). Cyberlibertarianism. In *Oxford research encyclopedia of communication.* Retrieved July 31, 2023, from https://oxfordre.com/communication/view/10.1093/acrefore/9780190228613.001.0001/acrefore-9780190228613-e-70

Dempere, J., & Grassa, R. (2023, June 16). The impact of COVID-19 on women's empowerment: A global perspective. *Journal of Global Health, 13,* 06021. https://doi.org/10.7189/jogh.13.06021

Dimmock, M., & Fisher, A. (2017). Utilitarianism. In *Ethics for A-level: For AQA philosophy and OCR religious studies.* Open Book Publishers.

Driver, J. (2014). The history of utilitarianism. In E. N. Zalta (Ed.), *Stanford encyclopedia of philosophy.* https://plato.stanford.edu/archives/win2014/entries/utilitarianism-history/

Eke, H. N., Omekwu, C. O., & Odoh, J. N. (2014). The use of social networking sites among the undergraduate students of University of Nigeria, Nsukka. *Library Philosophy and Practice (e-journal), 1195.*

Elsesser, K. (2021). Here's how Instagram harms young women according to research. *Forbes.* www.forbes.com/sites/kimelsesser/2021/10/05/heres-how-instagram-harms-young-women-according-to-research/?sh=110557f3255a

Fasae, J. K., & Adegbilero-Iwari, I. (2016). Use of social media by science students in public universities in Southwest Nigeria. *The Electronic Library, 34*(2), 213–222.

Graca, M. (2022). COVID-19 and the impact on African women: All responses must respect the gendered impacts of the pandemic. *The Elders.* https://theelders.org/news/covid-19-and-impact-african-women-all-responses-must-respect-gendered-impacts-pandemic

Hare, R. M. (1981). *Moral thinking: Its levels, method, and point.* Academic. Retrieved July 26, 2023.

Hospers, J. (1971). *Libertarianism: A political philosophy for tomorrow.* Nash Pub.

Jason, C. (2022). How social media affects women's mental health: Negatives vs. positives. *Thriveworks.*https://thriveworks.com/blog/how-social-media-affects-womens-mental-health-negatives-vs-positives/

Kingsley, O. (2021). *Five (5) 5 Nigerian female celebrities who have been blackmailed with their video.* www.boomplay.com/buzz/2629440

Lasisi, W. O. (2022). A Mill-Kantian ethical evaluation of the incessant sociopolitical violence in Nigeria. *LASU Journal of African Studies, 10*(3), 79–88.

Lenhart, A., Purcell, K., Smith, A., & Zickuhr, K. (2010). *Social media & mobile Internet use among teens and young adults.* Pew Internet and American Life Project.

Leon-Guerrero, A. (2009). *Social problems: Community, policy, and social action.* Pine Forge Press.

Loades, M. E., Chatburn, E., Higson-Sweeney, N., Reynolds, S., Shafran, R., Brigden, A., Linney, C., McManus, M. N., Borwick, C., & Crawley, E. (2020, November). Rapid systematic review: The impact of social isolation and loneliness on the mental health of children and adolescents in the context of COVID-19. *Journal of the American Academy of Child and Adolescent Psychiatry, 59*(11), 1218–1239, e3. https://doi.org/10.1016/j.jaac.2020.05.009. Epub June 3, 2020. PMID: 32504808; PMCID: PMC7267797.

Loum, J. (2022). *Cultural African norma limiting women and girls: The Gambia norm and culture Vis-à-vis women and girls.* Matriarchal/Patriarchal Society. www.saggfoundation.org/blog/cultural-african-norms-limiting-women-and-girls

Madhavi, L., & Hima, B. (2019). Role of social media in women's health boon or bane. *Koneru International Journal of Management Research, 1*(2), 3–7.

Menkiti, I. A. (1984). Person and community in African traditional thought. In R. Wright (Ed.), *African philosophy: An introduction* (3rd ed., pp. 171–181). University Press of America.

Mill, J. S. (2007). *Utilitarianism, liberty, and representative government.* Wildside Press.

Nealon, J., & Giroux, S. (2011). *The theory toolbox: Critical concepts for the humanities, arts, and social sciences.* Rowman & Littlefield Publisher.

Nozick, R. (1974). *Anarchy, state, and utopia.* Basic Books.

Nwaolikpe, O. N. (2021). Women, social media, and culture in Africa. In O. Yacob-Haliso & T. Falola (Eds.), *The Palgrave handbook of African women's studies.* Palgrave Macmillan. https://doi.org/10.1007/978-3-319-77030-7_148-1

Nwosu, A. (2021, June 5). Twitter ban: Nigerians opt for VPN as Twitter stops working. *Daily Post.* https://dailypost.ng/2021/06/05/twitter-ban-nigerians-opt-for-vpn-as-twitter-stops-working/

Okorie, S. E. (2021). Social media invasion of African moral space. *The Guardian Newspaper.* https://guardian.ng/opinion/social-media-invasion-of-african-moral-space/

Olusola, K. (2023). Subverting women's subjugation in West African society: The roles of popular music KIU. *Journal of Humanities, 8*(1), 81–88.

Parsitau, D. S. (2021). *Invisible lives, missing voices: Putting women and girls at the center of post-COVID-19 recovery and reconstruction.* Brookings. www.brookings.edu/blog/africa-in-focus/2021/01/28/invisible-lives-missing-voices-putting-women-and-girls-at-the-center-of-post-covid-19-recovery-and-reconstruction/

Price, A. (2019). Richard Mervyn Hare. In E. N. Zalta (Ed.), *The Stanford encyclopedia of philosophy* (Summer ed.). https://plato.stanford.edu/archives/sum2019/entries/hare/

Princewill, N., & Busari, S. (2021, June 5). Nigeria bans Twitter after company deletes President Buhari's tweet. *CNN.* https://edition.cnn.com/2021/06/04/africa/nigeria-suspends-twitter-operations-intl/index.html

Rah, N., Masduki, M., & Ellyanawati, N. (2021). Women entrepreneurs and the usage of social media for business sustainability in the time of Covid-19. *Research Square.* https://doi.org/10.21203/rs.3.rs-907854/v1

Rodger, E., & Dietz, C. (2014). *Ethics of social media behavior: Act versus rule utilitarianism.* www.mckendree.edu/academics/scholars/rodgers-issue-24.pdf

Samples, J. (2019). *Why the government should not regulate content moderation of social media* (Policy Analysis No. 865). Cato Institute.

Statistica. (2018). *Number of social media users worldwide from 2010 to 2021.* www.statista.com/statistics/278414/number-of-worldwide-social-network-users/

Teich, A. H. (Ed.). (1972). *Technology and man's future.* St Martin's Press.

Tomchak, A.-M. (2014, May 6). #BBCtrending: How a million people called to #BringBackOurGirls. *BBC News.* www.bbc.com/news/blogs-trending-27298696

Turel, O., Poppa, T., & Gil-Or, O. (2018). Neuroticism magnifies the detrimental association between social media addiction symptoms and wellbeing in women, but not in men: A three-way moderation model. *Psychiatric Quarterly, 89.* https://doi.org/10.1007/s11126-018-9563-x

TwongyeirweI, H. (2012). *Dare to say: African women share their stories of hope and survival.* Chicago Review Press.

Uduigwomen, A. F. (2006). *Introducing ethics: Trends, problems and perspectives.* Jochrissam Publishers.

United Nations. (2020). *Policy brief: The impact of Covid-19 on women.* www.un.org/sexualviolenceinconflict/wp-content/uploads/2020/06/report/policy-brief-the-impact-of-covid-19-on-women/policy-brief-the-impact-of-covid-19-on-women-en-1.pdf

Van der Vossen, B. (2019). Libertarianism. In E. N. Zalta (Ed.), *Stanford encyclopedia of philosophy.* https://plato.stanford.edu/archives/spr2019/entries/libertarianism/

Venditto, B., Beatha Set, B., & Amaambo, R. N. (2022). Sexualization and dehumanization of women by social media users in Namibia. *Sexes, 3*(3), 445–462.

West, H. R., & Duignan, B. (2023, June 8). Utilitarianism. In *Encyclopedia britannica.* www.britannica.com/topic/utilitarianism-philosophy

Wolff, J. (2006). Libertarianism, utility, and economic competition. *Virginia Law Review, 92*(7), 1605–1623.

World Health Organization. (2020). *COVID-19 and violence against women: What the health sector/system can do.* Retrieved October 28, 2020, from www.who.int/reproductivehealth/publications/emergencies/COVID-19-VAW-full-text.pdf

World Health Organization. (2022). *Strengthening mental health promotion* (Fact Sheet No. 220). World Health Organization.

Young, C. (2014). HarassMap: Using crowdsourced data to map sexual harassment sin Egypt. *Technology Innovation Management Review, 4*, 7–19.

Zainal, R. (2022). *Sexualisation, harassment and objectification of women on social media: Towards gender inequality.* www.researchgate.net/publication/358187181_ SEXUALIZATION_HARASSMENT_AND_OBJECTIFICATION_OF_ WOMEN_ON_SOCIAL_MEDIA_TOWARDS_GENDER_INEQUALITY

13 Intersections Among Vaccine Hesitancy, Mental Health, and COVID-19

Jones Hamburu Mawerenga

13.1 Introduction

The triad of the COVID-19 pandemic, vaccination hesitancy, and mental health in Southern Africa is a conspicuous phenomenon. The chapter aims to discuss the triad of the COVID-19 pandemic, vaccination hesitancy, and mental health in Africa. In line with the aim of the study, the chapter is divided into three parts: the COVID-19 pandemic in Africa, vaccination hesitancy in Africa, and mental health in Africa. Dzinamarira et al. (2020) affirm that COVID-19 has affected many countries worldwide and that Africa has not been exempted. Anjorin (2020) indicates that the African continent confirmed its first case of COVID-19 in Egypt on 14 February 2020, and in sub-Saharan Africa, the first case was reported in Nigeria on 27 February, in an Italian patient who flew to Nigeria from Italy on 25 February 2020. South Africa is the leading country with the highest number of confirmed COVID-19 cases on the African continent (Kinfu et al., 2020). For instance, on 29 November 2022, over 21,308,365 COVID-19 tests had been conducted, 4,034,234 COVID-19 positive cases were confirmed, 3,923,661 recoveries were reported, 102,395 deaths were reported, and 37,898,854 vaccines were administered in South Africa (see DHSA, 2022).

Nuwagira and Muzoora (2020) report that the epidemiology of the COVID-19 pandemic in Africa was due to infection with the SARS-CoV-2 virus, which had evolved. There were several variants of the original virus causing COVID-19 infections in Africa and globally. Zoa-Assoumou et al. (2021) observed that some of the notable variants that were associated with high infection rates, morbidity, and mortality were the beta (SARS-CoV-2 variant: B.1.351), Delta (SARS-CoV-2 variant: B.1.617.2) and Omicron (SARS-CoV-2 variant: B.1.1.529), which were discovered in South Africa on the 24 November 2021 (Banerjee et al., 2021). Chenchula et al. (2022) relate that symptoms and signs of patients presenting with the omicron variants were milder than those of the Delta variant. More docile symptoms have been reported, such as headache, slight fever, rhinorrhoea (an excessively runny nose), and sore throat resembling the common cold. It was also speculated that the Omicron variant was more transmissible than Delta.

DOI: 10.4324/9781003425861-16

Lone and Ahmad (2020) contend that the weak healthcare system in Africa exposed its vulnerability to the COVID-19 pandemic. Elhadi et al. (2020) maintain that the healthcare capacity of a country plays a vital role in a pandemic situation in terms of management and control. Elebesunu et al. (2021) argue that, from most regions globally, Africa appeared to be the least prepared regarding the pandemic response, and most African countries demonstrated vulnerability in handling the COVID-19 pandemic. COVID-19 brought to the fore the limited capacity of most African countries to respond to health emergencies, highlighted by studies emphasising the deficiencies in health systems across the African continent (Adebisi et al., 2021).

Lone and Ahmad (2020) suggest that the ongoing COVID-19 pandemic has exposed many shortfalls of African healthcare systems, that is, limited testing capacity, shortage of trained staff required for diagnostics and intensive care units (ICU), inadequate ventilators and ICU facilities (required in severe cases of COVID-19), a lack of personal protective equipment (PPE) for healthcare workers, and a scarcity of funds for the health sector. These are some of the core healthcare-related issues on the continent, which make it more susceptible to the COVID-19 pandemic.

Malawi is one of the many countries whose healthcare system was overstretched by the COVID-19 pandemic. Patel et al. (2020) suggest that the Malawian health sector, which battled the epidemic, was already challenged by inadequate funding, insufficient staffing, dilapidated infrastructure, and a lack of essential medicines and equipment. Mandala and Changadeya (2021) report that the decrepit Malawian healthcare system rendered frontline health personnel incapable of mounting an adequate response to critically ill COVID-19 patients who required ventilation during the peak of the epidemic, which was experienced from January to February 2021.

Following the declaration of COVID-19 as a public health emergency of international concern (PHEIC) and pandemic on 30 January 2020 (World Health Organization [WHO], 2020), the WHO (2020) issued several recommendations that were adopted by different countries to prevent the spread of COVID-19. The non-pharmaceutical recommendations included physical distancing, wearing a mask, keeping rooms well-ventilated, avoiding crowds, and cleaning hands with alcohol-based hand rub or soap and water. Multiple communication platforms, from social media to radio, television, and messaging, were used to conduct mass health education and sensitise the public to COVID-19.

The governments of several African countries, including Uganda, Kenya, Malawi, South Africa, Rwanda, Nigeria, and Ghana, implemented containment measures to curb the transmission of COVID-19. These included the closure of international airports, closing of ground crossing points for passengers except cargo drivers, closure of schools and other high congregation points, freezing of public and private transport, outlawing all mass gathering events, overnight curfew, and nationwide lockdowns (Verani et al., 2020). Contact tracing, quarantine, and isolation of confirmed COVID-19 cases were also implemented to minimise the spread of infection (Nachega et al., 2021a).

The implementation of the COVID-19 prevention measures was fiercely challenged in Malawi. The pandemic developed in sociopolitical turmoil connected with the country's 2019 tripartite elections and the 2020 Fresh Presidential Elections (FPE) (Tengatenga et al., 2021). Nyasulu et al. (2021) observed that the Malawian response to the COVID-19 pandemic was initially resisted for three reasons:

- Political altercations were augmented by a constitutional court ruling in February 2020 for an FPE due to irregularities observed in the May 2019 elections.
- The announcement of the first COVID-19 cases escalated the pre-existing mistrust Malawians had in the then government that was presumed to be running away from holding the FPEs. Consequently, the majority of the population's mistrust towards the government negatively affected the efforts to contain the spread of the COVID-19 pandemic.
- The people rejected a national lockdown aimed at preventing the further spread of COVID-19 because the government failed to announce any measures to cushion the poor during the lockdown (Kaunga, 2020).

While most African countries agreed with the WHO on COVID-19 prevention measures, Tanzania was peculiar in declaring itself as a COVID-19-free country in June 2020, and prayers were advised as a remedy for the COVID-19 pandemic (Saleh, 2020). However, on 20 February 2021, the WHO Director-General, Tedros Ghebreyesus, urged Tanzania to share data, take robust action against the pandemic, and accept vaccination (Buguzi, 2021). By April 2020, Tanzania had stopped releasing official COVID-19 statistics, and at that time, the country had reported 509 positive cases, 21 deaths, and 183 recoveries (Makoni, 2021). It is noted that the absence of scientific data on the extent of COVID-19 infections in the country rendered the fight against the pandemic ineffective (Patterson, 2022).

The discussion demonstrates that African countries developed multisectoral plans, ensuring preparedness and timely, consistent, and coordinated response to the COVID-19 pandemic. The engagement of partners, including the private sector, was critical in the response efforts. Strengthening surveillance systems, increasing the number of responders – including epidemiologists and community health workers – improving the prevention of hospital-acquired infection and control, improving diagnostic testing capabilities, strengthening critical care, and revising public health legislature to fast-track authorisations were crucial in the COVID-19 response in Africa (Bwire et al., 2022).

13.2 COVID-19 Vaccination Hesitancy in Africa

A theoretical foundation is critical in understanding why people engage in or fail to engage in health-enhancing behaviour (Glanz & Bishop, 2010). Consequently, theoretical evidence can help implement successful public health interventions (Sharma, 2021). Sharma et al. (2021) identify four stages of the progression of theory-based health behaviour research, namely knowledge – attitude – practices (KAP) surveys, skill-based intervention planning, single-theory interventions, and the current "fourth-generation multiple-theory precision interventions" (Sharma, 2021, p. 1273). Linke et al. (2014) mention the multi-theory model (MTM) of health behaviour change as an example of the fourth-generation theory utilised as a framework in this chapter. Therefore, this chapter aims to discuss the triad of the COVID-19 pandemic, vaccination hesitancy, and mental health in Africa. Further, the chapter discusses the factors influencing COVID-19 vaccine hesitancy in Africa.

Marti et al. (2017) define vaccine hesitancy as the delay in the acceptance or an outright refusal of vaccines despite the availability of vaccine services. Carcelen et al. (2022) posit that, at the time, mass vaccination or immunisation proved to be the most effective intervention against the spread of communicable diseases. Consequently, several countries adopted and implemented vaccination programmes to curb the spread of the COVID-19 pandemic. However, contrary to the fact that the administration of vaccines has prevented innumerable deaths and the demonstrated efficacy of vaccines in curbing the spread of COVID-19, an increase in global vaccine hesitancy has been observed (Ackah et al., 2022). Vaccine hesitancy thus became a viable research topic worth investigating in view of its implications associated with the COVID-19 pandemic in Africa (Sallam, 2021).

The current chapter discusses eleven causes of COVID-19 vaccine hesitancy in Africa.

- a lack of confidence in the safety of the vaccines;
- a lack of confidence in the effectiveness of the vaccine;
- complacency regarding the individual risk of getting infected with COVID-19;
- a lack of time to go out and get vaccinated (Wiysonge et al., 2022);
- The COVID-19 pandemic has contributed to developing an infodemic that hindered an adequate public health approach to managing the crisis. Dash et al. (2021) define an infodemic as an overabundance of information, some accurate and some false, that occurs during an epidemic. Afolabi and Ilesanmi (2021) argue that fake news, myths, propaganda, and conspiracy theories, pervasive in both social media and mainstream media, have spread since the beginning of the COVID-19 pandemic and have negatively affected vaccination efforts across Africa.
- African governments failed to make the necessary effort to demystify conspiracy theories on both social and traditional media, which purported that the African continent was immune to COVID-19 due to its climatic conditions (Dinga et al., 2021).
- Some African governments intentionally introduced policies that promoted COVID-19 vaccine hesitancy. For instance, Tanzania initially denied the existence of COVID-19 and suggested that the pandemic could be

eradicated by divine intervention through prayer. Moreover, key government officials propagated anti-vaccine sentiments, and the country refused to join the accessible COVAX vaccine facility (Kamazima et al., 2020). Even after the COVID-19 vaccine was introduced in August 2021, it was, therefore, challenging to demystify COVID-19 untruths despite various government efforts, including hosting a national-level launch of the COVID-19 vaccination campaign (Kabakama et al., 2022).

- Some African governments, such as Uganda and Tanzania, exonerated themselves from COVID-19-related adverse effects by insisting that the programme was optional and voluntary. Moreover, the requirement of written consent before vaccination absolved the government from any blame for any adverse effects but negatively increased fear and suspicion in the population. Nevertheless, some affluent groups of people, such as the rich and diplomats in Tanzania and Kenya, countered the government's hesitancies by importing the vaccines ahead of the government. Inevitably, this led to various vaccine brands in these countries negatively affecting the provision of the desirable vaccination schedule and regulatory oversight (Kabakama et al., 2022).

- Religious beliefs were identified as one of the causes of vaccine hesitancy in Africa. Some faith-based groups in Africa resist healthcare, including vaccines (Dzinamarira et al., 2020). Moreover, religious leaders were divided on the decision to vaccinate. On the one hand, some religious leaders openly received vaccination on national TV. On the other hand, others used religious gatherings to advance anti-vaccine campaigns in Ghana, Kenya, South Africa, Tanzania, and Zimbabwe (Dzinamarira et al., 2020).

- The prioritisation of particular groups of people to be the first ones to receive vaccination contributed to the COVID-19 vaccine hesitancy by making the rest of the population think that the vaccine was not for them. For instance, most African countries prioritised the following groups: healthcare workers, immigration officers, national defence forces, prison warders, prisoners, teachers, those 60 years old and above, and people with underlying health conditions (Kayode et al., 2022).

- Some African countries promoted herbal medicine and steam inhalations as protective against and curative for COVID-19. Therefore, most African countries' populations valued herbal medicines and steaming more than the COVID-19 vaccine (Shumba et al., 2022).

The current chapter reflects five high-level interventions to address COVID-19 vaccine hesitancy and improve vaccine uptake in sub-Saharan Africa at the time:

- A multifaceted framework tailored explicitly to sociopolitical contexts, social groups, and individuals can help combat COVID-19 vaccine hesitancy. Policymakers, public health officials, vaccine developers, healthcare workers, researchers, advocates, communicators, the media, traditional leaders, religious leaders, and other stakeholders must collaborate to create and sustain public confidence in COVID-19 vaccines (Aborode et al., 2021).

- African governments, policymakers, health workers, and all other stakeholders should have basic knowledge of the scientific basis of the COVID-19 vaccination interventions. They should be able to deconstruct the rumours and myths using scientific data. For instance, in Africa, it became imperative to address concerns about the hasty development of COVID-19 vaccines, the introduction of the vaccines according to priority groups, and reassuring the public about the effectiveness and safety of the vaccine (Sato, 2022).
- African governments should strive to resolve the mistrust of COVID-19 vaccines by instilling and maintaining public confidence in the safety and effectiveness of the vaccines and having competent and reliable institutions to deliver these (Van de Walle et al., 2008).
- African governments should initiate a context-tailored approach to COVID-19 vaccine awareness initiatives by partnering with community-based organisations. The COVID-19 vaccination campaigns should be integrated into the already existing community structures and programmes, including involving religious and traditional-cultural leaders (Mutombo et al., 2022).
- Public health experts in sub-Saharan Africa should counter COVID-19 misinformation, mainly targeting the youth who are the majority on the African continent and the heaviest social media users (Ogunleye et al., 2022).

13.3 COVID-19 and Mental Health in Africa

According to the WHO, mental health is defined as a "state of well-being in which the individual realises their abilities, can cope with the normal stresses of life, can work productively and fruitfully, and can contribute to his or her community" (WHO, 2001, p. 1). Later, some factors that influence mental health problems or disorders in Africa are presented, specifically those related to COVID-19. Ojeahere et al. (2020) observe that the SARS-CoV-2 virus was initially considered to be restricted to the respiratory system, mainly affecting the lungs; however, recent studies have demonstrated its multisystem involvement with the brain tissue (see Mukherjee & Pahan, 2021; Banerjee et al., 2021). A correlation has been established between COVID-19 disease and some mental health problems, such as post-traumatic stress disorder (PTSD), obsessive-compulsive disorder (OCD), anxiety, delirium, and depression. In addition, COVID-19 has the potential to either worsen previous mental health issues or generate new psychiatric disorders (Giorgi et al., 2020).

Jaguga and Kwobah (2020) state that various efforts to contain the spread of COVID-19, such as restricting physical and social interactions, have increased mental health problems in Africa. Inevitably, people had limited access to social support structures, vital in the African communitarian way of life (Chigangaidze et al., 2022). Moreover, the restricted access to religious institutions and religious leaders due to the ban on social gatherings deprived people of receiving faith-based mental health care (De Backer, 2021). COVID-19 prevention measures, for example, physical distancing, quarantine, curfews, and lockdowns, physically isolated people from friends, family, and community networks. This subsequently increased the experience of uncertainty, unrest, loneliness, job losses, grief, gender-based violence, substance abuse and post-traumatic distress (Magamela et al., 2021).

Semo and Frissa (2020) claim that the following direct effects of the disease heightened the predisposition to mental health problems in Africa:

- a near-death experience during COVID illness;
- stress as a result of news about high death rates among the very ill and the highly exposed (e.g., healthcare workers);
- loss of loved ones or parents or guardians; and
- stigma and discrimination among survivors and affected families.

Uncertainty and stress resulting from losing jobs and livelihoods brought many mental health challenges to African people. Posel et al. (2021) estimate that between 2.2 and 2.8 million adults in South Africa lost their jobs between February 2020 and April of that year due to the lockdown. This loss of employment had significant implications for people's access to economic resources and activities, leading to increased depressive symptoms among South Africans.

Laurance (2005) established a correlation between fear concerning the COVID-19 disease and mental health. Fear was singled out as one of the drivers of contemporary mental health. Rwafa-Ponela et al. (2022) mention the following fears and anxieties related to the pandemic: perceived risk of infection, the possibility of severe illness, financial insecurity, hospitalisation, and death.

Additionally, fear and uncertainty were heightened because of people's inability to visit family and churches during the lockdowns.

Semo and Frissa (2020) argue that mental health services will need to be prioritised during a future pandemic such as COVID-19 in sub-Saharan Africa. Mental health has been given less priority during this pandemic and received little attention from most African governments than other diseases. Worse still, mental health policies have not been given priority in some countries, that is, Botswana, Sierra Leone, Ethiopia, Zambia, and Zimbabwe (Molebatsi et al., 2021). Mental health is thus underprioritised in Africa. Monteiro (2015) identifies low funding for mental health in Africa as one of the major setbacks in the region. There is therefore an urgent need for African governments to increase funding for mental health. Even without the influence of the COVID-19 pandemic, the mental health system in sub-Saharan Africa is already overstretched and insufficient with challenges related to the economic and development inequalities and sociocultural contexts.

Despite the lack of focus on mental health needs in sub-Saharan Africa, some countries have taken some steps to address the issue. For instance, countries such as Cameroon, Kenya, South Africa, Tanzania, and Uganda all had mental health guidelines or a mental health component in their health guidelines. Kenya and Cameroon, in particular, initiated training of mental health and lay providers in psychological first aid (PFA) to help manage the needs of health-care workers, and to identify COVID cases, their families as well as the public (Molebatsi et al., 2021). According to the WHO (2011), PFA is humane, supportive, and practical assistance to fellow human beings who have recently suffered exposure to serious stressors. Molebatsi et al. (2021) assert that PFA is a non-professional framework that works to provide comfort and practical support, focusing on mental and psychosocial response during and after a crisis. Shah et al. (2020) remark that PFA is crucial in managing the mental stress emanating from the COVID-19 pandemic. Horn et al. (2019) recall that PFA was pivotal in mounting psychological responses during the 2014 Ebola virus disease outbreak in Liberia and Sierra Leone. The training-of-trainers (ToT) model, as well as the PFA guidelines provided by the WHO, enabled the education of healthcare workers, community leaders, teachers, and social workers in responding to the epidemic. PFA thus proved to be a significant tool in mounting psychological intervention during a crisis because it enhanced the mental well-being of trauma-stricken populations.

Gispen and Wu (2018) recommend that African governments should train adequate personnel with PFA skills to facilitate psychological intervention in hospitals and trauma centres. McCabe et al. (2014) convey that approaches – such as the training-the-trainer (TTT) and just-in-time (JIT) models – can be rewarding by escalating training exercises to increase the number of providers capable of rendering psychological intervention during a future pandemic in Africa. Mashaphu et al. (2021) highlight the need to incorporate spirituality and religion to address African mental health issues. Spirituality and religion play a crucial role in organising the institutional features of faith traditions and practices, which are common in African society. Moreover, spirituality and religion also provide a framework of meaning for people in their daily interactions with the natural environment and in their interpretation and coping with the disruptions occurring in the universe (see De Backer, 2021). For instance, people's access to places of worship needs to be enhanced to maintain social support systems and promote mental health resilience during future pandemics.

13.4 Conclusion

In conclusion, I present the threefold implications of the phenomenon of the triad of the COVID-19 pandemic, vaccination hesitancy, and mental health in Africa. First, the COVID-19 pandemic served as a wake-up call to African governments to invest more in their healthcare systems to fulfil Aspiration 1 of Agenda 2063 (see Nkengasong & Tessema, 2020). The achievement of the 2063 Agenda is contingent on ensuring that African citizens are healthy and well-nourished and that African governments invest adequately to expand access to quality healthcare services for all people (Ufomba, 2020). Second, given the reported vaccine hesitancy and misinformation throughout the COVID-19 pandemic, it was incumbent upon African governments to combat COVID-19 vaccine hesitancy and increase demand for possible vaccination in future. The provision of accurate information, demystifying myths about COVID-19-like illnesses, and ensuring an integrated community engagement strategy that includes everyone and leaves no one behind when introducing vaccinations are some of the ways that could help combat vaccine hesitancy in Africa. Third, mental health and psychosocial support must be integrated into future pandemic responses in Africa. Addressing the mental health effect of the COVID-19 pandemic demands prioritisation and a sense of urgency in dealing with the current and post-COVID-19 situation in Africa.

References

Aborode, A. T., Fajemisin, E. A., Ekwebelem, O. C., Tsagkaris, C., Taiwo, E. A., Uwishema, O., & Yunusa, I. (2021). Vaccine hesitancy in Africa: Causes and strategies to the rescue. *Therapeutic Advances in Vaccines and Immunotherapy*, *9*, 1–5.

Ackah, M., Ameyaw, L., Gazali Salifu, M., Afi Asubonteng, D. P., Osei Yeboah, C., Narkotey Annor, E., . . . Boakye, H. (2022). COVID-19 vaccine acceptance among health care workers in Africa: A systematic review and meta-analysis. *PLoS One*, *17*(5), e0268711

Adebisi, Y. A., Alaran, A. J., Okereke, M., Oke, G. I., Amos, O. A., Olaoye, O. C., & Lucero-Prisno, D. E., III. (2021). COVID-19 and antimicrobial resistance: A review. *Infectious Diseases: Research and Treatment*, *14*, 1–9.

Afolabi, A. A., & Ilesanmi, O. S. (2021). Dealing with vaccine hesitancy in Africa: The prospective COVID-19 vaccine context. *Pan African Medical Journal*, *3*.

Anjorin, A. A. (2020). The coronavirus disease 2019 (COVID-19) pandemic: A review and an update on cases in Africa. *Asian Pacific Journal of Tropical Medicine*, *13*(5), 199–203.

Banerjee, I., Robinson, J., Banerjee, I., & Sathian, B. (2021). Omicron: The pandemic propagator and lockdown instigator – what can be learnt from South Africa and such discoveries in future. *Nepal Journal of Epidemiology*, *11*(4), 1126–1129.

Buguzi, S. (2021). Covid-19: Counting the cost of denial in Tanzania. *British Medical Journal*, *373*, 1–2.

Bwire, G., Ario, A. R., Eyu, P., Ocom, F., Wamala, J. F., Kusi, K. A., & Talisuna, A. O. (2022). The COVID-19 pandemic in the African continent. *BMC Medicine*, *20*(1), 1–23.

Carcelen, A. C., Prosperi, C., Mutembo, S., Chongwe, G., Mwansa, F. D., Ndubani, P., & Truelove, S. A. (2022). COVID-19 vaccine hesitancy in Zambia: A glimpse at the possible challenges ahead for COVID-19 vaccination rollout in sub-Saharan Africa. *Human Vaccines & Immunotherapeutics*, *18*(1), 1–6.

Chenchula, S., Karunakaran, P., Sharma, S., & Chavan, M. (2022). Current evidence on efficacy of COVID-19 booster dose vaccination against the omicron variant: A systematic review. *Journal of medical virology*, *94*(7), 2969–2976. https://doi.org/10.1002/jmv.27697.

Chigangaidze, R. K., Matanga, A. A., & Katsuro, T. R. (2022). Ubuntu philosophy as a humanistic – existential framework for the fight against the COVID-19 pandemic. *Journal of Humanistic Psychology*, *62*(3), 319–333.

Dash, S., Parray, A. A., De Freitas, L., Mithu, M. I. H., Rahman, M. M., Ramasamy, A., & Pandya, A. K. (2021). Combating the COVID-19 infodemic: A three-level approach for low and middle-income countries. *BMJ Global Health*, *6*(1), e004671.

De Backer, L. M. (2021). COVID-19 lockdown in South Africa: Addiction, Christian spirituality and mental health. *Verbum et Ecclesia*, *42*(1), 1–9.

DHSA. (2022). *COVID-19 online resources and news portal*. Department of Health. https://sacoronavirus.co.za/

Dinga, J. N., Sinda, L. K., & Titanji, V. P. (2021). Assessment of vaccine hesitancy to a COVID-19 vaccine in Cameroonian adults and its global implication. *Vaccines*, *9*(2), 175–175.

Dzinamarira, T., Dzobo, M., & Chitungo, I. (2020). COVID-19: A perspective on Africa's capacity and response. *Journal of Medical Virology*, *92*(11), 2465–2472.

Elebesunu, E. E., Oke, G. I., Adebisi, Y. A., & Nsofor, I. M. (2021). COVID-19 calls for health systems strengthening in Africa: A case of Nigeria. *The International Journal of Health Planning and Management*, *36*(6), 2035–2043.

Elhadi, M., Msherghi, A., Alkeelani, M., Alsuyihili, A., Khaled, A., Buzreg, A., & Alghanai, E. (2020). Concerns for low-resource countries, with under-prepared intensive care units, facing the COVID-19 pandemic. *Infection, Disease & Health*, *25*(4), 227–232.

Giorgi, G., Lecca, L. I., Alessio, F., Finstad, G. L., Bondanini, G., Lulli, L. G., & Mucci, N. (2020). COVID-19-related mental health effects in the workplace: A narrative review. *International Journal of Environmental Research and Public Health*, *17*(21), 7857–7875.

Gispen, F., & Wu, A. W. (2018). Psychological first aid: CPR for mental health crises in healthcare. *Journal of Patient Safety and Risk Management*, *23*(2), 51–53.

Glanz, K., & Bishop, D. B. (2010). The role of behavioral science theory in development and implementation of public health interventions. *Annual Review of Public Health*, *31*, 399–418.

Horn, R., O'May, F., Esliker, R., Gwaikolo, W., Woensdregt, L., Ruttenberg, L., & Ager, A. (2019). The myth of the 1-day training: The effectiveness of psychosocial support capacity-building during the Ebola outbreak in West Africa. *Global Mental Health*, *6*, e5.

Jaguga, F., & Kwobah, E. (2020). Mental health response to the COVID-19 pandemic in Kenya: A review. *International Journal of Mental Health Systems*, *14*(1), 1–6.

Kabakama, S., Konje, E. T., Dinga, J. N., Kishamawe, C., Morhason-Bello, I., Hayombe, P., & Dzinamarira, T. (2022). Commentary on COVID-19 vaccine hesitancy in sub-Saharan Africa. *Tropical Medicine and Infectious Disease*, *7*(7), 130.

Kamazima, S. R., Kakoko, D. C., & Kazaura, M. (2020). Manifold tactics are used to control and prevent pandemics in contemporary Africa: A case of Tanzania's fight against COVID-19. *International Journal of Advanced Scientific Research and Management*, *5*(11), 20–33.

Kaunga, S. B. (2020). *How have Malawi's courts affected the country's epidemic response?* The London School of Economics and Political Science. https://blogs.lse.ac.uk/africaatlse/2020/11/13/how-have-malawis-courts-law-affected-epidemic-response/

Kayode, O. R., Obidiro, O. P., Lawrence, U. S., Oyetola, A. B., Hasan, M. M., Olajide, A., . . . Aderonke, O. M. (2022). Obstacles and policy measures toward COVID-19 vaccination: Creating a sustainable road map for Malawi. *Saudi Pharmaceutical Journal*, *30*(7), 1060–1063.

Kinfu, Y., Alam, U., & Achoki, T. (2020). COVID-19 pandemic in the African continent: Forecasts of cumulative cases, new infections, and mortality. *MedRxiv*, 2020–2024. https://www.medrxiv.org/content/10.1101/2020.04.09.20059154v3

Laurance, J. (2005). *Pure madness: How fear drives the mental health system*. Routledge.

Linke, S. E., Robinson, C. J., & Pekmezi, D. (2014). Applying psychological theories to promote healthy lifestyles. *American Journal of Lifestyle Medicine*, *8*(1), 4–14.

Lone, S. A., & Ahmad, A. (2020). COVID-19 pandemic: An African perspective. *Emerging Microbes & Infections*, *9*(1), 1300–1308.

Magamela, M. R., Dzinamarira, T., & Hlongwa, M. (2021). COVID-19 consequences on mental health: An African perspective. *South African Journal of Psychiatry*, *27*(1), 1–2.

Makoni, M. (2021). Tanzania refuses COVID-19 vaccines. *The Lancet*, *397*(10274), 566.

Mandala, M., & Changadeya, W. (2021). The fight against corona virus in Malawi: A review of challenges and opportunities in the health sector. *Malawi Journal of Science and Technology*, *13*(1), 1–10.

Marti, M., De Cola, M., MacDonald, N. E., Dumolard, L., & Duclos, P. (2017). Assessments of global drivers of vaccine hesitancy in 2014: Looking beyond safety concerns. *PLOS One*, *12*(3), e0172310.

Mashaphu, S., Talatala, M., Seape, S., Eriksson, L., & Chiliza, B. (2021). Mental health, culture and resilience: Approaching the COVID-19 pandemic from a South African perspective. *Frontiers in Psychiatry*, *12*, 1–5.

McCabe, O. L., Everly, G. S., Jr., Brown, L. M., Wendelboe, A. M., Abd Hamid, N. H., Tallchief, V. L., & Links, J. M. (2014). Psychological first aid: A consensus-derived, empirically supported, competency-based training model. *American Journal of Public Health*, *104*(4), 621–628.

Molebatsi, K., Musindo, O., Ntlantsana, V., & Wambua, G. N. (2021). Mental health and psychosocial support during COVID-19: A review of health guidelines in sub-Saharan Africa. *Frontiers in Psychiatry*, 1–10.

Monteiro, N. M. (2015). Addressing mental illness in Africa: Global health challenges and local opportunities. *Community Psychology in Global Perspective*, *1*(2), 78–95.

Mukherjee, S., & Pahan, K. (2021). Is COVID-19 gender-sensitive? *Journal of Neuroimmune Pharmacology*, *16*, 38–47.

Mutombo, P. N., Fallah, M. P., Munodawafa, D., Kabel, A., Houeto, D., Goronga, T., & Kanamori, B. (2022). COVID-19 vaccine hesitancy in Africa: A call to action. *The Lancet Global Health*, *10*(3), e320–e321.

Nachega, J. B., Atteh, R., Ihekweazu, C., Sam-Agudu, N. A., Adejumo, P., Nsanzimana, S., & Kilmarx, P. H. (2021a). Contact tracing and the COVID-19 response in Africa: Best practices, key challenges, and lessons learned from Nigeria, Rwanda, South Africa, and Uganda. *The American Journal of Tropical Medicine and Hygiene*, *104*(4), 1179–1187.

Nkengasong, J. N., & Tessema, S. K. (2020). Africa needs a new public health order to tackle infectious disease threats. *Cell*, *183*(2), 296–300.

Nuwagira, E., & Muzoora, C. (2020). Is sub-Saharan Africa prepared for COVID-19? *Tropical Medicine and Health*, *48*(1), 1–3.

Nyasulu, J. C. Y., Munthali, R. J., Nyondo-Mipando, A. L., Pandya, H., Nyirenda, L., Nyasulu, P. S., & Manda, S. (2021). COVID-19 pandemic in Malawi: Did public sociopolitical events gatherings contribute to its first-wave local transmission? *International Journal of Infectious Diseases*, *106*, 269–275.

Ogunleye, O. O., Godman, B., Fadare, J. O., Mudenda, S., Adeoti, A. O., Yinka-Ogunleye, A. F., & Meyer, J. C. (2022). Coronavirus disease 2019 (COVID-19) pandemic across Africa: Current status of vaccinations and implications for the future. *Vaccines, 10*(9), 1–28.

Ojeahere, M. I., De Filippis, R., Ransing, R., Karaliuniene, R., Ullah, I., Bytyçi, D. G., & Da Costa, M. P. (2020). Management of psychiatric conditions and delirium during the COVID-19 pandemics across continents: Lessons learned and recommendations. *Brain, Behavior, & Immunity-Health, 9*, 1–9.

Patel, P., Adebisi, Y. A., Steven, M., & Lucero-Prisno, D. E. III. (2020). Addressing COVID-19 in Malawi. *The Pan African Medical Journal, 35*(Suppl. 2), 1–2.

Patterson, A. S. (2022). *The Tanzanian state response to COVID-19*. https://ideas.repec.org/p/unu/wpaper/wp-2022-34.html

Paul, E., Steptoe, A., & Fancourt, D. (2021). Attitudes towards vaccines and intention to vaccinate against COVID-19: Implications for public health communications. *The Lancet Regional Health-Europe, 1*, 1–10.

Posel, D., Oyenubi, A., & Kollamparambil, U. (2021). Job loss and mental health during the COVID-19 lockdown: Evidence from South Africa. *PLOS One, 16*(3), e0249352.

Rwafa-Ponela, T., Price, J., Nyatela, A., Nqakala, S., Mosam, A., Erzse, A., & Goldstein, S. (2022). "We were afraid": Mental health effects of the COVID-19 pandemic in two South African districts. *International Journal of Environmental Research and Public Health, 19*(15), 1–18.

Saleh, M. (2020). Impact of COVID-19 on Tanzania political economy. *International Journal of Advanced Studies in Social Science & Innovation, 4*(1), 24–36.

Sallam, M. (2021). COVID-19 vaccine hesitancy worldwide: A concise systematic review of vaccine acceptance rates. *Vaccines, 9*(2), 1–14.

Sato, R. (2022). COVID-19 vaccine hesitancy and trust in government in Nigeria. *Vaccines, 10*(7), 1–7.

Semo, B. W., & Frissa, S. M. (2020). The mental health impact of the COVID-19 pandemic: Implications for sub-Saharan Africa. *Psychology Research and Behavior Management, 13*, 713–720.

Shah, K., Kamrai, D., Mekala, H., Mann, B., Desai, K., & Patel, R. S. (2020). Focus on mental health during the coronavirus (COVID-19) pandemic: Applying learnings from the past outbreaks. *Cureus, 12*(3), 1–6.

Sharma, M. (2021). *Theoretical foundations of health education and health promotion* (4th ed.). Jones & Bartlett Learning.

Sharma, M., Batra, K., & Batra, R. (2021, September). A theory-based analysis of COVID-19 vaccine hesitancy among African Americans in the United States: A recent evidence. *Healthcare, 9*(10), 1–18.

Shumba, S., Nyangari, E., & Mpofu, M. (Eds.). (2022). African indigenous knowledge and the management of COVID-19 pandemic. In *Knowledge production and the search for epistemic liberation in Africa* (pp. 179–199). Springer.

Tengatenga, J., Tengatenga Duley, S. M., & Tengatenga, C. J. (2021). Zimitsani Moto: Understanding the Malawi COVID-19 response. *Laws, 10*(2), 1–14.

Ufomba, H. U. (2020). The African Union development agenda 2063: Can Africa get it right? *Brazilian Journal of Development, 6*(8), 62626–62648.

Van de Walle, S., Van Roosbroek, S., & Bouckaert, G. (2008). Trust in the public sector: Is there any evidence for a long-term decline? *International Review of Administrative Sciences, 74*(1), 47–64.

Verani, A., Clodfelter, C., Menon, A. N., Chevinsky, J., Victory, K., & Hakim, A. (2020). Social distancing policies in 22 African countries during the COVID-19 pandemic: A desk review. *The Pan African Medical Journal, 37*(Suppl. 1), 1–12.

Wiysonge, C. S., Ndwandwe, D., Ryan, J., Jaca, A., Batouré, O., Anya, B. P. M., & Cooper, S. (2022). Vaccine hesitancy in the era of COVID-19: Could lessons from the past help in divining the future? *Human Vaccines & Immunotherapeutics, 18*(1), 1–3.

World Health Organization. (2001). *The world health report 2001: Mental health: New understanding, new hope*. World Health Organization.

World Health Organization. (2011). *Psychological first aid: Guide for field workers*. World Health Organization.

World Health Organization. (2020). *COVID-19 public health emergency of international concern (PHEIC): Global research and innovation forum: Towards a research roadmap*. World Health Organization.

World Health Organization. (2021). *Advice for the public: Coronavirus disease. COVID-19*. World Health Organization.

Zoa-Assoumou, S., Ndeboko, B., Manouana, G. P., Houechenou, R. M. A., Bikangui, R., Mveang-Nzoghe, A., & Siawaya, J. F. D. (2021). SARS-CoV-2 emerging variants in Africa: View from Gabon. *The Lancet Microbe, 2*(8), e349.

Part 4

Digital Remedies or Poisons?

14 Health Worker Experiences of Using Digital Resources for the Improvement of Mental Well-Being

Tilinao Lamba, Edister S. Jamu, Demoubly Kokota, Limbika Maliwichi, Alex Zumazuma, Eckhard Kleinau, Katy Gorentz, Wanda Jaskiewicz, Donya Rahimi, and Michael Kapps

14.1 Introduction

Mental, neurological, and substance use disorders pose serious public health challenges in many countries (Whiteford et al., 2013). In Malawi, 28.8% of primary healthcare attendees have been reported to have a common mental disorder (Wright et al., 2013). In another study, the prevalence of depression among patients in two health centres in southern Malawi was 30.3% (Udedi, 2014). A weighted prevalence of 30.4% (95% CI 22.8–38.1%) was also found for any current depressive episode for Malawian rural women with infants (Stewart et al., 2010). All these studies show how prevalent mental illnesses are in Malawi.

People who experience various mental health problems are recommended to receive evidence-based psychological interventions with a trained psychotherapist (Claringbull, 2010). However, several barriers, such as the exorbitant costs of face-to-face therapy, a lack of trained staff, and time and caseload pressures mean that timely support access is not always available (Fisher et al., 2016). In Malawi, access to mental health services is even more limited than in other countries, with only 0.02 psychologists and 0.01 psychiatrists per 100,000 Malawian population (WHO, 2018). In addition to only having successfully trained three psychiatrists, most Malawian mental health professionals, such as psychiatric nurses, are usually deployed to other services within the healthcare system (Kauye, 2008). According to the Malawi Ministry of Health (MOH), mental health facilities constitute just 0.3% of the health facilities available in the country (Udedi, 2016). This has had a cumulative negative effect on the mental health of frontline healthcare workers by raising anxieties regarding on-the-job risks, infrastructural and technological deficits, human-capital deficits, and public stigma – particularly during the COVID-19 crisis (Munyenyembe & Ying-Yu, 2021).

Using digital technologies to combat mental health challenges is a viable option for low-resource areas (Berry et al., 2019). Malawi has seen recent digital mental health innovations, such as the Malawi Quick Guide to Mental

DOI: 10.4324/9781003425861-18

Health, produced by the Scotland Malawi Mental Health Education Project to provide practical information for assessing and managing mental disorders in Malawi (Scotland Malawi Mental Health Education Program, 2021). The main target user of the guide is the busy primary healthcare provider working at first- and second-level healthcare facilities in Malawi (Scotland Malawi Mental Health Education Program, 2021). This resource was translated into Chichewa (the primary local language in Malawi), printed and distributed to all district health offices (DHOs) and over 600 health facilities in the country. Another non-profit organisation promoting mental health awareness through digital innovation is the Mental Lab app, developed by Sparc Systems Limited (Africa) and Caring Hands (Chiyembekeza, 2021). It also shares information about various mental challenges with therapy video content and a platform where users can access experts in mental issues (Chiyembekeza, 2021).

However, there is a lack of empirical evidence on the effectiveness or usability of these digital resources, particularly from the users' perspective. It is this knowledge gap that the current study aimed to fill. The study supports the Malawi mental health policy 2020 priority area 3, which seeks to provide comprehensive, integrated, and responsive mental health services to all individuals, families, and communities at all levels (see The Government of the Republic of Malawi, 2000). This study explored the effectiveness of one such digital mental health innovation used by Malawian health workers named Vitalk.

Originally from Brazil, the Vitalk app is an automated chatbot that delivers mental health content to users using a conversational format to improve well-being by reducing stress, anxiety, and depression using a preventive approach to mental health (Daley et al., 2020). Vitalk functions with three language options: Portuguese, Spanish, and English. For the trial conducted in Malawi, the participants used Vitalk in English.

14.2 Theoretical and Methodological Considerations

Conceptually, the findings were broadly anchored in the technology adoption model (TAM) by Davis (1989), which was later modified by Holden and Karsh (2010). Specifically, the focus was perceived usefulness (PU) and perceived ease of use (PEOU) as predictors of behavioural intentions, predicting actual use. In their review of TAM, Holden and Karsh (2010) found that the model predicts a substantial portion of the use or acceptance of health information technology. We theorised that participants' experience using Vitalk regarding PU and PEOU during the trial period would influence compliance.

The study was a two-arm, parallel, randomised controlled trial (RCT) to investigate the hypothesis that Vitalk is more effective in improving mental health and resilience outcomes than passive Internet resources. A total of 1,584 participants enrolled in the study, based on the projected number of 640 participants initially required per study arm (treatment and control), calculated using STATA 17 and making provisions for an up to 75% dropout rate, as well as 20% not meeting the inclusion criteria for the study (Kleinau et al.,

2023). The study participants were health workers from eight professional cadres working in public and private healthcare facilities in Lilongwe and Blantyre districts in Malawi, comprising doctors, nurses, laboratory technicians, physiotherapy technicians, pharmacists, physiotherapists, medical assistants, and clinical officers.

The participants were recruited from Blantyre and Lilongwe districts. Study participants were randomly assigned to either the Vitalk app treatment group or the control group. This latter group was provided with links to Internet resources about mental health issues. Participants were informed of their assigned mental health resource, whether Vitalk or the website, through an email with their unique trial ID number and a link to either Vitalk or the website. Each participant used their unique trial ID number to log into their allocated mental health resource throughout the trial, thus, ensuring that each engaged only with their intended content. The study was single-blinded, with only the researchers blinded to the participants' allocations. The participants in both study arms were aware of the intervention they were using. Later during the trial, they may have discovered that others used a different mental health resource, either Vitalk or the website (Kleinau et al., 2023).

All participants began the eight-week trial by taking a baseline assessment, a midterm assessment at week four, and an end-line assessment to test the hypothesis that an app like Vitalk could improve mental health outcomes. The assessments provided outcome measures for anxiety (GAD-7), depression (PHQ-9), burnout (OLBI), loneliness (ULCA), resilience (RS-14), and resilience-building activities. The effectiveness of Vitalk was analysed using mixed-effects linear models, effect-size estimates, and reliable change in risk levels (Kleinau et al., 2023). The results of the quantitative analysis supported the hypothesis: the use of Vitalk is effective in improving various mental health indicators for the treatment group, reducing depression (-0.68 [95% CI -1.15–0.21]), anxiety (-0.44 [95% CI -0.88–0.01]), and burnout (-0.58 [95% CI -1.32–0.15]). Additionally, changes in resilience (1.47 [95% CI 0.05–2.88]) and resilience-building activities (1.22 [95% CI 0.56–1.87]) were significantly more significant in the treatment group than in the control group (Kleinau et al., 2023).

At the end of the 8-week trial period, closing workshops and a digital post-study survey were conducted with the participants to gain feedback about their experiences. The aim of this qualitative exploration was (1) to learn which features of Vitalk or the website resources were liked or disliked by the participants; (2) to gain suggestions to improve the effectiveness of the Vitalk app; and (3) to see if user experience drives compliance (continued use of the app). The findings from these post-study feedback workshops provided the data presented in this chapter.

A total of 1,138 participants of the 1,584 initially enrolled in the study took part in the post-study feedback workshops conducted in Lilongwe and Blantyre. Participants were divided into focus groups based on their study allocation of treatment and control groups. Each focus group had between

7 and 10 participants. In addition to the FGDs, 820 participants completed a digital post-study survey, accessed on their smartphones by following a link to a Google Docs questionnaire. This questionnaire was completed anonymously by the participants. It comprised four demographic questions, 17 user experience questions with responses set to a five-point Likert-type scale, six multiple-choice questions, three open-ended feedback questions, and one linear scaling question recommending the Vitalk app or website resources to others. Responses to this digital post-study survey were disaggregated by study group (treatment vs. control). The treatment group questionnaire also included an additional Vitalk-specific question regarding how the participants would rate their experience using the app.

The audio recordings of the FGDs were reviewed alongside the flip charts and participants' notes, and data analysis used interpretive phenomenological analysis (IPA) to identify recurrent themes and sub-themes within the responses. Descriptive analysis was used for the quantitative data collected by the post-study survey. Ethical approval was granted by the University of Malawi Research Ethics Committee (UNIMAREC) (Protocol No. P09/21/84) and the University Research Co. (URC) in the United States of America. All participants provided written consent before participating in the study, the FGDs, and the digital post-study survey.

14.3 Knowledge of Mental Health Challenges

Health workers were classified as essential workers at a high risk of infection, particularly those caring for COVID-19 patients. This increased their experiences of anxiety, as they worried about their health and welfare, as well as those close to them.

> [I feel] anxiety because of worrying if I'm going to catch COVID-19.
> [Y]ou even worry about your family . . . what if they get it if you infect them.
> [T]here is a fear of the unknown.

Several studies identify anxiety as one of the most common mental health challenges affecting health workers (Aly et al., 2021; Motahedi et al., 2021). A systematic review found a range of 22.2 to 33.0% in the global prevalence of anxiety in all healthcare workers (Fernandez et al., 2021). One study found COVID-19-related anxiety and functional impairment in Malawi in 25.5% and 48% of nurses, respectively (Chorwe-Sungani, 2021). Factors such as fears of contagion, fear of bringing the virus home, changing protocols, caring for very sick patients, and personal protective equipment (PPE) have all contributed to anxiety in health workers (Hall, 2020; Walton et al., 2020). Those health workers who had been quarantined were found to face additional fears of living with the illness and guilt about contributing to an understaffed frontline (Brooks et al., 2020).

In Malawi, additional fears of stigma and discrimination and inadequate training for the COVID-19 response have also been found (Mpasa et al., 2021). Health workers' constant mental health challenges can potentially cause post-traumatic stress symptoms, suicidal ideation, and poor care delivery (Søvold et al., 2021). One study found thoughts of self-harm and suicide in up to 13% of health workers working in COVID-19 intensive care units (ICUs) (see Spoorthy et al., 2020).

Participants also reported experiencing burnout. Burnout among health workers increased during COVID-19, as health workers are exposed to life-threatening situations, increased workload, and workplace changes because of the pandemic (Denning et al., 2021).

> I felt burnout because of short staffing at my facility.
> We work very long hours. At my facility, there are only three of us [nurses] and one was sick.
> This job is very stressful; it's not an easy job at all.

Burnout rates among various types of health workers during COVID-19 have been reported as 66.2% in the United States (see Stone et al., 2021), 82.1% in Singapore (see Lum et al., 2021), and 47.9% in Kenya (see Ali et al., 2021) and in other developing countries (El Dabbah & Elhadi, 2023). In Malawi COVID-19 added to an already prevailing lack of health resources such as personnel and equipment (Makwero, 2018), putting low- or middle-income countries (LMICs) high on the list of infections (Kola et al., 2021). All this, plus a lack of psychosocial support for health workers, increased burnout symptoms (Sultana et al., 2020).

Depression was also named one of the common mental health challenges experienced by health workers, with varied triggers and probable causes.

> Depression is also not far from you because people are dying.
> Losing a loved one, you can get depressed . . . or patients are dying.

This finding is consistent with other studies looking at depression during the COVID-19 pandemic (see Fond et al., 2022; Motahedi et al., 2021). A systematic review found the global prevalence of depression during COVID-19 in all healthcare workers to range from 17.9% to 36% (Fernandez et al., 2021). A different systematic review and meta-analysis found a pooled global prevalence of depression to be at 24% among healthcare workers, 24% among medical doctors, 25% among nurses, and 43% among frontline health workers (Olaya et al., 2021). In Kenya and Saudi Arabia, up to 53.6% and 54.69% of frontline healthcare workers were found to suffer from depression (Almalki et al., 2021; Shah et al., 2021).

In some African countries, factors such as fear of death due to COVID-19, and inadequate resources or training have been found to contribute to depression among health workers (Elgohary et al., 2021). Inadequate resources correlate with increased depression in countries outside Africa (Ang et al., 2021). Malawi is one of the countries ranked as poor worldwide, with a lack of health resources. This could contribute to mental health conditions, including depression, especially during the COVID-19 pandemic.

14.4 Benefits of Utilising Vitalk as a Mental Health Resource

The Vitalk app presents its users with a virtual mental health assistant named Viki, who refers to herself in the first person and describes herself as a robot that intends to assist users in improving their mental health. Viki communicates with users in an interactive format. She presents psychoeducation, CBT recommendations, emotional check-ups, self-improvement exercises, and mental health assessments in a conversational mode that engages the user, which participants found enjoyable. Participants also enjoyed Viki's companionship, mainly because the interaction with the app was a back-and-forth conversation.

Overall, users of Vitalk enjoyed the interactive nature of the experience, which is consistent with other study findings that have shown a user preference for a positive, fun, practical, and interactive method for self-management of mental health matters (Berry et al., 2019). This approach to digital mental health interventions helps provide a substitute for human-based interaction (Ahmed et al., 2021), including the conversational tone during user interactions and the variety of assessments and exercises available to users (Alqahtani & Orji, 2020).

> I like Viki – she is so friendly.
> It felt like I was talking to a real person. Sometimes I would be bored during my shift at night, and there's nobody to talk to on WhatsApp. I could talk to Viki.

Conversely, most of the positive reviews from the control group participants centred on the mental health information to which they had access. However, there was no mention of enjoyable interaction or additional pleasurable experiences.

> It gave us information about mental health that we didn't know.
> The thing I liked about the website was the mental health assessments.

Some participants in the control group also expressed interest and curiosity in using Vitalk upon hearing of the experiences of their colleagues from the treatment group.

> Now I'm so curious about this Viki . . . I never got greeted by my name on that website!
> Ours was boring! We didn't have any chats . . . just these textbooks with difficult words!

Aside from the sense of companionship and friendly interactions with Viki, Vitalk users reported that they could improve their self-awareness and incorporate new self-care techniques.

> I enjoyed the mindfulness exercise; I still use it in my free time.
> The relaxation exercises are very helpful . . . the breathing exercises . . . it helps when you're stressed.

Vitalk use also fostered self-awareness. Users reported learning more about some of their mental health challenges and healthy habits that they could incorporate to safeguard their mental health.

> I thought it was normal – at least now I know I'm facing burnout.
> Viki taught me to be more assertive . . . to say no . . . take time out.

The psychoeducation that was presented through Vitalk was also appreciated, with many people stating that they shared the information they learned with others so that their learning had a trickle-down effect.

> I look very knowledgeable when talking to my friends about mental health challenges, I can tell someone that "this is anxiety, you should try deep breathing" or "take a walk."

Mental health apps are widely known for their ability to assist users in various wellness-focused activities, such as relaxation, mood-tracking, practising mindfulness and self-care (Thach, 2019). These benefits were available to the users of the Vitalk app, in addition to improved sleep patterns, an increase in forming healthy habits (e.g., exercising), and conflict resolution. In comparison, while members of the control group stated that they also had access to copious amounts of mental health information, there was a poor show of practical incorporation of that information into their everyday lives.

Compliance refers to a user's propensity to continually access a product due to previous positive experiences with it (Carlo et al., 2020). The users of Vitalk described numerous positive and enjoyable experiences with using the app and expressed interest in accessing additional content. In addition to Viki's interactive and friendly nature as a significant contributor to compliance, others commented on how the conversations with Viki were brief yet effective.

> I expected that the app will take up too much of my time, but it didn't.
> Viki doesn't take much time; she chats with you for just a few minutes then she says "bye" . . . I can go doing other things.

This appreciation of being able to access the benefits of the app without spending excessive amounts of time on it is consistent with other studies of mental health apps, where user compliance was indicated when user experiences were not time-consuming, inflexible, or too involving (see Dederichs et al., 2021). Overall, current research points to the efficacy of mental health apps in reducing mental health challenges, such as depression, anxiety, and suicidal ideation, as the most significant contributors to user compliance (Huckvale et al., 2020; Lecomte et al., 2020).

14.5 Challenges of Using Vitalk as a Mental Health Resource

While reported usage of both types of mental health resources remained high, some challenges hampered the consistent use of the platforms. Of the participants, 49.5% in the treatment arm reported actively using the Vitalk app for 29 or more days during the study period, compared to only 21% of participants in the control arm using the resource website. The top five reasons for not using the Vitalk app more often were (1) not having time to use the app (45.2%); (2) the app taking too long to work with (27.8%); (3) the app being challenging to use (13.4%); (4) not being comfortable completing mental health assessments (8.3%); and (5) content being difficult to understand (7%).

Time-related constraints topped the list of reasons why participants did not use the app (78.8%) or the website (81.5%) consistently. About 20% of the Vitalk app users complained that the app was too difficult to use or the content was too difficult to understand. Other content-related reasons were the repetitiveness of the content, which made it boring, and content that users deemed irrelevant. This was common among those who accessed the resources through the website.

Digital illiteracy was also a major challenge to using the Vitalk app. Most participants (90%) thought the Vitalk app was generally easy to use, but many had challenges installing the Vitalk app (26.9%), signing in (76.3%), and finding the mental health assessments (24.5%). Additionally, participants implied that the unfamiliarity with digital technology might be considered a generational barrier.

> I struggled to download the app, I had to ask a colleague of mine to do it for me.
> [M]ost of the people who struggled were older members, and they usually are not very knowledgeable on using such things . . . sometimes they can't even use WhatsApp.

Participants also identified the exorbitant Internet data costs as a significant barrier to Vitalk use. Since the functions of Vitalk are accessed on an active Internet connection, this study made provision for all participants to receive allocations of 4 GB of mobile data bundles per month throughout this study. This provision was made because engaging with the Vitalk app would require steady and reliable Internet, a significant expense in Malawi.

> I doubt I'll use it [Vitalk] again; [Internet] bundles are expensive.
> We got our second bundles late . . . so I didn't use Vitalk for a while.

With the cost of Internet connectivity, research participants stated that they would likely not use the app again after the termination of the study.

14.6 Improvements Suggested by Users

Studies identify out-of-pocket costs as a significant barrier to adopting digital apps in many countries (Roland et al., 2020; Zhou et al., 2019). Participants recommended increased accessibility of Vitalk by using alternative platforms that do not require an Internet connection, such as through a USSD-supported format.

> Vitalk should be improved by allowing offline access; it should not require [data] bundle.

A few participants complained about the unavailability of Vitalk on App Store, and proposed that it should be made available for iPhone and iPad users as well.

Participants also observed that their interactions with Viki were limited to a selection of predetermined responses provided on the Vitalk app, leading participants to feel that the app was controlling the direction of conversations unlike what happens in real counselling settings.

> It should have open-ended questions in some parts where we can express ourselves or our thoughts and that Vitalk should give us a chance to give ideas and ask questions.

Another cumbersome quality of the app was the failure of the users to continue a session from where they had previously stopped and having to repeatedly enter their login details, which some participants found tedious. This points to the importance of user testing to ensure the user experience is smooth – even if the interaction is cut off (due to poor Internet access or other pressing demands on the healthcare worker's time, etc.)

Vitalk users also stated that they wanted to have the freedom to alter their response selections on the app, proposing that the app should not automatically lock user responses.

> Sometimes we could mistakenly press or click a response that we needed to reverse or change but this was not possible.

Finally, participants felt that the app would be more beneficial if it contained the contact details of local mental health professionals with whom they could get in touch. Although participants found the app beneficial, it was felt that as a tool – "a robot" – it was not possible to deal satisfactorily with all challenges that participants were experiencing. Directing users to the appropriate or specialised service providers within their geographical locations would therefore be a welcome addition to the functionality of the app.

> Linking the individuals who have mental health problems with the right person, such as therapists, in real-time.
> There should be a provision for a toll-free telephone line which they can call when they encounter a problem.

Other studies that focused on mental health app user experience found that users are happy with mental health tools that can be integrated with traditional services (Povey et al., 2016; Roland et al., 2020) or hybrid models of care that combine face-to-face, telehealth, and digital health approaches (Balcombe & De Leo, 2020).

14.7 Conclusion

Considering the low availability of mental health services in Malawi, it is essential to diversify the mental health support options available to people. The current study explored the experiences, including the various highlights and challenges, of users who have utilised a mental health chatbot to improve their mental health. These findings could help to inform other innovative digital mental health efforts with factors that should be considered to enhance user experience and the effectiveness of said innovations. Improved digital literacy would help users of such digital mental health resources benefit from their use, particularly with the incorporation of a more interactive format that allows users to express themselves freely and get responses to their questions. Noteworthy is that Malawi's high data cost significantly limits the freedom of using these resources when the user cannot access the Internet. Such insights can go a long way in informing further digital mental health innovations in Malawi to produce an effective service that provides lasting solutions to people's mental health problems.

Acknowledgements

This material is made possible by the generous support of the American people through the United States Agency for International Development (USAID) under the terms of cooperative agreement no. AID-OAA-A-15–00046 (2015–2022) in partnership with The US President's Emergency Plan for AIDS Relief. The contents are the responsibility of the University of Malawi and the Kamuzu University of Health Sciences and do not necessarily reflect the views of USAID or the United States government.

References

Ahmed, A., Ali, N., Aziza, S., Alaa, A. S., Hassana, A., Khalifah, M., Bushra, E., Ali Siddig Ahmed, M. M., & Househ, M. (2021). A review of mobile chatbot apps for anxiety. *Computer Methods and Programs in Biomedicine Update, 1*, 1–8. https://doi.org/10.1016/j.cmpbup.2021.100012

Ali, S. K., Shah, J., & Talib, Z. (2021). COVID-19 and mental well-being of nurses in a tertiary facility in Kenya. *PLOS One, 16*(7), e0254074. https://doi.org/10.1371/journal.pone.0254074

Almalki, A. H., Alzahrani, M. S., Alshehri, F. S., Alharbi, A., Alkhudaydi, S. F., Alshahrani, R. S., Alzaidi, A. H., Algarni, M. A., Alsaab, H. O., Alatawi, Y., Althobaiti, Y. S., Bamaga, A. K., & Alhifany, A. A. (2021). The psychological impact of COVID-19 on healthcare workers in Saudi Arabia: A year later into the pandemic. *Frontiers in Psychiatry, 12*, 797545. https://doi.org/10.3389/fpsyt.2021.797545

Alqahtani, F., & Orji, R. (2020). Insights from user reviews to improve mental health apps. *Health Informatics Journal, 26*(3), 2042–2066. https://doi.org/10.1177/1460458219896492

Aly, H. M., Nemr, N. A., Kishk, R. M., & Elsaid, N. M. (2021). Stress, anxiety and depression among healthcare workers facing COVID-19 pandemic in Egypt: A cross-sectional online-based study. *BMJ Open, 11*, e045281. https://doi.org/10.1136/bmjopen-2020-045281

Ang, Y., Lu, L., Chen, T., Ye, S., Kelifa, M. O., Cao, N., Zhang, Q., Liang, T., & Wang, W. (2021). Healthcare worker's mental health and their associated predictors during the epidemic peak of COVID-19. *Psychology Research and Behaviour Management, 14*, 221–231. https://doi.org/10.2147/PRBM.S290931

Balcombe, L., & De Leo, D. (2020). An integrated blueprint for digital mental health services amidst COVID-19. *JMIR Mental Health, 7*(7), e21718.

Berry, N., Lobban, F., & Bucci, S. (2019). A qualitative exploration of service user views about using digital health interventions for self-management in severe mental health problems. *BMC Psychiatry, 19*(1), 35. https://doi.org/10.1186/s12888-018-1979-1

Brooks, S. K., Webster, R. K., Smith, L. E., Woodland, L., Wessely, S., Greenberg, N., & Rubin, G. J. (2020). The psychological impact of quarantine and how to reduce it: Rapid review of the evidence. *Lancet, 395*(10227), 912–920. https://doi.org/10.1016/S0140-6736(20)30460-8

Carlo, A. D., Ghomi, R. H., Renn, B. N., Strong, M. A., & Areán, P. A. (2020). Assessment of real-world use of behavioral health mobile applications by a novel stickiness metric. *JAMA Network Open, 3*(8). https://doi.org/10.1001/jamanetworkopen.2020.11978

Chiyembekeza, C. (2021, August 24). Sparc systems partners NGO on mental health app. *The Nation.* https://mwnation.com/sparc-systems-partners-ngo-on-mental-health-app/

Chorwe-Sungani, G. (2021). Assessing COVID-19-related anxiety and functional impairment amongst nurses in Malawi. *African Journal of Primary Health Care & Family Medicine, 13*(1), e1–e6. https://doi.org/10.4102/phcfm.v13i1.2823

Claringbull, N. (2010). *What is counselling and psychotherapy?* T. J. International.

Daley, K., Hungerbuehler, I., Cavanagh, K., Claro, H. G., Swinton, P. A., & Kapps, M. (2020). Preliminary evaluation of the engagement and effectiveness of a mental health chatbot. *Frontiers in Digital Health, 2*. https://doi.org/10.3389/fdgth.2020.576361

Davis, F. D. (1989). Perceived usefulness, perceived ease of use, and user acceptance of information technology. *MIS Quarterly, 13*, 319–340.

Dederichs, M., Weber, J., Pischke, C. R., Angerer, P., & Apolinario-Hagen, J. (2021). Exploring medical students' views on digital mental health interventions:

A qualitative study. *Internet Interventions, 25,* 100398. https://doi.org/10.1016/j. invent.2021.100398

Denning, N., Goh, E. T., Tan, B., Kanneganti, A., Almonte, M., Scott, A., Martin, G., Clarke, J., Sounderajah, V., Markar, S., Przybylowicz, J., Chan, Y. H., Sia, C., Chua, Y. X., Sim, K., Lim, L., Tan, L., Tan, M., Sharma, V. . . . Kinross, J. (2021). Determinants of burnout and other aspects of psychological well-being in healthcare workers during the Covid-19 pandemic: A multinational cross-sectional study. *PLOS One, 16,* e0238666. https://doi.org/10.1371/journal.pone.0238666

El Dabbah, N. A., & Elhadi, Y. A. M. (2023). High levels of burnout among health professionals treating COVID-19 patients in two Nile basin countries with limited resources. *Scientific Reports, 13*(1), 6455. https://doi.org/10.1038/s41598-023-33399-2

Elgohary, H. M., Sehlo, M. G., Bassiony, M. M., Youssef, U. M., Elrafey, D. S., & Amin, S. I. (2021). Depression among health workers caring for patients with COVID-19 in Egypt. *The Egyptian Journal of Neurology, Psychiatry and Neurosurgery, 57,* 139. https://doi.org/10.1186/s41983-021-00394-1

Fernandez, R., Sikhosana, N., Green, H., Halcomb, E. J., Middleton, R., Alananzeh, I., Trakis, S., & Moxham, L. (2021). Anxiety and depression among health-care workers during the COVID-19 pandemic: A systematic umbrella review of the global evidence. *BMJ Open, 11*(9), e054528. https://doi.org/10.1136/bmjopen-2021-054528

Fisher, A., Manicavasagar, V., Kiln, F., & Juraskova, I. (2016, July). Communication and decision-making in mental health: A systematic review focusing on bipolar disorder. *Patient Education and Counseling, 99*(7), 1106–1120. https://doi.org/10.1016/j.pec.2016.02.011. Epub February 23, 2016. PMID: 26924609.

Fond, G., Fernandes, S., Lucas, G., Greenberg, N., & Boyer, L. (2022). Depression in healthcare workers: Results from the nationwide AMADEUS survey. *International Journal of Nursing Studies, 135,* 104328. https://doi.org/10.1016/j.ijnurstu.2022.104328

The Government of the Republic of Malawi. (2000). *National mental health policy.* Ministry of Health. https://extranet.who.int/mindbank/collection/country/malawi/mental_health_policies

Hall, H. (2020). The effect of the COVID-19 pandemic on healthcare workers' mental health. *JAAPA: Journal of the American Academy of PAS, 33*(7), 45–48. https://doi.org/10.1097/01.JAA.0000669772.78848.8c

Holden, R. J., & Karsh, B. T. (2010). The technology acceptance model: Its past and its future in health care. *Journal of Biomedical Informatics, 43*(1), 159–172.

Huckvale, K., Nicholas, J., Torous, J., & Larsen, M. E. (2020). Smartphone apps for the treatment of mental health conditions: Status and considerations. *Current Opinion in Psychology, 20,* 65–70.

Kainja, J. (2019). *Digital rights: How expensive is the Internet in Malawi?* Media Institute of Southern Africa. https://malawi.misa.org/2019/02/23/digital-rights-how-expensive-is-the-internet-in-malawi/#:~:text=The%20current%20average%20monthly%20income,mobile%20data%20is%20in%20Malawi.

Kauye, F. (2008). Management of mental health services in Malawi. *International Psychiatry: Bulletin of the Board of International Affairs of the Royal College of Psychiatrists, 5*(2), 29–30.

Kleinau, E. F., Lamba, T., Jaskiewicz, W., Gorentz, K., Hungerbuehler, I., Rahimim, D., Kokota, D., Maliwichi, L., Jamu, E. S., Zumazuma, A., Negrão, M., Mota, R.,

Khouri, Y., & Kapps, M. (2023). *COVID-19 SARS-CoV-2 preprints from medRxiv and bioRxiv.* https://doi.org/10.1101/2023.01.24.23284959; https://connect.medrxiv.org/relate/content/181

Kola, L., Kohrt, B. A., Hanlon, C., Naslund, J. A., Sikander, S., Balaji, M., Benjet, C., Cheung, E. Y. L., Eaton, J., Gonsalves, P., Hailemariam, M., Luitel, N. P., Machado, D. B., Misganaw, E., Omigbodun, O., Roberts, T., Salisbury, T. T., Shidhaye, R., Sunkel, C., . . . Patel, V. (2021). COVID-19 mental health impact and responses in low-income and middle-income countries: Reimagining global mental health. *Lancet Psychiatry, 8*, 535–550. https://doi.org/10.1016/S2215-0366(21)00025-0

Lecomte, T., Potvin, S., Corbière, M., Guay, S., Samson, C., Cloutier, B., Francoeur, A., Pennou, A., & Khazaal, Y. (2020). Mobile apps for mental health issues: Meta-review of meta-analyses. *JMIR mHealth uHealth, 8*(5), e17458. https://doi.org/10.2196/17458. PMID: 32348289; PMCID: PMC7293054.

Lum, A., Goh, Y. L., Wong, K. S., Seah, J., Teo, G., Ng, J. Q., Abdin, E., Hendricks, M. M., Tham, J., Nan, W., & Fung, D. (2021). Impact of COVID-19 on the mental health of Singaporean G.P.s: A cross-sectional study. *British Journal of General Practice, 5*(4), https://doi.org/10.3399/BJGPO.2021.0072

Makwero, M. T. (2018). Delivery of primary health care in Malawi. *African Journal of Primary Health Care & Family Medicine, 10*(1), e1–e3. https://doi.org/10.4102/phcfm.v10i1.1799

Motahedi, S., Aghdam, N. F., Khajeh, M., Baha, R., Aliyari, R., Bagheri, H., & Mardani, A. (2021). Anxiety and depression among healthcare workers during COVID-19 pandemic: A cross-sectional study. *Heliyon, 7*(12), e08570. https://doi.org/10.1016/j.heliyon.2021.e08570

Mpasa, F., Baluwa, M., Lungu, F., Chipeta, M. C., Munthali, G., Mhango, L., Chimbe, E., & Konyani, A. (2021). COVID-19 related fears among Mzuzu University's nursing students during clinical practice. *Nursing: Research and Reviews, 11*, 31–39. https://doi.org/10.2147/NRR.S331137

Munyenyembe, B., & Ying-Yu, C. (2021). COVID-19 anxiety-coping strategies of frontline health workers in a low-income country Malawi: A qualitative inquiry. *Journal of Workplace Behavioural Health, 37*(1), 47–67. https://doi.org/10.1080/15555240.2021.2011303

Olaya, B., Pérez-Moreno, M., Bueno-Notivol, J., Gracia-García, P., Lasheras, I., & Santabárbara, J. (2021). Prevalence of depression among healthcare workers during the COVID-19 outbreak: A systematic review and meta-analysis. *Journal of Clinical Medicine, 10*(15), 3406. https://doi.org/10.3390/jcm10153406

Povey, J., Mills, P. P. J. R., Dingwall, K. M., Lowell, A., Singer, J., Rotumah, D., Bennett-Levy, J., & Nagel, T. (2016). Acceptability of mental health apps for Aboriginal and Torres Strait Islander Australians: A qualitative study. *Journal of Medical Internet Research, 18*(3), e5314.

Roland, J., Lawrance, E., Insel, T., & Christensen, H. (2020). *The digital mental health revolution: Transforming care through innovation and scale-up.* World Innovation Summit for Health.

Scotland Malawi Mental Health Education Program. (2021). *Press launch of the Malawi quick guide to mental health.* www.smmhep.org.uk/content/press-launch-malawi-quick-guide-mental-health

Shah, J., Monroe-Wise, A., Talib, Z., Nabiswa, A., Mohammed Said, M., Abdulaziz Abeid, A., Mohamed, M. A., & Mohamed, S. (2021). Mental health disorders among healthcare workers during the COVID-19 pandemic: A cross-sectional survey from three major hospitals in Kenya. *BMJ Open, 11*(6), e050316. https:// doi.org/10.1136/bmjopen-2021-050316

Søvold, L. E., Naslund, J. A., Kousoulis, A. A., Saxena, S., Qoronfleh, M. W., Grobler, C., & Münter, L. (2021). Prioritising the mental health and well-being of health-care workers: An urgent global public health priority. *Frontiers in Public Health, 9,* 679397. https://doi.org/10.3389/fpubh.2021.679397

Spoorthy, M. S., Pratapa, S. K., & Mahant, S. (2020). Mental health problems faced by healthcare workers due to the COVID-19 pandemic: A review. *Asian Journal of Psychiatry, 51.* https://doi.org/10.1016/j.ajp.2020.102119

Stewart, R. C., Bunn, J., Vokhiwa, M., Umar, E., Kauye, F., Fitzgerald, M., Tomenson, B., Rahman, A., & Creed, F. (2010). Common mental disorder and associated factors amongst women with young infants in rural Malawi. *Social Psychiatry and Psychiatric Epidemiology, 45*(5), 551–559.

Stone, K. W., Kintziger, K. W., Jagger, M. A., & Horney, J. A. (2021). Public health workforce burnout in the COVID-19 response in the U.S. *International Journal of Environmental Research and Public Health, 18*(8). https://doi.org/10.3390/ ijerph18084369

Sultana, A., Sharma, R., Hossain, M. M., Bhattacharya, S., & Purohit, N. (2020, October–December). Burnout among healthcare providers during COVID-19: Challenges and evidence-based interventions. *Indian Journal of Medical Ethics, V*(4), 1–6. https://doi.org/10.20529/IJME.2020.73

Thach, K. S. (2019). A qualitative analysis of user reviews on mental health apps: Who used it? For what? And why? In *2019 IEEE-RIVF international conference on computing and communication technologies (RIVF).* IEEE. https://doi.org/10.1109/ RIVF.2019.8713726

Theu, J. A., Kabaghe, A. N., Bello, G., Chitsa-Banda, E., Kagoli, M., Auld, A., Mkungudza, J., O'Malley, G., Bangara, F. F., Peacocke, E. F., Babaye, Y., Ng'ambi, W., Saussier, C., MacLachlan, E., Chapotera, G., Phiri, M. D., Kim, E., Chiwaula, M., Payne, D., . . . Public Health Institute of Malawi COVID-19 Surveillance Committee. (2022). SARS-CoV-2 prevalence in Malawi based on data from survey of communities and health workers in 5 high-burden districts, October 2020. *Emerging Infectious Diseases, 28*(13), S76–S84. https://doi.org/10.3201/eid2813.212348. PMID: 36502413. PMCID: PMC9745213.

Udedi, M. (2014). The prevalence of depression among patients and its detection by primary health care workers at Matawale Health Centre (Zomba). *Malawi Medical Journal, 26*(2), 34–37.

Udedi, M. (2016). *Improving access to mental health services in Malawi.* Ministry of Health. https://doi.org/10.13140/RG.2.1.3996.9524

Walton, M., Murray, E., & Christian, M. (2020). Mental health care for medical staff and affiliated healthcare workers during the COVID-19 pandemic. *European Heart Journal: Acute Cardiovascular Care, 9*(3), 241–247.

Weilenmann, S., Ernst, J., Petry, H., Pfaltz, M. C., Sazpinar, O., Gehrke, S., Paolercio, F., Von Känel, R., & Spiller, T. R. (2021). Health care workers' mental health during the first weeks of the SARS-CoV-2 pandemic in Switzerland: A cross-sectional study. *Frontiers in Psychiatry, 18*(12). https://doi.org/10.3389/fpsyt.2021.594340. PMID: 33815162; PMCID: PMC8012487.

Whiteford, H. A., Degenhardt, L., Rehm, J., Baxter, A. J., Ferrari, A. J., Erskine, H. E., Charlson, F. J., Norman, R. E., Flaxman, A. D., Johns, N., Burstein, R., Murray, C. J. L., & Vos, T. (2013). Global burden of disease attributable to mental and substance use disorders: Findings from the global burden disease study 2010. *Lancet, 382,* 1575–1586.

World Health Organization. (2018). *Mental health atlas 2017.* www.who.int/publications/i/item/9789241514019

Wright, J., Common, S., Kauye, F., & Chiwandira, C. (2013). Integrating community mental health within primary care in southern Malawi: A pilot educational intervention to enhance the role of health surveillance assistants. *International Journal of Social Psychiatry, 60*(2). https://doi.org/10.1177/0020764012471924

Zhou, L., Bao, J., Watzlaf, V., & Parmanto, B. (2019). Barriers to and facilitators of the use of mobile health apps from a security perspective: Mixed-methods study. *JMIR mHealth and uHealth, 7*(4), e11223. https://doi.org/10.2196/11223

15 Online COVID-19 Discourse and Mental Health Impacts in Malawi

Rachel Chimbwete-Phiri

15.1 Introduction

This chapter reports on some of the linguistic strategies which individuals who were affected by social isolation due to COVID-19 used to negotiate distress evoked by the pandemic and their presence on social network sites (SNSs), particularly Facebook and WhatsApp, during the peak of the three waves of the COVID-19 pandemic in Malawi. The devastation of COVID-19 on the physical, emotional, and mental health of patients and those whose family members were affected, and also for society, in general, was considerable (Deng et al., 2022; Gao et al., 2020; Kainja et al., 2022). Moreover, preventive measures, such as physical and social distancing, isolations, quarantines, and closures of social institutions at different points during the pandemic, heightened the effects of the pandemic on individuals' psychological well-being. Naturally, the pandemic caused periods of uncertainty, and people were seeking answers. Social media was one of the avenues that helped mitigate anxieties and confusion and where individuals learned survival strategies (Ugbo et al., 2022).

The role of SNSs during the peak of COVID-19 was vast. Apart from situation updates, individual experiences and treatment plans, some jokes and memes made the distressful moments lighter (Ngwira, 2022). The sites were a source of connection with others when physical and social distance restrictions were prevalent (Saud et al., 2020). Social media played a crucial role in spreading information about the virus and ways to prevent it. For many, however, it was also a source of panic due to information overload and misinformation. This state of overload of information has been termed an infodemic, – "too much information including false or misleading information in digital and physical environments during a disease outbreak" (WHO, n.d., p. 1), such that the World Health Organization (WHO, 2020) called on its partners to not only focus on fighting the coronavirus but also the infodemic.

There was a proliferation of fake news from when the coronavirus was first discovered in China in late 2019. Over time, there was no control over the nature of COVID-19 information circulating (Bukhari, 2020). With panic and confusion, for example, there are dangers of inaccuracies and deceptions and a lack of limited literacy in social media use during such times. The coming

DOI: 10.4324/9781003425861-19

of smartphones and social media proliferated "citizen journalism" as ordinary people started to act as journalists to post, comment, and discuss news ordinarily handled by mainstream media (Ugbo et al., 2022). Citizen journalism thus brought challenges and opportunities for health and risk communication.

In the wake of fake news, misinformation and information overload, it was therefore of interest to examine how individuals who were directly or indirectly affected by COVID-19 responded to SNSs – not only as the most readily available source of information but also as a source of social contact with those outside their physical location – and the ways they navigated its effects. This chapter considers qualitative data to discuss how patients and individuals whose families suffered from COVID-19 constructed the effects of COVID-19 on their mental wellness. The chapter further presents the experiences of users of social media. More specifically, the focus is on how social media – as a communication platform during periods of isolation – is portrayed in how people talk and how users negotiate social media's effects on their mental well-being. The current study provided critical insights not only on the nature of health communication in Malawi but also on efforts to curb misinformation and disinformation around health issues and ways to curb the effects of infodemics and pandemics on mental health.

15.2 Effects of Social Media on Users' Mental Health During COVID-19

The use of social media has been associated with positive and negative outcomes on users' mental health during the COVID-19 pandemic. A study by Saud et al. (2020) done in Indonesia presented specific ways in which SNSs such as Facebook, Twitter, and WhatsApp were vital for psychosocial healing. Family, friends, colleagues, and other social groups supported each other by sending encouraging messages, religious texts, and health information for them to remain positive in the situation. However, in public risk communication, social media may lead to an overload of (mis)information, increasing fear, anxiety, and stigma among the population. Banerjee and Meena (2021) describe COVID-19 as the evolution of an infodemic, and social media as the main medium that has had both negative and positive effects on the masses during the pandemic.

Social media is believed to have intensified negative effects of the COVID-19 pandemic for some users. A quantitative survey of social media use during the first wave in Wuhan (January – February 2020) indicated that mental health problems, such as anxiety and depression, were prevalent among those who had frequent exposure to social media during the outbreak (Gao et al., 2020). Similarly, Valdez et al.'s (2020) longitudinal study of a corpus of COVID-19 tweets and user timelines in the United States illustrated how social media use heightened users' negative emotions during this time. The negativity was felt by both patients and healthy citizens; nevertheless, patients are said to have experienced the effects more intensely (Deng et al., 2022; Son et al., 2021). Furthermore, excessive exposure to social media during the pandemic was associated with psychological ill-being, such as social media burnout and fatigue in young people in the United Kingdom (Liu et al., 2021).

Information overload can heighten anxieties, as users are not sure what to believe or how to handle the situation best, amidst the ostensibly conflicting information. While a number of studies have shown the effects of this information overload in other contexts, very few studies have given a detailed analysis of the effects of social media on mental health during COVID-19 in the Malawian context.

15.2.1 COVID-19 and Mental Health in Malawi

COVID-19 presented challenges in various degrees to many Malawians' mental health. Like in other parts of sub-Saharan Africa, in Malawi, communities play a crucial role in individuals' psychological well-being during illnesses. Malawians have a spirit of communitarianism: they are used to caring for one another, being together and visiting one another during illnesses, and even more during hospitalisation. This aspect of communitarianism – *umunthu* – was challenged during the COVID-19 pandemic, when social isolation and quarantine of the infected were recommended (Kainja et al., 2022). According to Kainja et al. (2022), the spirit of *umunthu* plays a commendable role in reducing stress in patients and is central to the fight against mental health issues, such as anxiety, trauma, and stress that arose from COVID-19 and its effects. Religion is also believed to play a pivotal role in public health concerns and during pandemics because Malawians have a strong religious affiliation, which is part of their wholesomeness. The restrictions of physical visits were, therefore, seen as a contributing factor to the distress experienced by the affected groups (Tengatenga et al., 2021). Previous studies observed that the absence of essential community responses, such as conducting funeral rites and offering support for the ill through hospital and home visits, caused traumatic experiences for the affected (Kainja et al., 2022; Tengatenga et al., 2021). In this case, social media were the channel of psychosocial support by many who accessed it (see Ngwira, 2022).

Conventional media were being promoted as the only source of information about the COVID-19 pandemic, and it was not easy to control posts on social media, as many users actively participated in sharing and receiving news about the pandemic. This had its dangers (see Jiyajiya & Mtenje-Mkochi, 2022; Manda, 2021). Additionally, social media are linked to problems of mental health in young people because of the need to fit in socially, and this could cause much pressure that might affect their mental health negatively (Jumbe et al., 2022).

Although there was official communication by public health communicators, who had to control what was communicated about the pandemic, its effectiveness in reaching the masses is not clear. Jiyajiya and Mtenje-Mkochi (2022) observe that the messages were imbalanced as the channels and language used seemed to target the urban and rich populace, particularly those with access to social media. Similarly, others felt there were information gaps that resulted due to second-hand information and myths about the pandemic (Manda, 2021). Information about the pandemic was existent, but the excess quantity and myriad sources somehow problematised its effects on the masses. Malawi thus struggled with the infodemic, and social media was one of its prolific avenues.

Against this background, this chapter addresses some of these issues by isolating a few individuals' experiences to have an in-depth look at their experiences and feelings associated with accessing SNSs during the COVID-19 pandemic in this under-researched context. It was imperative to understand how citizens utilised social media, its role on their lives, and individual users' experiences, especially those affected by physical isolation. While several studies have shown how COVID-19 affected people's mental health in Malawi (Kainja et al., 2022) and the effects of infodemics on Malawians during COVID-19 (Manda, 2021), a discourse analysis of the personal lived experiences with regard to using social media, its effects on their mental health and a focus on the micro details of their talk was needed to add to this repertoire of studies.

A critical discourse analytical approach was used to explore narratives of 15 Malawians – who had either experienced a period of social isolation or had suffered from COVID-19 – on their lived experiences and their use of social media. In addition, social media posts of selected participants were also examined to understand how the participants oriented themselves to the effects of the pandemic in their interactions with others. The social media chats were collected between January and February 2021, particularly during the peak of the second wave of COVID-19 in Malawi.

This study emanated from the author's involvement in radio broadcasting at the University of Malawi as a programme producer and presenter of COVID-19 health programmes during the peak of the first and second waves of COVID-19 in 2020 to 2021. Part of the data was sought as an extension of research conducted when developing radio content for episodes on mental health and coping with COVID-19, which were aired during school closures and physical distance restrictions. The personal narratives were obtained from in-depth interviews with 15 participants purposively selected in Malawi (eight male and seven female). The participants were recruited from various social media forums to which the researcher belonged at the time, and some using the snowball sampling technique from a network of friends and family. The selection criteria were those who indicated to have experienced moments of isolation because they had a family member infected by COVID-19, or those who were infected by COVID-19. An informed consent sheet was electronically shared with all participants, and a phone interview was arranged when they gave their consent. The interviews were mainly conducted in English according to the interviewee's choices, although Chichewa was also an option.

Four participants were recruited because of their posts on the WhatsApp and Facebook social groups to which the researcher belonged at the time and/or by seeking consent privately. In-depth interviews followed these. In the examples of social media posts, the texts were retyped into a regular font to preserve the poster's anonymity. All data were analysed using a critical discourse analytical approach.

15.3 Critical Discourse Analysis of Narratives and Social Media Posts

Critical discourse analysis was employed in the study as a theoretical and analytical framework (see Van Leeuwen, 2008). Critical discourse analysis is about closely studying the use of language along with other textual resources, which speakers employ to construct meaning and related social structures in a text. Critical discourse analysts are interested in how language represents social structures and social practices (see Gill, 2000). Discourse holistically means using language in action in particular social contexts, with the understanding that language creates realities (see Gill, 2000). Therefore, the study of discourse is the study of language as a social practice occurring within a sociocultural context, reflective of ideologies and social constructs (see Baker & Ellece, 2011). These social practices are "socially regulated ways of doing things" formulated by various elements, inter alia, social actors, social actions, social identities, and context (Van Leeuwen, 2008, p. 6).

Mental and psychological states were identified from their talking as participants narrated their experiences. Personal narratives emanating from interviews is valuable data in examining the discourse of mental health (e.g., Galasiński, 2013) because people use language to describe their world, and language itself is understood as a reflection of that world, in other words, people use language "to do things" (Gill, 2000, p. 174). Speakers will employ different discoursal features in a text to make meaning, represent social practices and social actors, and construct themselves and their world (Van Leeuwen, 2008). The respondents' texts are therefore not understood in isolation; text is closely tied to its context.

From the narratives, the participants' construction of their world was inferred. Their construction of themselves as social actors in the discourse of mental health and the COVID-19 pandemic and their social practices on matters concerning their mental well-being are therefore reflected.

Section 5 presents the analysis, which involved transcribing the interview data, coding thematic areas, and identifying linguistic resources used by the respondents. For all data excerpts, code **PF** means female participant, **PM** male participant; and **SGP** means social group participant.

15.4 Psychological Distress Evoked by COVID-19 and Social Isolation

One common aspect in all narratives was an explicit or implicit reference to the participants' emotions. The participants referred to their feelings in relation to the effects of COVID-19 and their experiences of physical and social distance restrictions. Where studying mental health discourse is concerned, narratives are linguistic forms that contain information of the individual's mental states (see Hong et al., 2015). Use of certain descriptive linguistic features, such as emotional words with certain frequencies, marks a speaker's psychological state of mind (for example, feelings of boredom, loneliness, anxieties, irritability, emotional distress, insomnia, grief, panic) (see Deng et al., 2022). Extracts 1 and 2 are presented here because they are representative of the informants' feelings of isolation and being infected by COVID-19.

1. PF4: The days were dark; it was a bit like there was a high wall ahead of you . . . As others were describing the stages of the COVID disease, how it progresses in the body; talking about seventh or ninth day as the worst in terms of symptoms . . . or to say those who have died have mostly died between day this and that. And you look at yourself, and wonder, which day is my husband on? Which day am I on? I don't know . . . it was scary.
2. PM2: It was kind of depressing, I mean like . . . you feel like isolated and you feel like everyone who gets close to you is going to catch COVID, and you just feel like you are alone. And I think that triggers also issues . . . mmm . . . as I said, the feeling of Africanness . . . you feel like you should be doing everything together with others, and then you are being told, "no" . . . you should stay alone in your bedroom. I had to stay in my own bedroom, something that as Africans, we are not used to, and I kept on thinking . . .

In Extracts 1 and 2, speakers PF4 and PM2 explicitly used emotive language to signal negative emotions pertaining to their experiences of getting infected by COVID-19: "it was scary," "depressing," "disturbed," feeling "alone,", and feeling "isolated." Another participant (PF2, not quoted here) said, "it was nasty" and "it was tough." Direct reference to manifestations of physical signals of distress was made by another female patient (PF6, not quoted here), "I cried," which explicitly constructed panic-stricken and distressed states. It was observed by Valdez et al. (2020) that such feelings of negativity were common during the pandemic as the language that was expressive of positivity largely declined when figures of those affected with the pandemic started rising. Furthermore, use of words that reflected such negative emotions were said to be common in those who became infected by the pandemic compared to those who were healthy (Deng et al., 2022) and such language reflects the mood of mental confusion and distress among the affected people.

A noteworthy linguistic strategy that was employed in at least seven of the narratives was the metaphor, which is a notable device in language of emotions. Some of the metaphors in the quoted extracts were, "the days were dark," "a high wall" (Extract 1), another informant said, "it was a battle" and "one would feel buried." In these narratives the negative emotions evoked by the pandemic were communicated using these metaphors of emotional pain, trauma, feelings of uncertainty, and loneliness. Metaphors are said to be significant in communication and cognition, "they express, reflect, and reinforce different ways of making sense of particular aspects of our lives" and by using them, speakers frame their experiences (Semino et al., 2017, p. 621). In this regard, Semino (2021) notes that metaphors about fighting and fire were commonly used in referring to COVID-19, which was indicative of the state of emotions as those of being in a battle, and their use could have been productive in depicting inner strength to fight, or it might have been counterproductive to suggest losing.

There were also instances of vivid anecdotes to denote the distressing facets of the pandemic. Storytelling devices by PF4 (Extract 1), a female informant who was a patient while caring for her seriously infected husband during the peak of the second wave. In her narration, she creates an imagery of a suffering patient and caretaker to depict her anxieties, ". . . and you look at yourself, and wonder, which day is my husband on? Which day am I on? . . . It was scary." These were stated in reference to her fear of death in relation to the information that was circulated about the progression of COVID-19 symptoms vis-à-vis the phase or day when death was likely to occur. Her reference to the effects of the information to which she was exposed, and her own mental suffering significantly reflected the negative effects of this particular kind of information on the patients.

While there were reports that many people had their mental health negatively affected, these expressions of negative emotions and feelings evoked by COVID-19 effects as told by the participants are noteworthy because they vividly detailed the mental states of some of those who suffered from the effects of isolation, the illness, or those whose loved ones had suffered from the illness.

15.4.1 Social Media as a Threat to Psychological Well-Being

One of the critical questions during the interviews was, "[w]hat were the benefits of being on social media at that time?" It was noted that all participants responded to this by presenting the positive side of social media; yet, these were immediately followed by a conjunction that pointed to the negative aspects. Each participant found accessing social media useful, albeit only to a certain extent, as stated by one participant, ". . . **but at the same time**, while it was positive, it also required a bit of strength" (PM3). Presented next are excerpts of posts from a WhatsApp group, illustrative of expressions of distress by some members of the group when topics about COVID-19 were raised.

SGP1:   I think it is time to curtail the discussion . . . Let us revert to the purpose of the group.

SGP2:   Yes, please let's not start again, please. We have agreed no more of these issues here.

SGP3:   Information or updates are important we may not know which one is vital as long as it won't harm us.

SGP1: Agreed but we need to stick to the purpose of this group.

SGP3: Yes, but sometimes protocol is broken due to the situation we are in.

SGP6: Enough of this Covid. Let's talk about something other than Covid, please.

Two days later, as updates and discussions about COVID ostensibly continued, the participant posted the message that follows:

SGP6: I just want to say I will not be around for a while. I will be back when there are other topics to talk about. Bye for now.

The posts by SGP1, SGP2, SGP3, and SPG6, excerpts from a social media group, are illustrative of ambivalences of belonging to social media groups as experienced by some users. Three of the four participants take a strong stance to suggest that they should change the topic of discussion. This resistance to discussions on the topic was opposed by SGP3, who believed that information and updates shared on the forum, although breaking the group's protocol, were important for them to be equipped with full information. SGP2's discomfort in terms of the topic was strengthened by a pleading word, "please," which was repeated within one sentence, perhaps to enforce the message. By resisting this, the posters illustrated how discomforting the topic was to them in spite of being part of the group. Negative sentiments such as these, expressed in posts of resistance, are seen as an indication of a user's attention to their mental well-being (e.g., Valdez et al., 2020).

User self-regulation is illustrated in the extract when one member, SGP6, decided to leave the group temporarily as a way of resisting the incessantness of the discussions about COVID-19. SPG6 indicated, in a follow-up interview, that she had moments of social isolation when she was diagnosed with COVID-19. She, therefore, initially tried to remain within this social network by suggesting that the topic should be avoided, but upon being ignored, she decided to leave the group. Exiting the group was noteworthy; it indicated an individual's exercise of self-control and self-protection from distressing situations created by their presence on SNSs. These reactions are noteworthy in that, although jokes and memes in relation to the COVID-19 pandemic were shared in such spaces, and some of the humour might have served to depict the distressful moments that some people were experiencing, the humour sometimes made fun of the lived experiences (Ngwira, 2022).

The members' resistance to the COVID-19 topics on these forums also shows that they were agentive. By speaking up, they enacted their power as users to control what is posted on the group. Being agentive is about individuals' power to control a situation or having some capacity to act in a situation (Van Leeuwen, 2008). It was observed that after SPG6's exit, the members of the relevant WhatsApp group did not stop sharing information, remedies, and updates about COVID-19, which attests to the inevitability of the topic during this period. The effects of COVID-19 were obviously ubiquitous to many lives, and perhaps not easy for a single member to entirely avoid being exposed to the topic in a social media group.

Social media were mainly described in strong terms as a source of negativity to the users' emotions. Extracts 3, 4, and 5 illustrate some of the participants' reactions to use of social media during periods of physical suffering from the pandemic.

3. PM3: . . . because some people would post something that was a bit scary, at the same time, I think . . . it was something that was depressing or hysterical . . . it was so depressing. But it needed one who is a critical thinker, otherwise, it would . . . it could weigh you down . . . people commenting . . . yes . . . "some here are positive and they do not want to disclose," and others said, "it's their prerogative don't force them" . . . and people hovering over it; and knowingly that they are talking about me . . . I would still post something else and comment on other issues but nothing about Covid.

4. PF6: I was having heart palpitations, and I realized these were worst in the mornings, when I wake up . . . then I realized later on that it was because of the messages I was getting on Whatsapp . . . In the end, I decided to be offline. I was okay to be cut off from all that, and from the people, and focused on how to get better.

5. PM7: More especially on WhatsApp groups those I completely ignored, no interaction with those, but with individuals I could talk . . . discuss other things that would give me hope and morale or talk . . . some light moments . . . laugh or things of that sort . . . yah . . . to keep me away from messages that I feel would affect my confidence and hope . . . if you look at the messages, they weren't messages that would give you hope, at that time messages are supposed to give you hope.

These excerpts signal how being online and subsequently on wider social media networks, was seen as detrimental to the much-needed positivity during the period of isolation, and is portrayed as "depressing," "devastating," "cause of anxiety," "scary." These feelings are confirmed by Gao et al. (2020) and Valdez et al. (2020) who observed an increase in messages of negativity on social media and its correlation on mood of users during pandemics.

As they talked about social media, the participants constructed various social actors or "doers of action" as they also positioned themselves as actors in that context (e.g., Van Leeuwen, 2008, p. 148). One aspect that was repeated by participants was the role played by different referents, "the messages," "the news," "WhatsApp," "the people," or "them." Various actors in the social activity of conversing about COVID-19 could be isolated from the narratives, namely those who developed the messages, those who posted or forwarded them, which seemed to be in opposition with the self or the individual user.

The speaker's self is seen to be in an emotional struggle with various other actors in the social media contexts. It is observed from the narratives that the social relations of the actors were linguistically differentiated between "I" and "them" – with referents, such as "they," "them," "people," or "WhatsApp groups." For example, PM3 who experienced stigma after testing positive for the coronavirus presented this "I and them" dichotomy, "people hovering over it and knowingly that they are talking about me" (Extract 3). The speaker demonstrated the negative emotions of isolation on the one hand, and how this was heightened by the stigma on social media, on the other. His narrative indicated how isolation was not only physical – when physical distancing as a patient – but was also experienced when castigated in a social media group when singled out as a carrier of the coronavirus (see Extract 2).

The narratives indicated mixed feelings, not wanting to entirely miss out, but also not wanting to be emotionally disturbed. Common references in narratives were to the supportive role of friends and family who directly contacted them, even when offline, and seen as very helpful, for instance PM7 indicates how he used social media only to interact with friends, "to discuss other things that would give [me] hope and morale . . . some light moments . . ." (Extract 5). For those who suffered from COVID-19, interaction with close friends and family on social media was deemed more supportive than that of wider groups and networks from which emanated feelings of fear, stigma, and uncertainties (Son et al., 2021). In addition, most of the participants indicated how selective they were of those with whom they interacted and of the topics they discussed on social media in cases where using it was inevitable.

The participants' reactions to social media signalled dialectics that people might experience when relating with others: the need to isolate themselves and avoid anxieties or stigma, at the same time having the need to connect with others, in this case through social media, to mitigate the feeling of "being scared," "buried," "depressed," and "anxious." These dichotomies of using social media were also observed by other researchers when some users of social media dreaded the information about COVID-19 while others feared accessing the platforms, yet there was also a need to connect with family and friends (Liu et al., 2021; Saud et al., 2020; Valdez et al., 2020). Indeed, from the participants' perceptions, the extensive social media networks and social groupings were sometimes too heterogeneous to offer meaningful support to individuals suffering from the emotional effects of the pandemic, while a smaller and more supportive community of close family and friends seemed to be the most desirable during periods of isolation.

As the participants narrated the negative effects of social media upon their emotions, most of them positioned themselves as having agency to cope with the effects of social media. For instance, PM3 described how being on social media at that time "needed one who is a critical thinker" (Extract 3). Despite using the impersonal form "one" perhaps to not put himself explicitly in that category, this formulation might have included himself and others in his situation. The participants indicated taking various actions in relation to their presence on social media networks to avoid the ensuing negative emotions, for instance, "I just made a decision that I will not be as active as I used to be" (PF2), "I decided to be offline" (Extract 4), "What I really did was to reduce my interaction on WhatsApp . . . WhatsApp groups those I completely ignored" (Extract 5).

The use of the pronoun "I" by the speakers is significant in narratives as the speaker makes a direct reference to him- or herself as an actor or doer of action and construct him- or herself as having control (Galasiński, 2013, p. 51). The speakers in these instances thus constructed themselves as having the ability to take control of the situation by filtering what was received on social media for positive well-being as they grappled with the sources of negativity – "people," "WhatsApp groups," or "the messages."

In the data, social media are depicted as an abused social context during the pandemic. The social actors in that space are seen to have erred, and the social practice of posting or forwarding messages on COVID-19 is seen to have been done wrongly by many actors. User self-regulation on social media was demonstrated by the participants as most of them explicitly explained the actions they took to avoid negativity on social media to "[focus] on how to get better" (Extract 4).

15.5 Conclusion

This chapter has shown how individuals negotiated the effects of the pandemic and social media during physical isolation. Using critical discourse analytical approaches to examine their narratives, it was observed that the participants experienced negative emotions due to the effects of the pandemic and the physical distancing restrictions. These negative emotions were exacerbated by their presence on SNSs.

The data extracts indicated distressful feelings and negative emotions caused by social isolation and information overload on social media. Based on their use of emotional language, conceptual metaphors of COVID-19 and storytelling devices to express their lived experiences, it could be concluded that the individuals experienced anxieties, fears, and distress during social isolation. However, they had family members within that physical space. Furthermore, they had little control over the situation of being in physical isolation and the negative emotions that ensued. However, where social network sites (SNSs) as an external source of negative emotions were concerned, the participants oriented themselves to the notion of positive psychological and mental well-being. They positioned themselves as agentive social actors in avoiding the negative effects of the pandemic on their psychological state. Paying attention to how people talk about their experiences with regard to illnesses, as done in this study, is significant in health communication, for it will help health professionals and health promoters to know the language that empowers or disempowers the affected groups and the emotions associated with certain language choices of illnesses (see Semino, 2021; Semino et al., 2017).

Critical actors in relation to individual mental health and SNSs were family and friends who were seen as supportive actors in this context. The analysis also showed that insensitive actors, such as friends and colleagues on prominent social media groups mainly intensified emotions of distress. The chapter argued that as social and behaviour change campaigns harness the use of SNSs for health promotion, they ought to pay attention to the roles of other actors who abuse the SNSs, and they should take a leading role in diffusing such SNSs with the appropriate messages.

The ambiguous feelings about being on SNSs demonstrated in the narratives indicate the need to promote healthy and responsible use of SNSs (i.e., SNS literacy) to overcome the negative effects of SNSs on individuals' mental health during pandemics. There is a need to create a synergy between official channels and citizen journalists if correct information is to be spread. Although social media sites are not easy to control, those in public health institutions have a duty to saturate the media with positive messages that pay attention to promotion of positive emotions during pandemics (see Gao et al., 2020; WHO, 2020). The insights provided in this chapter demonstrate the need to strengthen positive talk about illnesses in our societies and promote messages tailored to meet the needs of those affected by pandemics.

References

Baker, P., & Ellece, S. (2011). *Key terms in discourse analysis.* Continuum International.

Banerjee, D., & Meena, K. S. (2021). COVID-19 as an "infodemic" in public health: Critical role of the social media. *Frontiers in Public Health, 9*(610623), 1–9.

Bukhari, W. (2020). Role of social media in COVID-19 pandemic. *The International Journal of Frontier Sciences, 4*(2), 59–60.

Deng, Y., Park, M., Chen, J., Yang, J., Xie, L., Li, H., Wang, L., & Chen, Y. (2022). Emotional discourse analysis of COVID-19 patients and their mental health: A text mining study. *PLOS One, 17*(9), e0274247.

Galasiński, D. (2013). *Fathers, fatherhood and mental illness: A discourse analysis of rejection.* Palgrave Macmillan.

Gao, J., Zheng, P., Jia, Y., Chen, H., Mao, Y., Chen, S., Wang, Y., Fu, H., & Dai, H. (2020). Mental health problems and social media exposure during COVID-19 outbreak. *PLOS One, 15*(4), e0231924.

Gill, R. (2000). Discourse analysis. In M. W. Bauer & G. Gaskell (Eds.), *Qualitative researching with text, image and sound: A practical handbook* (pp. 172–190). Sage.

Hong, K., Nenkova, A., March, M. E., Parker, A. P., Verma, R., & Kohler, C. G. (2015). Lexical use in emotional autobiographical narratives of persons with schizophrenia and healthy controls. *Psychiatry Research, 225*(1–2), 40–49.

Jiyajiya, P. M., & Mtenje-Mkochi, A. (2022). Linguistic and communication exclusion in COVID-19 awareness campaigns in Malawi. *Journal of African Media Studies, 14*(3), 455–470.

Jumbe, S., Nyali, J., Simbeye, M., Zakeyu, N., Motshewa, G., & Pulapa, S. R. (2022). "We do not talk about it": Engaging youth in Malawi to inform adaptation of a mental health literacy intervention. *PLOS One, 17*(3), e0265530.

Kainja, J., Ndasauka, Y., Mchenga, M., Kondowe, F., M'manga, C., Maliwichi, L., & Nyamali, S. (2022). Umunthu, Covid-19 and mental health in Malawi. *Heliyon, 8*(11), e11316.

Liu, H., Liu, W., Yoganathan, V., & Osburg, V. S. (2021). COVID-19 information overload and generation Z's social media discontinuance intention during the pandemic lockdown. *Technological Forecasting & Social Change, 166*(120600), 1–12.

Manda, L. Z. (2021). Exploring COVID-19 infodemic in rural Africa: A case study of Chintheche, Malawi. *Journal of African Media Studies, 13*(2), 253–267.

Ngwira, E. (2022). Viral giggles: Internet memes and COVID-19 in Malawi. *Journal of African Media Studies, 14*(2), 209–229.

Saud, M., Mashud, M. I., & Ida, R. (2020). Usage of social media during the pandemic: Seeking support and awareness about COVID-19 through social media platforms. *Journal of Public Affairs, 20*(4), e2417.

Semino, E. (2021). "Not soldiers but fire-fighters": Metaphors and Covid-19. *Health Communication, 36*(1), 50–58.

Semino, E., Demjén, Z., Demmen, J., Koller, V., Payne, S., Hardie, A., & Rayson, P. (2017). The online use of violence and journey metaphors by patients with cancer, as compared with health professionals: A mixed methods study. *BMJ Supportive & Palliative Care, 7*(1), 60–66.

Son, H. M., Choi, W. H., Hwang, Y. H., & Yang, H. R. (2021). The lived experiences of COVID-19 patients in South Korea: A qualitative study. *International Journal of Environmental Research and Public Health, 18*(14), 1–3, 7419.

Tengatenga, J., Tengatenga Duley, S. M., & Tengatenga, C. J. (2021). *Zimitsani moto*: Understanding the Malawi COVID-19 response. *Laws, 10*(2), 20–29.

Ugbo, G. O., Chinedu-Okeke, C. F., & Ogbodo, J. N. (2022). Citizen journalism and health communication in pandemics' prevention and control. In C. A. Dralega & A. Napakol (Eds.), *Health crises and media discourses in sub-Saharan Africa* (pp. 183–199). Springer International.

Valdez, D., Ten Thij, M., Bathina, K., Rutter, L. A., & Bollen, J. (2020). Social media insights into US mental health during the COVID-19 pandemic: Longitudinal analysis of Twitter data. *Journal of Medical Internet Research, 22*(12), e21418.

Van Leeuwen, T. (2008). *Discourse and practice: New tools for critical discourse analysis.* Oxford University Press.

World Health Organization. (2020). *Director-General's remarks at the media briefing on 2019 novel coronavirus on 8 February 2020.* www.who.int/directorgeneral/speeches/detail/munich-security-conference

World Health Organization. (n.d.). *Infodemic.* www.who.int/health-topics/infodemic#tab=tab_1

16 The Complex Interplay of Technology and Mental Health During COVID-19

Foster Gondwe, Jimmy Kainja, and Yamikani Ndasauka

16.1 Introduction

The COVID-19 pandemic has significantly affected mental well-being worldwide, including in Africa (Gloster et al., 2020; M'manga et al., 2023). Technology played a complex role in influencing mental health during this unprecedented time, with positive and negative effects on the mental well-being of African people. For instance, technology has facilitated the dissemination of accurate information about COVID-19 – including preventive measures, symptoms, and available resources – through online platforms, social media, and mobile applications. This has helped raise awareness and knowledge about the virus, alleviating anxiety and fear associated with misinformation and uncertainty, thereby improving mental well-being. In addition, technology has facilitated digital connectivity and social connection during the pandemic, allowing people in Africa to stay connected with loved ones, friends, and communities. Social media, messaging apps, and video conferencing tools have been used to maintain social connections, share experiences, and provide emotional support, reducing feelings of loneliness, isolation, and depression.

Another platform in which technology blossomed during COVID-19 is telehealth and online mental health services (Chitungo et al., 2021). With lockdowns, social distancing measures, and limited access to physical healthcare facilities, technology enabled the provision of telehealth and online mental health services in Africa (Chitungo et al., 2021). This allowed individuals to access mental health support remotely, reducing barriers to care and increasing the availability of mental health services. In addition, online counselling, therapy sessions, and support groups have helped individuals cope with stress, anxiety, and other mental health challenges during the pandemic (Torous et al., 2020). Furthermore, technology has enabled remote work and online education during the pandemic, allowing individuals to continue their work and studies from home. This provided a sense of normalcy and routine, reducing the disruption caused by the pandemic and mitigating the negative outcome on mental well-being (Chitungo et al., 2021).

DOI: 10.4324/9781003425861-20

The centrality of information and communication technologies (ICTs) during the pandemic changed the narrative around the importance of ICTs on the continent, focusing on accessibility, affordability, infrastructure, and legal and regulatory frameworks (ITU, 2019). In 2019, the International Telecommunication Union (ITU), a United Nations agency responsible for ICTs, reported that Africa had the lowest Internet usage in the world (see ITU, 2019). The report noted that despite the increasing penetration of mobile devices, African countries still lagged in terms of human development rankings, for example, on the Human Development Index. Bakibinga-Gaswaga et al. (2020) found that few people are connected to the Internet in Africa. In countries with better connections, male Internet users outnumber their female counterparts in every region (Bakibinga-Gaswaga et al., 2020). They, therefore, argue that the gender digital divide also affects efforts to communicate critical public health (Bakibinga-Gaswaga et al., 2020).

Vurayai (2022) observed that the lack of reliable Internet and infrastructure, particularly in some parts of Africa, has also created inequalities in accessing remote work and education opportunities, which could negatively affect the mental well-being of marginalised people. The low access to the internet in Africa may exacerbate feelings of exclusion and inequality, affecting mental well-being (Turiansky, 2020). In addition, technology has also raised concerns about cybersecurity and privacy. Cyberattacks, data breaches, and online scams have increased (Salamon, 2021), leading to anxiety and stress among African individuals who rely on technology for various purposes. The lack of robust cybersecurity measures and privacy protection may compromise the mental well-being of individuals, leading to fear, distrust, and increased anxiety (Signé & Signé, 2021).

This chapter delves deep into the multifaceted effect of technology on mental well-being in Africa during the COVID-19 pandemic, employing the theoretical lens of Bernard Stiegler's *pharmakon* perspective of technology. The chapter is outlined as follows. First, Bernard Stiegler's *pharmakon* theory is presented. Discussions on social media, mental well-being, and the role of ICT in education during the pandemic follow this. After that, we show how the increase in ICT use may have affected Africans' mental well-being from two fronts: the overreliance on ICT and, for some, the deficiency of ICT in their lives.

16.2 Bernard Stiegler's *Pharmakon*

Pharmakon is a concept introduced by Jacques Derrida (1981). It is derived from the Greek source term φάρμακον (*phármakon*), a word that could mean either remedy, poison, or scapegoat. *Pharmakon*, as espoused by Plato (in his book, *Phaedrus*), suggests that writing is to be rejected as strictly poisonous to the ability to think for oneself in dialogue with others. Given Derrida's understanding and assessment of Plato, Stiegler adapts pharmakon in his seminal work, *Technics and Time*, to mean both poisonous and curative, implying that technology is a double-edged sword, good and bad. Stiegler (2012) discusses the toxic effects of technology, which contribute to the elimination of idiomaticity, and its curative effects, which allow the formation of the type of attention that makes the singularity of the citizen and democratic participation possible.

Stiegler is influenced by Aristotle and Heidegger, who classify humans as technological subjects. Based on Aristotle's four causes, Heidegger concludes that technology discloses itself when we trace instrumentality back to fourfold causality. To explain this, Heidegger (1977) uses the example of a silver chalice. Each element works together to create the chalice differently:

> The four ways of owing hold sway in the sacrificial vessel that lies ready before us. They differ from one another, yet they belong together . . ..
> The four ways of being responsible bring something into appearance. They let it come forth into presencing. They set it free to that place and so start it on its way, namely into its complete arrival.
> (Heidegger, 1977, p. 287)

When these four elements work together to create something into appearance, it is called "bringing forth." Modern technology, however, differs from this in that, according to Heidegger (1977), modern technology "is based on modern physics as an exact science." Therefore, the revealing of modern technology is not bringing forth, but rather challenging. The essence of modern technology is thus beyond humanity as it keeps on challenging the dictates of society.

From a similar understanding of technology, Stiegler (2017) envisions technology to have preceded humanity. He claims that the human species is initially technological and that to understand the evolution of human society, there first and foremost must be a need to have a thorough understanding of the relationship between human beings and technology (Stiegler, 2017). Technology is, therefore, essential to all human cultures. Stiegler (1998) establishes the "technological rooting of all relation to time and, through his radical deconstruction of hominisation, makes the notion indecipherable from difference" (p. 135). For Stiegler, the difference is not the process that conditions the unfolding of time and, therefore, the human-technology relationship, but rather this relationship constitutes the historical manifestation of difference and the givenness of time (Kouppanou, 2015). In other words, the transcendental aspects of experience exist because of technology.

The historicisation of difference, however, clearly suggests that the *pharmakon*'s undecidable nature is alterable. Stiegler (1998) classifies roles in the technological development world: humans are co-creators of knowledge while the selection criteria, rhythms, and desires of the market and the culture industries are imposed on it. This takes place through the processes of accelerated registration of events that produce the live time of the media and the real-time of programming or computer industries and distort profoundly, if not radically, what could be called "eventisation"; thus, they take the place of time as much as they take the place of space (Stiegler, 1998, p. 16). By rendering registration and broadcasting simultaneously, eventisation threatens to conflate consciousness and the temporal object that otherwise would allow consciousness to reflect on itself (Hansen, 2004).

Stiegler argues that technology brings out different human and societal organisations and produces poisonous and curative effects. Technology is human's inevitable poison with curative potential, and culture is curable from its colonisation by the digital – audio – visual processes of cognitive capitalism (Stiegler, 2017). Technology is, thus, a poison that affects present society and a cure through which humanity could be saved. Stiegler (2017) further posits that even technologies that now predominantly present poisonous effects can be checked to release their curative potential. In the case of digitisation, knowledge is exteriorised "into machines with no other pseudo-interiorisation than that by which the individual 'serves' the system' while individuals are locked into a recycled temporality" (Stiegler, 1998, p. 127).

Stiegler's thoughts on technology have not been immune to criticism. Many scholars have challenged Stiegler's philosophy, for instance, Ian James (2019), Oliver Davis (2013), and Serge Trottein (2013). These scholars observed that Stiegler's (2012) argument that there has been a philosophical repression of techne from the early Greeks is vague. It is through writing which threatens our memories that we have material support for cultural production and reproduction. One problem identified by these scholars is that the undecidability of the pharmakon in Derrida (198) becomes highly definite when it comes to specific technologies of the 21st century (Howells & Moore, 2013). Trottein (2013) challenges Stiegler (2012) for denying the vital role of aesthetics in Kant. In extending this thought, Crogan (2013) argues that Stiegler's charge about contemporary aesthetics springs from his view that media produce only inactiveness on the part of consumers (Howells & Moore, 2013). These criticisms, however, do not negate Stiegler's (2012) depiction of the pharmacological nature of technology, especially in the digital age.

16.3 Social Media and Mental Well-being During the COVID-19 Pandemic

Social media, emphasising the social, has grown significantly since the advent of Web 2.0, the second generation of websites. Unlike the first generation of the web (Web 1.0), Hall (2022, paragraph 5) notices that Web 2.0 "offers more opportunities for collaboration, functionality, various applications, and user-generated content." Social media thus emphasise the user experience. As an antithesis of traditional media, social media are decentralised, marked by an absence of gatekeepers, and enable users to communicate directly. Unlike traditional media, social media platforms are used for private and public communication. Conversational media resembles an online word-of-mouth forum (see Mutsvairo & Ragnedda, 2017).

To prevent the spread of COVID-19, countries worldwide imposed national lockdowns, closing socialisation spaces, such as workplaces, universities, colleges, schools, and business centres. These lockdowns also restricted access to traditional forums where people interacted and shared information at a time when information, especially about the COVID-19 pandemic, was mainly needed. Pandey et al. (2010) observed that information sharing helps reduce anxiety in the population in crisis, as people are in touch with their loved ones. For most people, social media platforms filled this critical information gap during the pandemic, allowing them to communicate with their loved ones and quickly access information about the pandemic.

Lee et al. (2022) remark that social media platforms, due to accessibility, their ease of use, and socialisation in controlled environments, attracted individuals with underlying depression to social media interactions rather than face-to-face ones, as they feared exposing themselves to the coronavirus during the pandemic. Additionally, Islam et al. (2020) noticed that social media enable the fast transfer of information and allow people to share news, personal experiences, and viewpoints in real time with family, friends, and work colleagues.

Having information and the ability to communicate with loved ones in times of crisis could save lives as it preserves good mental health and reduces anxiety. As noticed by Lee et al. (2022), the fear of COVID-19 may have been compounded by coexisting depression and anxiety disorders. However, too much information can also be problematic because it affects decision-making and could misinform the public. Longest and Kang (2022) argue that as people used social media extensively to access health information, they also exposed themselves to information that exceeded their ability to digest, causing information overload, which often triggered negative consequences, such as social media discontinuance or psychological shutdown. This could have caused feelings of helplessness and mental health deterioration.

The absence of gatekeepers on social media platforms means that most information is not subjected to rigorous fact-checking. This leaves much room for disinformation and misinformation. The difference between disinformation and misinformation is the intention. Disinformation is spreading false information to lie and deceive, while misinformation is sharing false information without the intent to mislead (see Lee et al., 2022). While disinformation and misinformation have not come with the COVID-19 pandemic, their rapid spread and global reach were enabled by social media platforms during the pandemic. This negatively affected people's adherence to recommended public health measures or engagement in non-recommended habits (Laato et al., 2020).

In Africa, a BBC study (2018) about fake news established that, among other issues, people shared false information because the sender of information was someone they trusted. People cared more about the person who had shared the information than about the truth of the information. In 2018, the World Economic Forum identified online misinformation as one of humanity's top 10 global threats (Laato et al., 2020). Likewise, the World Health Organization (WHO) warned of the grave threat of misinformation to COVID-19 response efforts (Laato et al., 2020). Swire-Thompson and Lazer (2020) found that misinformation concerning health severely affected people's quality of life and even their mortality risk.

While much of false information originates and is shared online, Oxford Analytica (2022) found that people who lack access to the Internet are more vulnerable to misinformation than those with access to the Internet. This can be looked at from the Malawian point of view. Although access to the Internet and social media in Malawi remains low, Kainja (2019) has shown that online disinformation and misinformation affect offline spaces. In Malawi, most people only have partial Internet access and can only afford to subscribe to specific services. For example, some people can only afford to subscribe to a weekly WhatsApp bundle (Kainja, 2019). This partial access encourages sharing screenshots and images on WhatsApp because people are limited to using WhatsApp only – sharing a website link is, therefore, futile, and people's bundled subscription is limited to WhatsApp. Kainja (2019) observed that sharing screenshots and images exposes people to misinformation, as partial access to the Internet means that people lack the means to verify the information (i.e., the screenshots and images). According to Nightingale and Farid (2022), most online people cannot distinguish between fake and real news.

Disinformation and misinformation lead to wrong decision-making and affect people's mental health and well-being. Longest and Kang (2022) found that negative information concerning increased numbers of COVID-19, social distancing, and increased death tolls emanating from COVID-19 led to anxiety and depression. Lee et al. (2022) established that false coronavirus information led to discrimination and stigma. In Malawi, these fears were amplified by the government directive that, for example, COVID-19 victims had to be buried using special measures and not traditional means where relatives and loved ones mourn the dead and are allowed to view the deceased body (see Kainja et al., 2022).

While this was the case, social media positively affected mental health, especially among the youth. Vaingankar et al. (2020, p. 11) found that social media is integral to "the lives of today's youth and indicate that social media can offer opportunities for positive influence, personal expression, and social support, thus contributing to positive mental health among youth." They found that the youth's use of social media to connect with family and friends and to participate in global movements is critical for creative, positive mental health. Their study suggested that three features could affect positive mental health among youth. These relate to friends and their global community, engagement with social media content, and the value of social media as an outlet for expression.

Vaingankar et al. (2020) further identify that these three features lead to five positive mental health components: "positive relationships and social capital; self-concept; coping; happiness, and other relevant aspects of mental health"

(p. 9). Consequently, the impact of social media usage on mental health is multifaceted, and understanding it requires more than a singular approach. While information overload and false information could lead to anxiety and depression, social media may also be used for positive mental health outcomes. This was particularly important during the COVID-19 pandemic when social interaction and freedom of movement were limited to mitigate the effects of the pandemic.

The link between mental well-being and social media highlighted previously mirrors the technology concept of *pharmakon* (Derrida, 1981). During the pandemic, many people used various social media platforms as a remedy or scapegoat for continued interaction with others during lockdowns. Social media consequently contributed to positive mental health among people regardless of age, gender, or geographical location. On the other hand, social media became poisonous as people were subjected to information overload, as both mainstream and social media were saturated with information on COVID-19, creating overload and fatigue for some people. Moreover, the varying levels of access to social media also meant that some people were excluded from the mental health benefits of social media. As Stiegler (2012) argues, technology brought out different human and societal organisations as they faced the pandemic.

16.4 ICT in Education and Mental Well-being in Sub-Saharan Africa During and After the Pandemic

Historically, research on ICT in education has primarily focused on teaching with technology, characterised by attaching high importance to ICT as an instructional resource for improving educational access and quality. Presenting a history of instructional media in the United States, Reiser (2001) reports that not all new educational media introduced in education delivered the highly anticipated change in education. Similarly, in sub-Saharan Africa (SSA), since the early 2000s, many countries have attempted to develop ICT policies to improve educational quality and access. The availability of resources shaped the development of ICT in education in Africa and other developing countries, ICT policy frameworks, and the influences of external actors, primarily through foreign aid (Kunyenje & Chigona, 2019). ICT in education has also been especially prominent in higher education institutions, open and distance learning (ODL), and project-based piloting of different ICTs. Despite advancing ICT policies (Muianga et al., 2013) and donor support to facilitate the development of educational ICT in SSA (Ezumah, 2020), there are mixed results on the impact of ICT on changing instructional practices.

For starters, the impact of ICT on education in sub-Saharan Africa mirrors Stiegler's (2012) view of technology as having both poisonous and curative effects. This can be illustrated by Chen et al.'s (2017) reflection on the question, "Will technology make schools smarter?" Chen et al. observe that perspectives on the impact of ICT in education can be placed on opposite poles of a spectrum. On the one end of the spectrum, some oppose the use of ICT in education, among others arguing that technology affects the functioning of the human brain. Furthermore, in the SSA region and other low-income contexts, ICT has not delivered the much-anticipated change in education, mainly because of the shortfalls in the processes involved in adopting ICT in education. For instance, critics argue that the implementation of educational ICT in these contexts has tended to overlook technology professional development for teachers; takes a non-participatory approach to implementing ICT in education; and overlooks necessities of user populations, such as food, shelter, and other teaching and learning resources (Ezumah, 2020).

On the other end of the spectrum are enthusiasts claiming that, under the right circumstances, ICT could benefit students regardless of age or subjects of study. Some factors that influence the adoption of ICT are teachers' beliefs, attitudes, and perceptions of the usefulness and ease of using ICT (Davis, 1989; Ertmer et al., 2012). These factors could enable or impede the adoption of ICT in education. It is also reported that, if used appropriately, ICT in education could motivate learners, promote both individualised and collaborative learning, help teachers explain abstract concepts, and improve students' achievements (Rosen & Manny-Ikan, 2011). In line with Stiegler's (2012) view, it can be said that technology makes the learners' democratic participation in education possible.

Further exploring the effect of ICT in education, other scholars have focused on "teaching about technology which might allow for the foregrounding of techno-ethical issues in everyday classroom uses of technologies" (Krutka et al., 2019, p. 555). Attention to techno-ethical issues might help to unveil long-standing and current limitations of the educational use of ICT by educators and students. Techno-ethical issues become prominent when we acknowledge Stiegler's (2012) argument that technology brings out different human and societal organisations. Instead of conceptualising ICT as a medium for facilitating teaching and learning, it is equally important to pay attention to human aspects of using ICT in education because education is, in essence, a human and emotional process (see Castañeda & Selwyn, 2018). Agreeing with Stiegler's position, Castañeda and Selwyn (2018) argue that educational use of technology could shape students' and staff's emotions, moods, and feelings. To illustrate this point, we focus on the experiences students and educators had with ICT in education during the COVID-19 pandemic.

The COVID-19 pandemic catalysed the shift to ICT in teaching and learning at all levels of education. While research on ICT in education was already being done before the pandemic, the transition to digital learning during the pandemic also generated interest in lesser-known aspects of digital learning, such as mental well-being. Before the pandemic, some studies had already reported the possible effect of educational ICT on the mental health of young adults. For example, Thomée et al. (2012) found that intensive use of emails and computers without breaks was associated with sleep disturbance. Porter et al. (2015) investigated the positive and negative aspects of phone use in educational contexts in SSA countries, focusing on Malawi, Ghana, and South Africa. The study found that the financial cost of phone use put learners under pressure to forego necessities, such as food, books and, in some cases, their bodies. Apart from online bullying and class disruption from learners' phone use, study participants also reported experiences of pornography as a result of sending and receiving sexually explicit photographs and messages via mobile phones (Porter et al., 2015).

During and after the pandemic, understanding the well-being of learners and teachers continued to be of research interest to generate insight into better ways of supporting learners' learning and the work of educators. Literature highlights how the use of ICT in education during and after the pandemic has been linked to the mental well-being of educators and learners. For instance, at the University of Botswana, educators had to grapple with the unforeseen challenges of having to catch up with building their technology competencies and sparing time to transform teaching resources from traditional face-to-face to online instruction (Ntshwarang et al., 2021). Related literature from contexts outside sub-Saharan Africa also highlights similar experiences of ICT in education during the pandemic. In Switzerland, Lischer et al. (2022) found that "students reported coping well during lockdown but indicated that lecturers were challenged by distance teaching, which created some stress for the students" (p. 589) – at the Universiti Brunei Darussalam in Brunei increased screen time led to computer-related physical stress and being stressed due to deadlines, unexpected disruptions, and an increased workload (Idris et al., 2021).

Other examples of students' mental well-being experiences during the pandemic referred to anxiety and depression. In Uganda, Najjuka et al. (2021) investigated the prevalence of stress and anxiety among university students. The study reported a high prevalence of symptoms of depression, anxiety, and stress among university students during the lockdown. The students' experiences of anxiety were associated with factors such as being male, having a leisure activity during the lockdown, and using addictive substances (Najjuka et al., 2021). Similar experiences were also reported in the Philippines, where students faced challenges in controlling their emotions, actions, and thoughts to learn and their emotional discomfort because of being lonely and secluded from their peers because of remote learning (Barrot et al., 2021). In South Africa and Botswana, the transition to remote teaching affected the progress of students and lecturers, as they could not access information from the university libraries (Mahlaba, 2020; Ntshwarang et al., 2021). This experience was stressful, mainly because the available resources could not meet the instructional needs of lecturers and students. The abrupt change to remote teaching using various educational ICTs also meant a shift in how lecturers and students viewed teaching and learning (Mahlaba, 2020).

On the other hand, ICT supported efforts to ensure continued learning amidst lockdowns during the pandemic. Students reported some opportunities that had come with distance learning. Despite some losing a sense of belonging to their educational institutions, they had to learn coping strategies, such as resource management and utilisation, help-seeking, technical aptitude enhancement, time management, and learning environment control (Barrot et al., 2021). Online learning also made staff members explore new options, thereby becoming creative and innovative in their pedagogy and assessment approaches (Idris et al., 2021). In South Africa, Mahlaba (2020) suggested the need for self-directed learning as students and lecturers attempted to cope with remote teaching with limited access to traditional instructional resources, such as laboratories.

Meanwhile, considering some limitations, the effect of ICT on education, as highlighted previously, should be understood. As other scholars' challenging views argue, it cannot be assumed that human beings are shaped by technology. Kerres and Buchner (2022) highlight some methodological flaws in empirical research that have reported the effect of ICT on education during the pandemic. For example, some comparative studies did not address how contextual conditions, such as culture and institutional setup, influenced the response of educational systems to the pandemic. This makes it difficult to explain whether educational provision and learning changes resulted from the pandemic, ICT, or other factors (Kerres & Buchner, 2022).

16.5 Conclusion

This chapter explored the two-sided nature of technology by emphasising and dealing with mental well-being during the COVID-19 pandemic. We used Bernard Stiegler's *pharmakon* to evaluate technology's positive and negative effects, specifically focusing on social media and ICT in education during the pandemic. We also considered how the educational use of ICT affected the mental well-being of educators and students during the pandemic. Accordingly, the current chapter contributes insights to theory development regarding the cultural, affective, spiritual, and emotional aspects of using ICT in education. We observed how social media created information overload and fatigue for some people. Overall, this chapter argued that the increase in ICT use might have affected the mental well-being of Africans on two fronts: the overreliance on ICT and, for some, the deficiency of ICT in their lives.

References

Bakibinga-Gaswaga, E., Bakibinga, S., Bakibinga, D. B., & Bakibinga, P. (2020). Digital technologies in the COVID-19 responses in sub-Saharan Africa: Policies, problems and promises. *The Pan African Medical Journal, 35*(Suppl. 2). https://doi.org/10.11604/pamj.supp.2020.35.2.23456

Barrot, J. S., Llenares, I. I., & Del Rosario, L. S. (2021). Students' online learning challenges during the pandemic and how they cope with them: The case of the Philippines. *Education and Information Technologies, 26*(6), 7321–7338.

BBC News. (2018). What we have learned about fake news in Africa. *BBC News*. www.bbc.com/news/world-africa-46138284

Castañeda, L., & Selwyn, N. (2018). More than tools? Making sense of the ongoing digitisations of higher education. *International Journal of Educational Technology in Higher Education, 15*(1), 1–10.

Chen, C., Souraya, R., & Wohlleben, K. (2017). Will technology make schools smarter? In P. Sahlberg, J. Hasak, & V. Rodriguez (Eds.), *Hard questions on global educational change: Policies, practices, and the future of education* (pp. 73–84). Teachers College Press.

Chitungo, I., Mhango, M., Mbunge, E., Dzobo, M., Musuka, G., & Dzinamarira, T. (2021). Utility of telemedicine in sub-Saharan Africa during the COVID-19 pandemic. A rapid review. *Human Behaviour and Emerging Technologies, 3*(5), 843–853. https://doi.org/10.1002/hbe2.297

Crogan, P. (2013). Experience of the industrial temporal object. In C. Howells & G. Moore (Eds.), *Stiegler and technics*. Edinburgh University Press.

Davis, F. D. (1989). Perceived usefulness, perceived ease of use, and user acceptance of information technology. *MIS Quarterly, 13*(3), 319–340.

Davis, O. (2013). Desublimation in education for democracy. In C. Howells & G. Moore (Eds.), *Stiegler and technics*. Edinburgh University Press.

Derrida, J. (1981). Plato's pharmacy. In *Dissemination* (B. Johnson, Trans., pp. 63–171). University of Chicago Press.

Draženović, M., Vukušić Rukavina, T., & Machala Poplašen, L. (2023). Impact of social media use on mental health within adolescent and student populations during COVID-19 pandemic: Review. *International Journal of Environmental Research and Public Health, 20*(4), 33–92. https://doi.org/10.3390/ijerph20043392

Ertmer, P. A., Ottenbreit-Leftwich, A. T., Sadik, O., Sendurur, E., & Sendurur, P. (2012). Teacher beliefs and technology integration practices: A critical relationship. *Computers & Education, 59*(2), 423–435.

Ezumah, B. A. (2020). *Critical perspectives of educational technology in Africa: Design, implementation, and evaluation*. Palgrave Macmillan.

Gloster, A. T., Lamnisos, D., Lubenko, J., Presti, G., Squatrito, V., Constantinou, M., Nicolaou, C., Papacostas, S., Aydın, G., Chong, Y. Y., Chien, W. T., & Karekla, M. (2020). Impact of COVID-19 pandemic on mental health: An international study. *PLOS One, 15*(12), e0244809. https://doi.org/10.1371/journal.pone.0244809

Hall, H. (2022). Web 2.0 explained: Everything you need to know. *History Computer*. https://history-computer.com/web-2-0/

Hansen, M. B. N. (2004). 'Realtime synthesis' and the différance of the body: Technocultural studies in the wake of deconstruction. *Culture Machine*. http://www.culturemachine.net/index.php/cm/article/view/9/8

Heidegger, M. (1977). *The question concerning technology*. Garland.

Howells, C., & Moore, G. (Eds.). (2013). *Stiegler and technics*. Edinburg University Press.

Idris, F., Zulkipli, I. N., Abdul-Mumin, K. H., Ahmad, S. R., Mitha, S., Rahman, H. A., Rajabalaya, R., David, S. R., & Naing, L. (2021). Academic experiences, physical and mental health impact of COVID-19 pandemic on students and lecturers in health care education. *BMC Medical Education, 21*, 1–13.

International Telecommunication Union. (2019). *Measuring digital development: Facts and figures, 2019*. www.itu.int/en/ITU-D/Statistics/Documents/facts/FactsFigures2019.pdf

Irwin, R. (2020). Heidegger and Stiegler on failure and technology. *Educational Philosophy and Theory, 52*(4), 361–375.

Islam, A. N., Laato, S., Talukder, S., & Sutinen, E. (2020). Misinformation sharing and social media fatigue during COVID-19: An affordance and cognitive load perspective. *Technological Forecasting and Social Change, 159*, 120201.

James, I. (2019). *The technique of thought: Nancy, Laruelle, Malabou, and Stiegler after naturalism.* University of Minnesota Press.

Kainja, J. (2019, March 9). High cost of Internet in Malawi vs fake images. *Nyasa Times.* www.nyasatimes.com/high-cost-of-internet-in-malawi-vs-fake-images

Kainja, J., Ndasauka, Y., Mchenga, M., Kondowe, F., M'manga, C., Maliwichi, L., & Simunye, N. (2022). Umunthu, Covid-19 and mental health in Malawi. *Heliyon, 8*(11), 1–6. https://doi.org/10.1016/j.heliyon.2022.e11316

Kerres, M., & Buchner, J. (2022). Education after the pandemic: What we have (not) learned about learning. *Education Sciences, 12*(5), 315.

Kouppanou, A. (2015). Bernard Stiegler's philosophy of technology: Invention, decision, and education in times of digitisation. *Educational Philosophy and Theory, 47*(10), 1110–1123.

Krutka, D. G., Heath, M. K., & Willet, K. B. S. (2019). Foregrounding techno-ethics: Toward critical perspectives in technology and teacher education. *Journal of Technology and Teacher Education, 27*(4), 555–574.

Kunyenje, G., & Chigona, W. (2019). External actors in formulating a national information and communication technology policy in developing countries such as Malawi. *African Journal of Information Systems, 11*(1), 1–23.

Laato, S., Islam, A. K., Islam, M. N., & Whelan, E. (2020). Why do people share misinformation during the COVID-19 pandemic? *ArXiv.* https://doi.org/10.1080/0960085X.2020.1770632; https://arxiv.org/abs/2004.09600

Lee, Y., Jeon, Y. J., Kang, S., Shin, J. I., Jung, Y. C., & Jung, S. J. (2022). Social media use and mental health during the COVID-19 pandemic in young adults: A meta-analysis of 14 cross-sectional studies. *BMC Public Health, 22*(1), 995.

Lischer, S., Safi, N., & Dickson, C. (2022). Remote learning and students' mental health during the Covid-19 pandemic: A mixed-method enquiry. *Prospects, 51*, 589–599. https://doi.org/10.1007/s11125-020-09530-w

Longest, K., & Kang, J. A. (2022). Social media, social support, and mental health of young adults during COVID-19. *Frontiers in Communication, 7*, 828135.

Luo, N., Verma, S., & Subramaniam, M. (2022). Social media-driven routes to positive mental health among youth: Qualitative enquiry and concept mapping study. *JMIR Pediatrics and Parenting, 5*(1), e32758.

Mahlaba, S. C. (2020). Reasons why self-directed learning is important in South Africa during the COVID-19 pandemic. *South African Journal of Higher Education, 34*(6), 120–136.

M'manga, C., Ndasauka, Y., Kainja, J., Kondowe, F., Mchenga, M., Maliwichi, L., & Nyamali, S. (2023). The world is coming to an end! COVID-19, depression, and anxiety among adolescents in Malawi. *Frontiers in Psychiatry, 13*, 1024793. https://doi.org/10.3389/fpsyt.2022.1024793

Muianga, X., Hansson, H., Nilsson, A., Mondlane, A., Mutimucuio, I., & Guambe, A. (2013). ICT in education in Africa – myth or reality: A case study of Mozambican higher education institutions. *The African Journal of Information Systems, 5*(3), 5.

Mutsvairo, B., & Ragnedda, M. (2017). Emerging political narratives on Malawian digital spaces. *Communicatio, 43*(2), 147–167.

Najjuka, S. M., Checkwech, G., Olum, R., Ashaba, S., & Kaggwa, M. M. (2021). Depression, anxiety, and stress among Ugandan university students during the COVID-19 lockdown: An online survey. *African Health Sciences, 21*(4), 1533–1543.

Nightingale, S. J., & Farid, H. (2022). AI-synthesised faces are indistinguishable from real faces and more trustworthy. *Proceedings of the National Academy of Sciences*, *119*(8), e2120481119. https://doi.org/10.1073/pnas.2120481119

Ntshwarang, P. N., Malinga, T., & Losike-Sedimo, N. (2021). eLearning tools at the University of Botswana: Relevance and use under COVID-19 crisis. *Higher Education for the Future*, *8*(1), 142–154.

Oxford Analytica. (2022). *African anti-misinformation steps miss offline spread: Expert briefings*. Oxford Analytica. https://doi.org/10.1108/OXAN-DB268786

Pandey, A., Patni, N., Singh, M., Sood, A., & Singh, G. (2010). YouTube is a source of information on the H1N1 influenza pandemic. *American Journal of Preventive Medicine*, *38*(3), e1–e3.

Porter, G., Hampshire, K., Milner, J., Munthali, A., Robson, E., De Lannoy, A., & Abane, A. (2015). Mobile phones and education in sub-Saharan Africa: From youth practice to public policy. *Journal of International Development*, *28*(1), 22–39. https://doi.org/10.1002/jid.3116

Reiser, R. A. (2001). A history of instructional design and technology: Part I: A history of instructional media. *Educational Technology Research and Development*, *49*(1), 53–64.

Rocha, Y. M., De Moura, G. A., Desidério, G. A., De Oliveira, C. H., Lourenço, F. D., & De Figueiredo Nicolete, L. D. (2021). The impact of fake news on social media and its influence on health during the COVID-19 pandemic: A systematic review. *Journal of Public Health*, *31*, 1–10. https://doi.org/10.1007/s10389-021-01658-z

Rosen, Y., & Manny-Ikan, E. (2011). *The social promise of educational technology: The case of the time to know program*. Paper presented at American Educational Research Association Annual Meeting, New Orleans, LA.

Salamon, A. (2021, August 31). Cybersecurity: Africa's race against time against attacks. *The Africa Report*. www.theafricareport.com/122950/cybersecurity-africas-race-against-time-against-attacks/

Signé, L., & Signé, K. (2021). *How African states can improve their cybersecurity*. Brookings. www.brookings.edu/techstream/how-african-states-can-improve-their-cybersecurity/

Stiegler, B. (1998). *Technics and time, 1: The fault of Epimetheus* (R. Beardsworth & G. Collins, Trans.). Stanford University Press.

Stiegler, B. (2012). Relational ecology and the digital pharmakon. *Culture Machine*, *13*, 1–19.

Stiegler, B. (2017). *General ecology, economy, and organology* (E. Hörl & J. Burton, Eds., D. Ross, Trans., pp. 129–150). Bloomsbury Publishing.

Stiegler, B. (2020). *Nanjing lectures 2016–2019*. Open Humanities Press.

Swire-Thompson, B., & Lazer, D. (2020). Public health and online misinformation: Challenges and recommendations. *Annual Review of Public Health*, *41*, 433–451. https://doi.org/10.1146/annurev-publhealth-040119-094127

Thomée, S., Härenstam, A., & Hagberg, M. (2012). Computer use and stress, sleep disturbances, and symptoms of depression among young adults: A prospective cohort study. *BMC Psychiatry*, *12*(1), 1–14.

Torous, J., Jän Myrick, K., Rauseo-Ricupero, N., & Firth, J. (2020). Digital mental health and COVID-19: Using technology today to accelerate the curve on access and quality tomorrow. *JMIR Mental Health*, *7*(3), e18848. https://doi.org/10.2196/18848

Trottein, S. (2013). Technics, or the fading away of aesthetics: The sensible and the question of Kant. In C. Howells & G. Moore (Eds.), *Stiegler and technics* (pp. 87–101). Edinburgh University Press.

Turianskyi, Y. (2020). *COVID-19: Implications for the "digital divide" in Africa*. Africa Portal. www.africaportal.org/features/covid-19-implications-of-the-pandemic-for-the-digital-divide-in-africa/

Vaingankar, J. A., Dam, R. M., Samari, E., Chang, S., Seow, E., Chua, Y. C., Torous, J., Jän Myrick, K., Rauseo-Ricupero, N., & Firth, J. (2020). Digital mental health and COVID-19: Using technology today to accelerate the curve on access and quality tomorrow. *JMIR Mental Health*, 7(3), e18848. https://doi.org/10.2196/18848

Vurayai, S. (2022). COVID-19 pandemic and the narrative of the digital divide gap in universities in sub-Saharan Africa. *African Identities*, 1–12. https://doi.org/10.1080/14725843.2022.2122398

17 Refocusing African Mental Healthcare Readiness for Future Pandemics

Yamikani Ndasauka

17.1 Introduction

The COVID-19 pandemic has had a profound impact on mental health in Africa. As the chapters in this book have shown, the pandemic and associated lockdown measures increased stress, anxiety, depression, loneliness, and other mental health challenges across the continent. However, analysing these impacts through a communitarian lens provides unique insights. Communitarianism is a philosophy that emphasises the importance of community and society over the individual (Etzioni, 2022). In the African context, this manifests in communal values, social solidarity, and a collective sense of identity. These communal support structures were vital in protecting mental health during the pandemic. For instance, community-based mental health campaigns can help reduce stigma and increase awareness (Chapter 1). Religious communities and support groups were invaluable in relieving psychological distress, especially for women (Chapter 3). Family and friends provided emotional support during isolation (Chapter 15). This aligns with communitarian ideals of mutual care and collective responsibility. However, individualism also impacted mental health. Social media usage drove individualistic tendencies like social comparison and self-promotion, exacerbating distress (Chapters 12, 15, 16). Neoliberal economic policies widened inequalities, increasing vulnerability (Chapter 2). The stigmatisation of marginalised groups reflected a neglect of communal obligations (Chapter 11). Hence, while communitarianism's communal ethos supported mental health, unrestrained individualism undermined it. A moderate communitarian approach balancing individual rights and social solidarity is optimal.

The African communitarian spirit also influenced interpretations of pandemic information. Framing COVID-19 through communal worldviews led to speculation, misinformation, and heightened anxiety (Chapters 8, 11). Global public health communication about the pandemic was often inconsistent, contradictory, and evolving, compounding confusion and uncertainty (Moran et al., 2021). However, communal knowledge systems also empowered critical dialogue on pandemic governance (Chapter 4). Integrating cultural paradigms with biomedical approaches can improve health information

DOI: 10.4324/9781003425861-21

efficacy and counter misinformation (Fofana, 2021). This exemplifies how communal epistemologies shape mental health experiences.

Furthermore, restrictive lockdown policies tested communitarian values. While lockdowns were necessary for infection control, they disrupted economic and social systems, increasing hardship through job losses, income declines, and social isolation (Chapters 5, 6, 7). African communities adapted through mutual aid initiatives like food banks and social support groups. However, state communitarian obligations to provide social assistance and equitable healthcare access were often unfulfilled due to inadequate investments in public services (Kola et al., 2021). Hence custodians of communitarianism, like religious and traditional leaders, faced additional burdens amid the lockdowns (Chapter 3). This reveals tensions between rigid state containment policies and communal realities, indicating that communitarian governance should adopt context-specific, flexible approaches.

The pandemic also exposed gaps in mental healthcare requiring communitarian redress. Individualistic biomedical paradigms focused on pharmaceutical interventions dominate much of Africa's mental health landscape, while endogenous communal psychosocial healing practices are often marginalised (Chapter 11). Integrating these communal strategies can make mental health services more holistic, participatory, and accessible, in line with calls for decolonising global health (Kola et al., 2021). Community participation in shaping mental health interventions also upholds communitarian self-determination.

Additionally, communitarian ethics compel expanded investment in public mental healthcare, which remains severely under-resourced and difficult to access for many Africans despite rising pandemic-linked demand (Chapters 13, 14). Private mental healthcare systems are often inaccessible to disadvantaged populations. Upholding communal solidarity and justice calls for universal mental health coverage funded through progressive taxation and reallocation from military budgets (Alemu et al., 2023). This elevates communal well-being over individualistic profit motives. Ultimately a communitarian pandemic recovery strategy entails collective action to build more equitable, resilient, and socially just societies.

Communitarian ideals of collective responsibility helped communities withstand challenges. Tensions between rigid state policies and complex communal realities manifested, indicating communitarian approaches must be flexibly adapted to the context. Integrating cultural paradigms in mental health systems and governance can render interventions more participatory, holistic, and productive. Realigning priorities and resources towards mental healthcare provision guided by communitarian ethics of solidarity and justice is imperative, as are broader reforms to strengthen communal well-being. Overall, moderate communitarian principles emphasising individual rights and collective obligations provide a constructive framework for protecting and promoting mental well-being in Africa in the post-COVID era.

17.2 Gaps Revealed in Africa's Mental Healthcare Systems

The book has also shed light on how the COVID-19 pandemic has exposed gaps in Africa's mental healthcare landscapes, including the dominance of Western biomedical approaches, marginalisation of indigenous communal practices, substantial financing deficiencies, and barriers to equitable access. This underscores the urgent need to re-envision mental healthcare guided by communitarian principles of social justice and collective well-being.

Across Africa, mental healthcare remains heavily centred around Western biomedical paradigms reliant on pharmaceuticals and individualised hospital-based psychiatry. This reflects colonial legacies that devalued African knowledge systems. Consequently, communal and psychosocial mental healthcare strategies rooted in indigenous cultures are often sidelined in policy and practice. For instance, traditional healers and communal therapy groups can be considered primitive or unscientific. However, these endogenous approaches aligned with communal values of collective healing can enhance access and efficacy, particularly when integrated with evidence-based care (Alemu et al., 2023). Communitarian principles call for democratising mental health governance to give communities greater self-determination in shaping locally-grounded, holistic services that leverage African cultural strengths (Kola et al., 2021). Platforms for knowledge exchange between biomedical and traditional practitioners can also foster synergistic models. Ultimately decolonising mental healthcare involves affirming African epistemologies and empowering communal healing capacities.

Furthermore, the pandemic amplified financing and accessibility challenges within Africa's mental health systems. Public spending on mental health remains extremely low, averaging less than 1% of health budgets across the continent (Alemu et al., 2023). This forces high out-of-pocket expenditures at private facilities, excluding disadvantaged groups. From a communitarian standpoint, such inequities violate the ethical obligations of social justice and solidarity with vulnerable members (Alemu et al., 2023). Boosting public investments to offer universal mental healthcare regardless of socioeconomic status is essential. African countries have the potential to fund decolonised, communal mental health systems that leave no one behind. This upholds communitarian principles of collective prosperity and communal self-determination.

17.3 Leveraging African Knowledge Systems in Pandemic Response

The book has also highlighted the need to leverage African knowledge systems to contextualise public health messaging and decolonise pandemic governance. Top-down health communications often lacked cultural relevance, inadvertently amplifying misinformation. Integrating African epistemologies can enhance contextual appropriateness and public trust. Moreover, prioritising

African voices in research and policymaking upholds communitarian ethics of self-determination.

As demonstrated in this book, early pandemic communications primarily employed Western biomedical models insensitive to African cultures, fuelling uncertainty and misinformation (Chapters 4, 9). For instance, explanations of disease transmission overlooked communal lifestyles, generating confusion about social distancing (Chapter 11). African collective values also clashed with dictates for the rapid burial of the dead, causing scepticism. Framing COVID-19 as doom and punishment from God resonated more deeply than technical warnings across religious communities (Chapter 11).

These experiences underscore the need to co-create messaging embedding African cosmologies, using knowledge brokers embedded in culture (Ndasauka & Kainja, forthcoming). For example, communal solidarity messaging aligned with values like Ubuntu could reinforce social distancing norms and convey collective responsibility for health. Efforts to counter misinformation must engage cultural and faith leaders leveraging the strength of oral traditions. Through dialogue, public health and African knowledge systems can complement each other to foster greater public acceptance.

Broader calls have emerged for decolonising pandemic governance by centres like the Africa CDC to uplift African voices and empower participatory health policymaking grounded in lived realities (Nkengasong & Mankoula, 2020). Enhancing community representation in COVID-19 response coordination bodies can ensure contextual appropriateness and public buy-in of policies. Equitably including African scientists and scholars in global decision-making forums allow African solutions to guide international strategies (Nkengasong & Mankoula, 2020).

Similarly, establishing Africa-based research collaborations is vital to set priorities aligned with regional needs. Leadership from African institutions, use of Afrocentric frameworks, participatory methodologies, and communication of findings in accessible ways can decentre Eurocentric norms. This upholds communitarian self-determination and collective prosperity principles. Ultimately pandemic governance and research guided by African voices and knowledge systems, while integrating global resources, will strengthen capacities to address current and future outbreaks through contextualised, culturally resonant strategies.

As this book has shown, the COVID-19 pandemic was characterised by rampant misinformation that posed barriers to effective public health communication in Africa. Across Africa, misinformation circulated widely on social media and messaging apps, often outpacing factual information (Chapter 11). Speculation about foreign conspiracies, dubious cures, and vaccines causing infertility abounded, amplified by sensitivities rooted in colonialism (Chapter 7). Such falsehoods bred fear, uncertainty, and non-compliance with protective measures, undermining pandemic containment, which may have led to distress among African populations.

Communitarian ethics emphasise transparent, participatory processes to foster shared understanding (Cordeiro-Rodrigues & Metz, 2021). Hence, centralised attempts to censor misinformation are insufficient. Instead, a two-way dialogue engaging communities as partners is required. This uplifts diverse voices while also identifying concerns driving misinformation acceptance. Reframing narratives via trusted community influencers can then promote collective well-being. For instance, religious leaders wield strong moral authority in countering misinformation across Africa (Ndasauka & Kainja, forthcoming). Guidance situating public health directives within communal values like custodianship of the body as a divine gift could increase compliance. Additionally, participatory radio shows or street theatre conveying public health messages using familiar cultural idioms resonate more deeply with oral traditions.

If underpinned by transparency and civil liberties, Africa's close-knit social fabric is an asset in collaborative approaches to contain infodemics. Communities are best positioned to judge what communication strategies uphold collective welfare and individual dignity. Beyond the pandemic, enduring structures for community consultation could strengthen oversight and accountability of public health programmes. From a communitarian standpoint, addressing health misinformation in Africa requires contextualised and grassroots strategies focused on participatory dialogue and reframing narratives via trusted voices. This collectivist approach aligns with communitarian principles by foregrounding communal knowledge-sharing, self-determination, and consensus-building for the greater good. The pandemic provides vital lessons on the urgency of investing in sociocultural health communication capacities as integral to African health systems.

17.4 Future Research on Pandemics and Mental Health in Africa

The book has also highlighted significant gaps in research on mental health burdens and the implications for health systems in Africa. Several priority areas for the region's future pandemic and mental health research can be identified. Firstly, there is a need for high-quality, population-based mental health surveillance across Africa to accurately determine the prevalence of pandemic-related issues like anxiety, depression, and post-traumatic stress. Most countries lack such systems, hampering real-time tracking of mental health impacts during crises. Investments in surveillance infrastructure can generate essential data to guide interventions.

Secondly, research should investigate mental health outcomes across socio-economic groups, genders, ages, and high-risk populations to identify disparities and vulnerable subgroups (Kola et al., 2021). Current knowledge gaps remain regarding differential mental health impacts on diverse communities. Intersectional analyses can inform targeted pandemic response strategies. Thirdly, more implementation research is warranted on scalable, culturally-appropriate mental health services in African contexts (Kola et al., 2021). Studies should assess interventions like psychosocial support groups, community health worker programmes, indigenous healing practices, and the use of digital technologies to strengthen systems. Evaluating combinations of approaches can guide integration for a more significant impact.

Fourthly, investigations of mental health knowledge, attitudes, and practices across cultures and communities are needed to shape awareness campaigns (Kola et al., 2021). Research partnerships with local stakeholders can design engagement strategies to address contextual barriers and misconceptions. Fifthly, health economics research should evaluate mental healthcare financing gaps, the cost-effectiveness of interventions, and policies to enable equitable access and universal coverage (Alemu et al., 2023). This evidence can mobilise political will and guide efficient resource allocation towards comprehensive, sustainably financed systems.

Finally, African scholars should call and aim for inclusive, decolonised mental health research guided by African priorities and perspectives. Community-based participatory methodologies, Afrocentric theoretical frameworks, and African leadership in setting research agendas are recommended to decentre Eurocentric norms and empower African knowledge production. Ultimately, collaborative, locally-driven African research will provide contextualised evidence to strengthen pandemic preparedness and mental healthcare systems for communal well-being. COVID-19 has revealed these pressing research needs and opportunities for African scholars to lead impactful studies rooted in lived realities.

17.5 Conclusion

This book on Africa's pandemic mental health experiences through a communitarian lens yielded essential insights. The communal ethos of values like Ubuntu allowed communities to support mental health amid challenges. However, neoliberal governance and individualism were also vital, revealing the importance of balanced, moderate communitarian approaches. Integrating cultural paradigms into mental healthcare can render interventions more appropriate and effective if guided by inclusive, participatory processes. The pandemic exposed systemic deficiencies in mental healthcare, requiring redress based on communitarian ethics of social justice and equitable access. Significant research gaps remain regarding mental health burdens, interventions, and outcomes across diverse groups. African knowledge production should be at the centre of addressing these gaps. Ultimately communitarian principles provide a valuable framework for mental health promotion in Africa after COVID-19. This will involve collective action to build more equitable societies, strengthened community resilience, and health systems anchored in African realities. The pandemic illuminated communal strengths while also revealing areas for growth. With visionary leadership and political will, its lessons can galvanise African mental health futures.

References

Alemu, R. E., Osborn, T. L., & Wasanga, C. M. (2023). The network approach: A path to decolonise mental health care. *Frontiers in Public Health*, *11*, 1052077. https://doi.org/10.3389/fpubh.2023.1052077

Cordeiro-Rodrigues, L., & Metz, T. (2021). Afro-communitarianism and the role of traditional African healers in the COVID-19 pandemic. *Public Health Ethics*, phab006. https://doi.org/10.1093/phe/phab006

Etzioni, A. (2022). Communitarianism revisited. *Journal of Political Ideologies*, *27*(3), 256–272. http://dx.doi.org/10.1080/13569317.2014.951142

Fofana, M. O. (2021). Decolonising global health in the time of COVID-19. *Global Public Health*, *16*(8–9), 1155–1166. https://doi.org/10.1080/17441692.2020.1864754

Kola, L., Kohrt, B. A., Hanlon, C., Naslund, J. A., Sikander, S., Balaji, M., Benjet, C., Cheung, E. Y. L., Eaton, J., Gonsalves, P., Hailemariam, M., Luitel, N. P., Machado, D. B., Misganaw, E., Omigbodun, O., Roberts, T., Salisbury, T. T., Shidhaye, R., Sunkel, C., Ugo, V., . . . Patel, V. (2021). COVID-19 mental health impact and responses in low-income and middle-income countries: Reimagining global mental health. *The Lancet, Psychiatry*, *8*(6), 535–550. https://doi.org/10.1016/S2215-0366(21)00025-0

Moran, C., Campbell, D. J. T., Campbell, T. S., Roach, P., Bourassa, L., Collins, Z., Stasiewicz, M., & McLane, P. (2021). Predictors of attitudes and adherence to COVID-19 public health guidelines in Western countries: A rapid review of the emerging literature. *Journal of Public Health*, *43*(4), 739–753. https://doi.org/10.1093/pubmed/fdab070

Ndasauka, Y., & Kainja, J. (forthcoming). Stewards or manipulators? Knowledge brokers' complex positionality in combating the Covid-19 "infodemic" in Malawi. *Journal of African Journalism Studies*, under review.

Nkengasong, J. N., & Mankoula, W. (2020). Looming threat of COVID-19 infection in Africa: Act collectively and fast. *Lancet (London, England)*, *395*(10227), 841–842. https://doi.org/10.1016/S0140-6736(20)30464-5.

Index

For Product Safety Concerns and Information please contact our EU
representative GPSR@taylorandfrancis.com
Taylor & Francis Verlag GmbH, Kaufingerstraße 24, 80331 München, Germany